CW01467998

Clinical Acupuncture

CLINICAL
ACUPUNCTURE

A Practical Japanese Approach

By Katsusuke Serizawa, M.D.
with Mari Kusumi

Japan Publications, Inc.

Published by JAPAN PUBLICATIONS, INC., Tokyo and New York

Distributors:

UNITED STATES: *Kodansha International/USA, Ltd., through Harper & Row, Publishers, Inc., 599 Lexington Avenue, Suite 2300, New York, N. Y. 10022.* SOUTH AMERICA: *Harper & Row, Publishers, Inc., International Department.* CANADA: *Fitzhenry & Whiteside Ltd., 195 Allstate Parkway, Markham, Ontario, L3R 4T8.* MEXICO AND CENTRAL AMERICA: *HARLA S. A. de C. V., Apartado 30–546, Mexico 4, D. F.* BRITISH ISLES: *Premier Book Marketing Ltd., 1 Gower Street, London WC1E 6HA.* EUROPEAN CONTINENT: *European Book Service PBD, Strijkviertel 63, 3454 PK De Meern, The Netherlands.* AUSTRALIA AND NEW ZEALAND: *Bookwise International, 54 Crittenden Road, Findon, South Australia 5007.* THE FAR EAST AND JAPAN: *Japan Publications Trading Co., Ltd., 1–2–1, Sarugaku-cho, Chiyoda-ku, Tokyo 101.*

First edition: November 1988

LCCC No. 84–80451
ISBN 0–87040–782–1

Printed in Japan

Foreword

Half a century has passed since I first began clinical work with acupuncture. Be that as it may, in my clinical work there are still times when I am not quite sure what to do with a patient. This could be because after all these years I am still not that skillful in handling patients, but more likely it is because acupuncture is a complex Oriental manual medicine that is based on experience, which requires a diagnostic format taking individual differences into full consideration and the selection of appropriate tsubo, not to mention the optimal amount of stimulation. Because of this complexity a wide variety of approaches to acupuncture have been developed in Japan. There is a group of acupuncturists who attempt to "adhere strictly to the principles in Chinese classics" and to apply this in their clinical practice. The majority of Japanese practitioners, however, use traditional principles as a reference point but base their clinical practice on modern medical knowledge. These practitioners apply the knowledge of the functional distribution of the autonomic nervous system in their selection of tsubo and treatment. Another group of acupuncturists known as the Ryōdōraku School have modified the traditional techniques of acupuncture and define points with low electrical resistivity as reactive points similar to traditional tsubo and use these points clinically for treatment.

Acupuncture and moxibustion are medical techniques originating in the Orient which were developed from accumulated experience. They were derived from the view that the structural and functional systems of the human body, as a microcosm, are intimately tied to the composition and cyclical changes in the natural environment. The concept of meridians and acupuncture points were developed and systematized based on this understanding and the pathological condition of the individual was expressed in terms of the complementary opposites of yin and yang, deficient and excess, cold and hot, and external and internal. This perception of disease is obviously very different from the modern medical perspective which emphasizes the pathophysiology of specific structures.

Naturally, acupuncture does not lend itself to the treatment of infectious or acute diseases and instead the emphasis is placed on a holistic treatment to "treat the patient instead of the disease." The focus in acupuncture is therefore to treat diseases before they appear, or to deal with diseases in the incipient stage while they are still minor. In other words, Oriental medicine's greatest strength lies in preserving health, improving physical condition, and increasing resistance to disease. Acupuncture is thus an ideal form of treatment for "building health," which has become an important theme for medicine in Japan today. Acupuncture is also seen as an effective method to deal with the many complaints associated with aging.

One of the main characteristics of acupuncture, as an individualized form of medicine, is that there are only very general standards for its application, such as "tonify when deficient and reduce when excess." From one standpoint this is an extremely vague rule on the amount of stimulation to be applied, but it shows how much depends on the experience of the practitioner in Oriental medicine. In the beginning I had some difficulties teaching this very experiential form of medicine to the younger generation, but I worked on ways of rationalizing the therapeutic methods of acupuncture based on my own clinical observations.

This book was written as a text for the modern approach to acupuncture which I developed. In Part I the meridians and points are presented as the foundation of acupuncture, and the other traditional concepts are also described to give the reader an understanding of the roots of Oriental medicine. Since acupuncture is no longer a unique Oriental therapy based on mysterious and incomprehensible principles, new perspectives are offered on how acupuncture can be understood in light of modern medicine. Acupuncture has thus been redefined as a valuable traditional method of physiotherapy from the Orient. In Part I the similarities between the pain killing effects of acupuncture and the analgesics used in modern medicine are also discussed. This is followed by the principles of acupuncture treatment which are widely applied among Japanese practitioners, and the special acupuncture techniques in use today are also described. Furthermore, the attitudes and precautions crucial to successful clinical practice have been outlined in detail.

Part II of this book focuses on the clinical application of the principles discussed in Part I, and practical information is offered on how to treat thirty-four different conditions most often encountered in the acupuncture clinics in Japan.

Mari Kusumi, the coauthor of this book is a very talented practitioner who has fifteen years of clinical experience in acupuncture. Presently she is the president of the Waseda College of Medical Arts and Sciences in Tokyo as well as a board member of the Oriental Medical Techniques Promotion Foundation, of which I am the chairman. Some years ago, when I taught at Tsukuba University, she did research and clinical work under my supervision as a graduate student majoring in Oriental medicine.

This book was in fact written mostly by Mari Kusumi and, although she did use many of my published works as a foundation, she compiled this text from her own specialized knowledge and wealth of clinical experience in acupuncture and moxibustion. Five years has passed since she first undertook this project, and I have supported this project and have guided and edited her work through this time. It could be said that I, rather than being coauthor of this book, was the chief editor. Whatever the case, the approach to clinical acupuncture which is succinctly presented in this book is founded on the principles and practices of acupuncture therapy which I developed over many years. Mari Kusumi presented my approach and added to this more recent scientific research substantiating the therapeutic effects of acupuncture and also outlined effective treatments for common conditions.

I am very impressed by her intense dedication in putting together this text even while being extremely busy with her duties as the president of an acupuncture college, a board member of our foundation, and a clinician and instructor at the Oriental Medical Techniques Training Center. Finally, we are most thankful to Mr. Iwao Yoshizaki, the president of Japan Publications, Inc., who made the publication of this book possible. We would be most gratified if this book would serve as a useful text and reference for those involved in research and clinical work in acupuncture.

Katsusuke Serizawa

Preface

My main purpose in writing this book was to have acupuncturists outside of Japan understand the actual clinical situation in the practice of acupuncture in Japan today and to thus enable all practitioners to apply these treatment methods. Currently I am the president of the Waseda College of Medical Arts and Sciences in Tokyo, and I compiled this text from the lecture notes I used to teach my dear students. This is information I have gathered over the years in my clinical practice. Being an educator as well as a clinician, I have been involved for many years in the whole process of training acupuncturists. I wrote this book with the student in mind and began from basic theory and gradually worked up to practical application. I did my best to present the information as clearly and concisely as possible, and to select material that would have the widest possible application. I am sure that a student can become a capable practitioner by studying this text thoroughly and by constantly practicing the techniques presented. As acupuncturists we must keep a broad perspective so as to encompass both Oriental and Western viewpoints. The traditional four examinations of looking, listening, questioning, and touching must be performed to get a thorough understanding of the patient's condition and thus render the best possible treatment. It is important that we continually add to our knowledge and hone our skills to develop as practitioners.

In Part I of this text, in order to give some background in Oriental medicine and acupuncture, I presented traditional concepts, the meridians and acupuncture points, scientific viewpoints, and various techniques and approaches. In Part II, as practical application of these concepts, I included common conditions with a description of each condition, which points to treat, and how to go about giving a treatment. I have thus presented general information and a standard acupuncture treatment for specific conditions. In applying this material, however, I trust that all readers will understand that every individual is unique and will remember to take individual differences into account. We must view each patient we see with compassion as a special person on this earth with unique human and biological traits. It is my wish that readers use this book as a reference to deal more effectively with difficult patients and continue to grow as practitioners. The essence of medical care, I feel, is for practitioners to assist patients in coping with their conditions so they can find greater comfort and fulfillment in life. In order to serve this role it is important to have a strong background in Western medical science, but just as important, one must have a firm foundation in the holistic philosophy of Oriental medicine, which allows a practitioner to have true respect for the uniqueness of each individual.

It is my hope that through this book practitioners can acquire greater knowledge and skills to deal more effectively with patients who entrust themselves in the care of acupuncturists. It is my heartfelt desire that acupuncture practitioners put all their enthusiasm, creativity, and love into the care of their patients. As to whether I have been able to fully convey the teachings of my beloved teacher Katsusuke

Serizawa, I still have some doubts, but I have done my best to communicate his wisdom. In addition, I owe a great deal to Dr. Shinichi Yamada, the late president of Waseda College of Medical Arts and Sciences, whose teachings are also reflected in my writing. Further, I am grateful to Mr. Stephen Brown, who is himself an acupuncturist, for doing such a fine job in translating this book. Also, I owe much to the editor Ms. Yotsuko Watanabe for her constant encouragement and valuable advice. Finally I would like to express my sincere gratitude to Mr. Iwao Yoshizaki the President of Japan Publications, Inc. for giving me this opportunity.

Mari Kusumi

Contents

Preface, 5
Foreword, 7

PART I: BASIC CONCEPTS OF ACUPUNCTURE, *13*

Chapter 1:   Oriental Medicine—A Historical Perspective, *15*
   1.   Western Medicine and Oriental Medicine, *15*
   2.   The History of Oriental Medicine, *18*
       (1)   Historical outline of acupuncture in China, 18
       (2)   Historical outline of acupuncture in Japan, 21
   3.   Principles of Chinese Medicine, *23*
       (1)   The yin-yang theory, 23
       (2)   The five element theory, 25
   4.   The Meridians (Energy Circulation System), *29*
   5.   Acupuncture Points (Tsubo), *31*

Chapter 2:   Meridians and Acupuncture Points, *34*
   1.   The Circulation of Energy in the Meridians, *34*
   2.   Symptoms Associated with the Meridians, *35*
   3.   Locations of Acupuncture Points, *36*
   4.   The Fourteen Major Meridians and Their Acupuncture Points, *37*
       Lung meridian, 37
       Large intestine meridian, 39
       Stomach meridian, 41
       Spleen meridian, 44
       Heart meridian, 46
       Small intestine meridian, 48
       Bladder meridian, 50
       Kidney meridian, 54
       Pericardium meridian, 57
       Triple heater meridian, 58
       Gallbladder meridian, 60
       Liver meridian, 64
       Governor vessel, 66
       Conception vessel, 68

Chapter 3:   The Scientific Rationale for Acupuncture Therapy, *71*
   1.   A Modern Perspective on Meridians and Acupuncture Points, *71*
       (1)   Viscerocutaneous reflex, 72
       (2)   Cutaneovisceral reflex, 72

2. Physiological Mechanisms at Work in Acupuncture, *79*
   (1)   The synergistic workings of the body, 79
   (2)   The homeostatic mechanism of the body, 80
   (3)   The stress theory, 81
   (4)   The principle of cybernetics, 82
   (5)   Reilly phenomenon, 83
3. The Mechanisms of Pain and the Analgesic Effect of Acupuncture, *84*
   (1)   Theories on the mechanism of pain, 84
   (2)   The gate control theory, 85
   (3)   The mechanism in the analgesic effect of morphine, 85
   (4)   Morphinelike substances in the brain, 86
   *(5)   The analgesic effect produced by electrical stimulation of specific
         areas of the brain, 87*
   (6)   The mechanism of the analgesic effect of acupuncture, 89

Chapter 4:   The Equipment and Techniques of Acupuncture and Moxibustion, *91*
1. The Tools of Acupuncture and Moxibustion, *91*
   (1)   The history of acupuncture needles, 91
   (2)   Japanese acupuncture needles, 92
   (3)   Insertion tubes, 93
   (4)   The production of moxa and its qualities, 94
2. Basic Skills of Acupuncture, *95*
   (1)   Needle insertion, 95
   (2)   Needle manipulation techniques, 99
   (3)   Angle and depth of insertion, 101
3. The Basic Skills of Moxibustion, *102*
   (1)   Scarring and non-scarring moxibustion, 102
   (2)   Application of penetrating moxibustion, 103
4. Diagnosis for Acupuncture and Moxibustion Treatments, *105*
   *(1)   Detecting reactions in the skin and superficial tissue (locating
         acupuncture points), 105*
   (2)   Standard procedure for palpatory examination, 107
   (3)   Deciding the treatment based on palpatory findings, 110
5. Tonification and Dispersion Techniques in Acupuncture and
   Moxibustion, *111*
6. Special Needling Methods, *113*
   (1)   Moxa needling, 113
   (2)   Scatter needling, 114
   (3)   Intradermal needling, 115
   (4)   Pediatric acupuncture, 116
   (5)   Micropuncture, 118
   (6)   Cupping, 119
   (7)   Carotid sinus stimulation, 120
   (8)   Stellate ganglion stimulation, 121
   (9)   Auricular acupuncture, 122
   (10) Electroacupuncture, 125

Chapter 5: Guidelines for the Clinical Application of Acupuncture and Moxibustion, *135*

1. Guidelines for the Application of Acupuncture, *135*
    (1) Amount of stimulation and sensitivity of the patient, 135
    (2) The therapeutic effects of acupuncture, 137
    (3) Indications for acupuncture, 138
    (4) Contraindications for acupuncture, 140
    (5) Sanitation and sterilization for acupuncture, 141
    (6) Body positioning for acupuncture, 141
    (7) How to avoid problems in acupuncture, 142
    (8) How to deal with needle breakage, 143
2. Guidelines for the Application of Moxibustion, *143*
    (1) Amount of stimulation in moxibustion, 143
    (2) The therapeutic effects of moxibustion, 144
    (3) The indications and contraindications for moxibustion, 145
    (4) Precautions in applying moxibustion, 145
    (5) How to prevent infection after moxibustion, 146
    (6) How to deal with infections, 146

PART II: CLINICAL APPLICATION, *147*

1. Occipital Neuralgia (Pain and Tension in Occipital Region), *149*
2. Trigeminal Neuralgia, *151*
3. Trauma to Cervical Vertebrae (Whiplash Injury), *154*
4. Scapulohumeral Periarthritis (Frozen Shoulder), *156*
5. Brachialgia (Tennis Elbow and Brachial Neuralgia), *158*
6. Intercostal Neuralgia, *160*
7. Osteoarthritis of the Lumbar Vertebrae, *162*
8. Herniated Disk in Lumbar Vertebrae (Slipped Disk), *165*
9. Sciatica, *166*
10. Osteoarthritis of the Knee Joint, *169*
11. Chronic Rheumatoid Arthritis, *171*
12. Headache, *173*
13. Vertigo, *175*
14. Tinnitus, *177*
15. Insomnia, *180*
16. Neck and Shoulder Tension, *181*
17. Chronic Bronchitis, *183*
18. Bronchial Asthma, *185*
19. Hypertension, *187*
20. Hypotension, *189*
21. Pyrosis and Eructation, *191*
22. Nausea and Vomiting, *193*
23. Constipation, *195*
24. Diarrhea, *197*
25. Chronic Gastritis, *199*

26. Hemorrhoids, *201*
27. Chronic Hepatitis, *203*
28. Eczema and Urticaria, *205*
29. Menstrual Irregularity and Dysmenorrhea, *207*
30. Increasing Vitality, *210*
31. Preventing the Ill Effects of Aging, *212*
32. Wrinkles in Facial Skin, *214*
33. Blemishes and Freckles, *216*
34. Beautifying Skin, *218*

Index, *221*

Part I

Basic Concepts of Acupuncture

Chapter 1
Oriental Medicine — A Historical Perspective

1. Western Medicine and Oriental Medicine

Among the variety of therapeutic methods practiced in Japan today, Western medicine and Oriental medicine are the most prominent. Western medicine, which is also known as modern medicine, has advanced dramatically in recent history to become the mainstream of health care. Oriental medicine in Japan is synonymous with Chinese medicine, which was subject to some cultural modification since its introduction in the sixth century. The differences between Western medicine and Oriental medicine are largely a result of the different cultural settings and world views from which they originated.

There is a fundamental difference between Western medicine and Oriental medicine in how disease is perceived. In Western medicine a mechanistic and compartmentalized view is adopted and the body has been finely divided into smaller and smaller organic units with the advancement of medicine. Minute components of the body were initially identified by the use of optical microscopes and today electron microscopes are used for this purpose. The main emphasis in Western medicine has become pathophysiology on a cellular or even on a molecular level. The basic assumption in Western medicine is that we can grasp the true nature of life by finely differentiating our physical components and their functions and then piecing all this data together. According to this reasoning, the only reason Western medicine is not totally effective in all cases is that research concerning some diseases has not yet been sufficient to reveal a physical cause and effect relationship. The solution, therefore, is considered to be the relentless pursuit of basic research. The result of such an approach is a value judgment in which, more than treating a suffering patient, the emphasis is placed on basic research as the most essential and important element in medicine.

In contrast to the mechanistic perspective of Western medicine, the emphasis in Oriental medicine is to view the human body as an integrated whole, inseparable from its environment. Thus great value has always been placed on personal experience and individual practices for health, and Oriental medicine developed as individualized form of medicine. It may be said that the basic approach in Oriental medicine is to prevent disease and to enhance health by encouraging people to correct unhealthy tendencies, be they mental or physical. This is precisely why so much attention is given to the subjective complaints of patients, which cannot be substantiated by anyone except the patient himself. In Oriental medicine the patient is carefully examined from both an objective and subjective standpoint to determine his *shō* (*xiang* in Chinese: a symptom complex or disease pattern), which directly leads to a specific treatment.

Table 1: Contrast of Tendencies in Western Medicine and Oriental Medicine

Oriental Medicine	Western Medicine
philosophical	scientific
holistic	compartmentalized
organic	mechanistic
internal medicine	surgical medicine
treatment for the pattern	symptomatic treatment
empirical	logical
preventive medicine	hygienic medicine
individualized medicine	social medicine
improving constitution	killing microorganisms
experience with patients	animal experiments
humoral pathology	cellular pathology
subjective symptoms	objective symptoms
natural herbal medicine	synthetic chemical medicine

The aim in Oriental medicine has always been to improve health and prolong life by correcting imbalances in the functions of the body. Since human beings are a part of nature, we are constantly under the influence of climatic conditions associated with the four seasons, including that of heat, cold, dampness, rain, wind, and storms. The workings of our body (the functions of the nervous system, musculoskeletal system, and internal organs) generally adjust to the given conditions to maintain a healthy state of equilibrium.

We human beings often live a life in society where interpersonal relationships can be very demanding. This causes a considerable fluctuation in our mental and emotional states. The "seven emotions" of Oriental Medicine which include joy, anger, sadness, pensiveness, grief, fright, and fear, are considered to be very important as causes of disease.

From the standpoint of Oriental medicine, therefore, a person becomes sick when extreme climatic conditions, abnormal psychological states, or fatigue and immoderation in eating and drinking continue beyond the body's tolerance. Disease is seen as a group of symptoms which arise from imbalances in physical functions. The basic principle of treatment is to control the function that is over-active and to promote the functions that is underactive. Even though the acupuncture points and the methods employed in acupuncture therapy do not vary a great deal, applying the right amount of stimulation for each patient is sufficient to alleviate a wide variety of complaints.

As mentioned before, one of the characteristics of acupuncture therapy is the thorough examination of each individual patient and treatment directed at the whole person rather than dealing with specific organ systems. An acupuncturist must inquire in detail about his patient's problems, physical ailments, and pains. Also he must take his patient's pulse to find out whether their basic constitution is strong or weak. Finally, he must inspect each patient by touch to precisely decide the "prescription" or the acupuncture points and needling methods to be used in the treatment. Based on this "prescription" the acupuncturist applies the appropriate acupuncture stimulation (either strong or mild) on the "tsubo" located on the skin surface. In this manner, an acupuncturist renders treatment in a manner unique to Oriental medicine. That is to say, a diagnosis immediately leads to a treatment.

The term *tsubo* has been mentioned as an important feature of acupuncture therapy. A vital concept in Oriental medicine is that, whenever there are dysfunctions in the internal organs (functional imbalances), certain reactions appear in associated skin areas. These sensitive areas are on vertical bands of skin which run from the head to the feet or from the chest to the arms. The points which tend to show a reaction are commonly called tsubo in Japan, and these are also known as acu-points or acupuncture points. The bands of skin on which these reactive points appear are called meridians, or channels and collaterals. There are fourteen major meridians in the body. In acupuncture the tsubos are stimulated to adjust functional imbalances of the body. But for now, let us return to the broader topic of comparing Western medicine and Oriental medicine and leave the detailed discussion of tsubo for a later chapter.

Thus far we have examined the contrast of tendencies in Western medicine and Oriental medicine as well as some of their strengths and weaknesses. In the present age with the breathtaking advancement in modern technological society and drastic changes in our living environment, illnesses of a nervous or psychosomatic origin are on the rise. Today we are affected by largely untraceable internal and external factors such as mental stress and environmental pollution. In many cases the rational reductionistic methods of diagnosis and treatment employed in Western medicine are not as effective as we might hope. A new concept in health care called primary care is now growing in which an attempt is being made to treat individuals in a more comprehensive manner. Along with this trend, modern medicine is going through a period of reexamination by the public in light of harmful drug side effects and other critical problems. This is also fueling the popular movement to reappraise the value of Oriental medicine.

Be that as it may, both Western medicine and Oriental medicine have their particular strengths and weaknesses, which in many ways are a result of differences in the cultural setting and world view in which they developed. The key problem today is how to go about developing a more complete form of medicine which includes elements of both Western and Oriental medicine based on an acceptance of their basic differences and a clear understanding of their scope of effectiveness and their limitations. In China an attempt is being made to develop a new form of medicine by integrating Western medicine and Chinese medicine. A similar attempt to combine modern and traditional elements of medicine is being made in a few other countries as well. Many studies and experiments are being conducted to this end and there have been some promising results. Nevertheless, there are still a host of problems which need to be resolved before such a synthesis can be achieved, and it will take many more years before such a new type of medicine becomes a reality.

2. The History of Oriental Medicine

Primitive medicine practiced in prehistoric times was derived from the instincts of self-preservation and preservation of the species. Medicine was therefore based on instinct and acquired experience. It is very likely that the first thing done in primitive times, whenever someone became ill, was to put one's hands on the affected part to relieve the suffering. Through instinct and experience people knew that placing one's hand on the ailing part has a soothing and healing effect. Many vital points useful for bringing relief simply by touch must have been found and passed on in this way. In the course of time this manual form of medicine became increasingly complex as more specific effects were sought, and it eventually developed into Dō-in (exercises) and Ankyō (manipulation). Further, with the advancement of civilization, it is thought that various implements came into use such as stone needles (flint stones for draining abscesses) and the nine metal needles of antiquity. Also methods of using moxa for cauterization and herbs for ointments and poultices were developed.

In the *Huangdi Nei Jing (The Yellow Emperor's Classic of Internal Medicine)*, the oldest medical text of China, it is written that stone needles came from the east, herbal medicine from the west, moxibustion from the north, the nine metal needles from the south, and Dō-in and Ankyō from the central region. This indicates that different forms of medicine developed in various regions according to the environment and culture. Some form of therapy similar to acupuncture and moxibustion was also practiced in ancient India because legend has it that the famous Indian physician Jivaka, a contemporary of Buddha (fifth century B.C.), held a needle and medicinal herbs in his hands at birth. Also there is occasional mention of acupuncture in various Buddhist scriptures. For this reason some scholars consider the origin of acupuncture to be in India, although it is generally thought to come from China. The issue is obscured in antiquity, but there is clear evidence of acupuncture being practiced in China several centuries before Christ. Also it was in China that acupuncture developed into an indispensable component of Oriental medicine and reached its zenith to become the foundation of a tradition which is alive to this day.

(1) Historical Outline of Acupuncture in China

Protohistoric Period (2383 B.C.–1123 B.C.)
Primitive medicine before historical times developed in various regions of China spontaneously according to the people's basic instinct of self-preservation. The early beginnings of Chinese medicine were in this period and these primitive forms of medicine were handed down from one generation to the next. According to Chinese legend, the Emperor Fuxi discovered the use of fire and formulated the basis for the *I-Ching*. Shen Nong is given credit for the invention of agriculture and is also held to be the first one to discover the use of medicinal herbs. The earliest text on herbs is *Shen Nong Ben Cao Jing* (Shen Nong's Herbal Classic). It is said that the *Huangdi Nei Jing (The Yellow Emperor's Classic of Internal Medicine)*

was compiled sometime later under the orders of the Yellow Emperor (Huangdi). The *Huangdi Nei Jing* was the first complete exposition of the principles of Chinese medicine. The medical principles in this text were probably formulated in the latter half of the Spring and Autumn period (320 B.C.–250 B.C.). The completed version of the *Huangdi Nei Jing* is estimated to date from the Qin Dynasty or the Early Han Dynasty (221 B.C.–A.D. 6).

The *Huangdi Nei Jing* is considered to be a summarization of the clinical experience of the physicians of the Han people who lived in Yellow River basin. This text takes a dialogue form with the Yellow Emperor asking his six ministers (physicians) various questions about health and disease. The contents of this text were edited and annotated in later periods and the two parts of this text which remain today are the *Su Wen* and *Ling Shu*. The *Su Wen* and *Ling Shu* consist of nine chapters each. *Su Wen* means a record of plain questions and answers. *Ling Shu* means writings on the vital knowledge of divine beings. The *Su Wen* includes discourse on matters related to physiology, pathology, and ways to foster health and prevent disease. The *Ling Shu* details various acupuncture techniques based on the theories about anatomy, physiology, and the system of organs and meridians. These volumes are prized as the oldest original texts of Chinese medicine.

Zhou and Qin Dynasties (1122 B.C.–207 B.C.)
The long period from the beginning of the Zhou Dynasty to the end of the Qin Dynasty was a period of fermentation in which the medical practices coming from prehistoric times were tested and systematized. The famous ancient physician Bianque (Qin Yueren) lived in this period. *Nan Jing*, the acupuncture text ascribed to Bianque, expanded on the principles laid down in the *Su Wen* and *Ling Shu* and explains in detail the concepts of pathology and the treatment principle in traditional Chinese medicine. This text also takes the question and answer form and consists of eighty-one sections. The *Nan Jing* is a valuable acupuncture text which is still studied by acupuncturists of this day.

Early and Late Han Dynasties (206 B.C.–A.D. 264)
Chinese culture and civilization blossomed and flourished during the centuries of the two Han dynasties and codification of Chinese medicine was among the major achievements in this period. Medical practices became systematized and more uniform and Chinese medicine reached new heights to become a complete medical system. In this period the oldest classics of Chinese herbology the *Shang Han Lun* (Treatise on Febrile Diseases) and *Jin Kui Yao Lue Fang Lun* (Synopsis of Pre-·scriptions in the Golden Chest) were written by Zhang Zhong Jing.

Jin and Sui Dynasties (A.D. 265–617)
The fall of the Han dynasty was followed by centuries of civil war and this slowed down advancement in Chinese society (as well as medicine). Nevertheless, in the early part of this period Wang Shuhe wrote *Mai Jing* (The Pulse Classic) and Huangfu Mi compiled *Zen Jiu Jia Yi Jing* (A Classic of Acupuncture and Moxibustion). These works contributed greatly to the clinical practice of acupuncture for many generations to come. In the latter part of this period Cao Yuanfung

compiled *Zhu Bing Yuan Hou Zong Lun* (General Treaties on the Etiology and Symptomology of Diseases).

Tang Dynasty (A.D. 618–951)

The practice of medicine reached new levels of development with the stability and prosperity of Chinese society during the Tang dynasty. Many famous medical texts were written in this period. Among the most famous ones are *Bei Jin Qian Jin Yao Fang* (Emergency Prescriptions Worth a Thousand Gold) and *Bei Ji Qian Jin Fang* (Supplement to Prescriptions Worth a Thousand Gold). Wang Tao's *Wai Tai Mi Yao* (Medical Secrets of an Officer) is a famous text of the Tang dynasty which is particularly significant to the practice of acupuncture.

Song Dynasty (A.D. 952–1278)

In the Song Dynasty the Neo-Confucian concept of Xingli (a theory of cosmology in which a portion of the ultimate principle is thought to reside in all things) and the principle of Ju Fang Xue (a systematization of uses of herbs) were developed. Also in this period the printing press was invented and medical publications became widely available for the first time. In term of developments in acupuncture, Wang Weiyi had two life-size hollow bronze figures cast with the meridians and points inscribed. Wang Weiyi also compiled the text *Tong Ren Shu Xue Zhen Jiu Tu Jing* as a manual for studying acupuncture points with these bronze figures.

Jin and Yuan Dynasties (A.D. 1115–1367)

Medicine advanced considerably during the Jin dynasty and the ensuing Mongolian Empire. Various schools of herbology were in contention during this period such as the so-called Cold School of Medicine, the School of Purgation, the School of Tonifying the Spleen and Stomach, and the School of Preserving Life. In the field of acupuncture, Hua Shou (Hua Bairen) wrote many excellent texts still useful to acupuncturists today. These works include *Shi si Jing Fa Hui* (Exposition on the Fourteen Channels), *Nan Jing Ben Yi* (The Genuine Meaning of the Difficult Classic), and *Zhen Jia Shu Yao* (Essentials for a Clinician).

Ming Dynasty (A.D. 1368–1661)

There were no dramatic new developments in medicine during the Ming dynasty; the traditions developed in former times were simply carried on. The important texts of acupuncture that were published in this period were *Lei Jing* (Systematic Compilation of *The Yellow Emperor's Classic of Internal Medicine*) by Zhang Jiebin and *Zhen Jiu Ju Ying* (Essentials of Acupuncture and Moxibustion) by Gao Wu.

Qing Dynasty (A.D. 1662–1871)

The Qing dynasty was a period of confusion for Chinese medicine. Various schools of traditional medicine were in conflict with one another and Western medicine began to gain acceptance among the upper class. In the field of herbal medicine, Chinese therapeutic concepts adopted in Japan were developed further and re-introduced into China.

Republic of China and People's Republic of China
After the revolution of 1911 and the founding of the Republic of China, Western influences became dominant and traditional medicine began to lose ground, but the majority of doctors treating the general population were still practitioners of traditional medicine. The communist revolution of 1949 and the formation of the People's Republic brought sweeping changes in Chinese society. In the beginning there was some conflict between doctors of Western medicine and practitioners of Chinese medicine, but today both parties work together under the policy of "Uniting Chinese and Western Medicine." Now under this new policy traditional therapies and prescriptions based on experience are being reconsidered and investigated from a scientific standpoint.

(2) Historical Outline of Acupuncture in Japan

Early Period (fifth to sixth century A.D.*)*
Acupuncture and moxibustion were introduced into Japan from Korea early in the fifth century as part of the great transfer of knowledge and culture from the East Asian subcontinent. Initially the immigrants from the Korean Peninsula brought acupuncture and other forms of Chinese medicine to Japan for their own sake. In 562 the first teacher of medicine, a Chinese monk and physician named Zhicong, immigrated to Japan with 160 volumes of Chinese medical texts. After direct contact was established between China and Japan in the sixth century, Japanese envoys including physicians travelled to China and returned with a wealth of Chinese medical knowledge.

*Nara and Heian Periods (*A.D.* 710–1185)*
When the Taiho Code, the first legal system in Japan, was promulgated in 701, great importance was placed on acupuncture and moxibustion. An official department of acupuncture and moxibustion was established and the ranks of doctor of acupuncture, acupuncturist, and acupuncture student were designated. Medical education was conducted in the Capital and acupuncturists were required to study for a period of seven years. In 753 an eminent Chinese Buddhist monk Jianzhen immigrated to Japan with thirty-five of his disciples. Several of his disciples were physicians and they transmitted their medical knowledge to Japanese monks and students.

All knowledge from China including Chinese medicine was actively assimilated in Japan during the Nara Period, but in the mid-ninth century contact with China was curtailed and Chinese medicine began to undergo independent development in Japan. In 984 Yasunari Tamba, a doctor of acupuncture, was commissioned by the emperor of Japan to compile a comprehensive medical text. Tamba's book, *Ishimpō* became the first Japanese medical text and a landmark in the medical history of Japan.

*Kamakura and Muromachi Periods (*A.D.* 1185–1574)*
In the Kamakura Period the official medical system was abandoned and the practice of acupuncture and moxibustion began to decline in Japan. Not much

advancement was seen in the field of medicine in the upheaval of the warring period during the fifteenth and sixteenth centuries, but the healing art of acupuncture and moxibustion survived among the common people.

Momoyama Period (A.D. 1575–1602)
Japan became unified again in the Momoyama Period and the stability created in society by the new order lead to new developments in many fields including the practice of acupuncture. In the Momoyama period Isai Misono developed a new acupuncture technique using gold and silver needles. This was known as the *dashin* technique, and small mallets were employed to insert needles into the abdominal area.

Edo Period (A.D. 1602–1868)
Early in the Edo Period a blind acupuncturist named Waichi Sugiyama developed a painless needle insertion technique using a guide tube. Sugiyama was awarded the highest official rank as an acupuncturist, and the Sugiyama School of acupuncture became the most prominent school. This school had a profound influence on Japanese acupuncture, and the use of guide tubes and thin needles became widespread in Japan. The Edo Period was the era when Western medical knowledge of anatomy and physiology reached Japan by way of the Dutch Trading Company and their physicians. Many Japanese physicians began to study Dutch medical texts with great enthusiasm and became pioneers in a new pragmatic approach to medicine. Sotetsu Ishizaka was a famous acupuncturist from the Sugiyama School who went on to establish his own school of acupuncture based on the new knowledge of anatomy and physiology. Ishizaka taught acupuncture to Phillip Siebold, an official Dutch physician invited to Japan in the early nineteenth century. All during the Edo period acupuncture flourished as never before and Japanese acupuncture showed truly unique developments.

Modern Era
The Meiji Restoration marked the end of the feudal era and the new government resolved to modernize Japan after the Western model. This brought monumental changes in Japanese society as well as in the field of medicine. All physicians were required to study and pass an examination in Western medicine, and thus practitioners of traditional medicine lost their status as physicians. Although acupuncture was not outlawed, it lost ground to Western medicine and was reduced to a folk medicine. In time, however, those physicians with an appreciation for acupuncture conducted scientific studies and supported the cause of acupuncture to gain government approval of acupuncture. Even though acupuncture once more became a legitimate practice, new standards for acupuncture education were established with a disregard of traditional theories, and acupuncture was defined as nothing more than a type of stimulation therapy.

The American occupation after the defeat in the Second World War brought sweeping changes to Japanese society and initiated a new wave of westernization. At one point just after the war the occupation government tried to impose a ban on acupuncture and moxibustion in the belief that these were barbaric practices. This rallied all those in favor of acupuncture and moxibustion, and a new law was passed to guarantee the right to practice traditional forms of medicine. Since that time a diversity of approaches to acupuncture, both traditional and modern, have developed and flourished in Japan.

3. Principles of Chinese Medicine

(1) The Yin-Yang Theory

The yin-yang and five element theories are the central concepts among the principles of Chinese medicine, and these concepts are explained in the *Su Wen* and *Ling Shu*, which are the two parts of the *Huangdi Nei Jing (The Yellow Emperor's Classic of Internal Medicine)*. The theories of yin-yang and five elements are regarded as a cosmological system created by the ancient Chinese to analyze, classify, and organize their experiences according to their perceived order of natural phenomenon. In other words, this was an attempt to explain and find some order among the varied phenomena of nature. The yin-yang theory and five element theory developed separately, but eventually they came to be used together to complement each other. The basic principles of the yin-yang theory are as follows:

The Yin-Yang and Five Element Theory
The yin-yang theory of Chinese medicine came from the *I-Ching*, the book of divination. In this theory Tai Ji (the formless state before heaven and earth separate) is transformed so that the active aspect becomes yang and the quiescent aspect becomes yin. All manifestations in nature are the result of the interaction of yin and yang, and yin and yang aspects can be traced in everything. Generally things in which activity is predominant are considered yang and things characterized by quiescence are considered yin. For example the heavens are in a constant state of flux so it is yang, and the earth in contrast is yin. Based on a similar analogy, men are regarded as being yang while women are yin. The division of meridians into yin meridians and yang meridians is based on this concept.

The theory of five elements or five phases first appears in *Shang Shu*, a classic attributed to Confucius. In this theory all things in nature are composed of the five elements of wood, fire, earth, metal, and water, and all things can be categorized as belonging to one of the five elements. The five elements can be understood either as basic elements or as a means of classifying all things by their essential nature. The theory of five elements is applied to the human body to categorize the five yin organs (liver, heart, spleen, lung, and kidney) and the five yang organs (gallbladder, small intestine, stomach, large intestine, and bladder). The yin-yang and five element theories were combined a few centuries before the Han Dynasty to become the main framework for Chinese cosmology.

The Opposition and Complementarity of Yin and Yang

Yin and yang is viewed as two complementary opposites such as day and night, or light and dark. The two opposite poles of yin and yang are otherwise expressed as the heaven and earth, the sun and the moon, up and down, front and back, and father and mother, with the former being yang and the latter being yin. Thus all manifestations are classified as being either more yang or more yin according to various criterion such as being more or less active, and more external or more internal.

The Inter-transforming Relationship of Yin and Yang

Yin and yang are not just viewed as two complementary opposites, but also as changeable conditions. Yin does not remain yin forever, and yang does not remain yang forever. This point is illustrated by the old saying: "Activity when reaching an extreme gives rise to quiescence, and quiescence when reaching an extreme produces activity. Within activity there is an element of quiescence and within quiescence there is an element of activity." It is also said that; "What is hard eventually becomes soft and what is soft eventually becomes hard. There is a softness within the hard and a hardness within the soft."

In this way, all things contain both a yin and a yang aspect and the dominance of one over the other depends upon the circumstances. A man is yang in contrast to a woman, but if the same man is compared to either of his parents, he is yin. Likewise, a woman is considered as being yin, but she is yang when compared to her children. Similarly, the front of something is yang compared to its back, but this front is yin when compared to something further in front. When a person is very active he is yang, but when he becomes inactive he is yin. Yin and yang are in a constant state of flux perpetually transforming from one into the other.

Yang represents the energy which produces action, that seeking to express itself, that which differentiates, and that which progresses. If this function of yang is carried to an extreme, however, activity brings exhaustion, expression becomes poor, differentiation leads to disorganization, and progress grinds to a halt. Yin energy is what keeps the yang functions from going too far. The function of yin is quiescence, drawing inward, unifying, and compensating. If yin functions become too dominant, however, there is atrophy, obsession, and stagnation, which all lead to an overall decline. Normal life activity is possible only when both yin and yang functions are in balance. The harmonious inter-transformation of yin and yang makes the creation of new life possible.

The yin-yang theory was devised as a way to come to terms with the complexities of phenomena in nature by explaining how antagonistic elements worked to complement each other and how opposing aspects become dominant and then subordinate in a cyclic manner. This principle of interaction between opposite forces was seen to operate in all spheres of life including the natural environment and society as well as a person's mental and physical composition. In this way, as the central concept of a complex cosmology, the yin-yang theory was applied to all aspects of Chinese society including medicine.

In Table 2, the basic yin-yang categories specially relevant to Oriental medicine are listed for the sake of reference.

Table 2

	YIN	*YANG*
Human Anatomy	lower half	upper half
	internal	superficial
	anterior	posterior
	medial	lateral
	zang	*fu*
	Xue	*Qi*
Functional Condition	inhibition	excitation
	hypoactive	hyperactive
Pathology	interior	exterior
	cold	heat
	deficiency	excess
Pulse	sinking	floating
	slow	rapid
	empty	full
	thin	big

(2) The Five Element Theory

In addition to the yin-yang theory, the ancient Chinese formulated the five element theory to categorize things in the natural environment. The things classified according to the five elements were all phenomena or objects which were important in people's lives. The five basic qualities (elements) of plant life, heat, soil, minerals, and liquid were considered to be the essence of all things, and these were expressed as wood, fire, earth, metal, and water. The five element theory outlines the inter-relationship of five types of essential *ki* (since all matter was thought to originate from *ki*). It is a system of classifying and interpreting all phenomena in terms of the basic elements.

In Oriental medicine a human being is viewed as a microcosm existing within the macrocosm of nature, and therefore all the laws of nature apply in some way to the body. All medical experience can be fit into the framework of the five elements to understand how various factors such as diet and environment affect the body. Also, the body's structural components, physiological functions, and pathology, as well as approaches to diagnosis and treatment are defined in a systematic way with the five elements.

The essential organic components that maintain life functions within the human body are said to be the five *zang* (yin organs), each of which corresponds to one of the five elements. The five *zang* are the liver, heart, spleen, lung, and kidney, and among these, the liver is associated with wood, the heart with fire, the spleen with earth, the lung with metal, and the kidney with water. Although the basic life functions of the body are maintained by the harmonious functioning of the five *zang*, this is made possible with the help of the five *fu* (yang organs). Among the *fu*, the gallbladder is associated with the liver, the small intestine with the heart, the stomach with the spleen, the large intestine with the lung, and the bladder with the kidney. In this way every *zang* and *fu* is paired in a yin-yang relationship.

There is a tendency when speaking about the *zang*, such as the liver or the spleen, for people to confuse them with the anatomical structures known in modern medicine. Even though most of the *zang* and *fu* of traditional Chinese medicine bear the same name as organs in modern medicine, this in no way means that they refer to the same things. It just so happens that the same names were adopted for organs in Western medicine as those of the *zang* and *fu*. In the case of Japan, Oriental medicine was the only kind of medicine during the feudalistic period in which there was almost no contact with the Western countries. When anatomy texts of Western medicine first arrived in Japan in the eighteenth century, the existing terms of Oriental medicine were used in the translation to describe similar organs. Thus unwittingly the traditional *zang* and *fu* came to be mis-construed as being nothing more than the anatomical structures known in modern medicine.

In any case, there are five *zang-fu* combinations which are each associated with one of the five elements. There is actually one more *zang-fu* combination which is the pericardium and the triple heater. This yin-yang pair belongs to the fire ele-ment, but this pair is in its own category distinct from the rest of the *zang-fu*. The pericardium is viewed as having the special function of protecting the heart, the most vital organ which must initiate a rhythmic impulse continually throughout our entire life. The triple heater is the *fu* associated with the pericardium, and its name implies three sources of heat. The body's ability to maintain a constant temperature regardless of the temperature outside was explained in Oriental medicine by designating three central areas in the body where heat is generated.

The concept of six *zang* and six *fu* may seem a little strange from the standpoint of modern medicine, but the human body is conceptualized in a totally different way in Oriental medicine. Rather than organs existing as anatomically distinct structures, the *zang-fu* are best understood as functional divisions of the human body, which is a complex and delicate interrelationship between structure and function. All life functions of the human body come under the control of the six *zang* and six *fu*, and if there is a disturbance in one of the *zang* or *fu*, the whole body is affected and various symptoms appear. Each of the six *zang* and six *fu* is related to one meridian, or channel of energy circulation. These twelve meridians together with the two meridians which travel up the center line on the front and back of the body make up the fourteen major meridians which will be discussed in detail in the next chapter.

All the *zang-fu* and meridians fit into the five element theory, since all things can be categorized by this theory. There is a long traditional list of five element correlations, and these were used for diagnosis in medicine. Table 3 lists some of the main five element correlations.

The five element correlations were sometimes applied in a very simplistic fashion. Concerning the color of food, it was thought that greens were good for the liver and gallbladder, red foods, for the heart and small intestine, and yellow foods,

Table 3: Five Element Correlations

Element	wood	fire	earth	metal	water	
Mother Element	water	wood	fire	earth	metal	
Zang	liver	heart	spleen	lung	kidney	The pericardium is fire.
Fu	gallbladder	small intestine	stomach	large intestine	bladder	The triple heater is fire.
Orifice	eyes	tongue	lips (mouth)	nose	ears	(excretory openings)
Tissue	tendons	vessels	flesh	skin	bone	controlled by the *zang*
Nourishes	nails	complexion	lips	body hair	scalp hair	nourished by the *zang*
Season	spring	summer	late summer	fall	winter	season *zang* is most active
Direction	east	south	center	west	north	direction of influence
Color	green	red	yellow	white	black	skin color of patient
Odor	rancid	burned	fragrant	fleshy	rotten	body odor of patient
Taste	sour	bitter	sweet	pungent	salty	preferred taste
Climate	windy	hot	damp	dry	cold	harmful climate
Emotions	anger	laughing	pensiveness	sorrow	fear	characteristic emotion
Fluids	tears	sweat	saliva	snivel	urine	origin of fluids
Abnormality	clenching	melancholy	hiccupping	coughing	shivering	sign of disease in the *zang*
Functions	sight	voice	taste	smell	fluids	function of the *zang*
Voice	shouting	chattering	singing	whining	groaning	voice quality of patient
Grain	wheat	millet	rye	rice	beans	beneficial grain
Meat	chicken	mutton	beef	horse	pork	beneficial meat
Vegetable	leeks	shallots	mallows	onions	course greens	beneficial vegetable
Fruit	plums	apricots	dates	peaches	chestnuts	beneficial fruit

(*Source:* primarily from the fifth chapter of *Su Wen*)

for the spleen and stomach. Likewise it was understood that in the case of kidney or bladder problems one's complexion would appear blackish, that with lung or large intestine problems the complexion became pale and white, and that with liver or gallbladder problems the complexion would turn bluish or greenish. Such correspondences were not clinically useful in all cases, but just as often it provided valuable clues when correlated with findings obtained with other diagnostic approaches.

The most important concepts in the five element theory is that of the productive relationship and the controlling relationship. In the productive cycle of the five elements, wood gives rise to fire, fire to earth, earth to metal, metal to water, and water to wood. The element which produces another is referred to as the mother, and the element which is produced is called the son. Two adjacent elements in this cycle of creation or production are therefore said to be in a mother/son relationship. Going in reverse of the productive cycle of wood, fire, earth, metal, and water, the element of water is compatible with that of metal, metal with earth, earth with fire, and fire with wood. This is known as the compatibility relationship.

The relationship of each of the five elements to the element subsequent to the next element in the productive cycle is called a controlling relationship. Thus wood controls earth, earth controls water, water controls fire, fire controls metal, and metal controls wood. This mutually controlling relationship of the five elements is explained in simple terms as trees taking their nourishment from the ground, the earth being used as dikes to control water, water quenching fires, fire being used to melt metals, and metal being used to cut wood. In the reverse of the controlling cycle, earth is subjugated by wood, wood by metal, metal by fire, fire by water, and water by earth. This is known as the subjugation relationship.

The productive cycle and the controlling cycles are shown below in a diagrammatic form.

Fig. 1   Productive Cycle

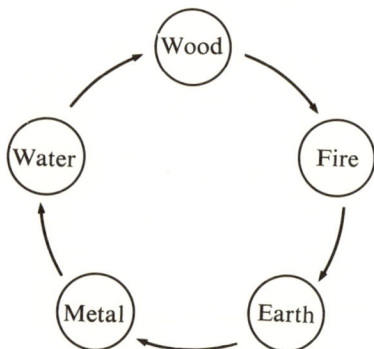

Fig. 2   Controlling Cycle

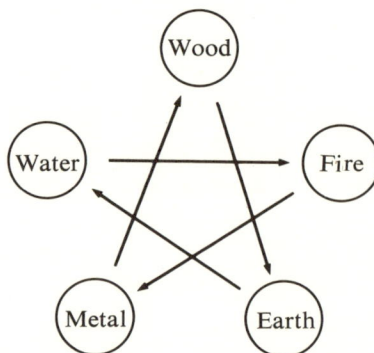

The five zang and five fu are listed according to their five element correlations in Fig. 3. The productive and controlling relationships of the five elements apply in the same manner to the corresponding five zang and five fu.

Fig. 3   **Yin-Yang Relationship of the Zang-Fu**

Yin (zang)   Yang (fu)

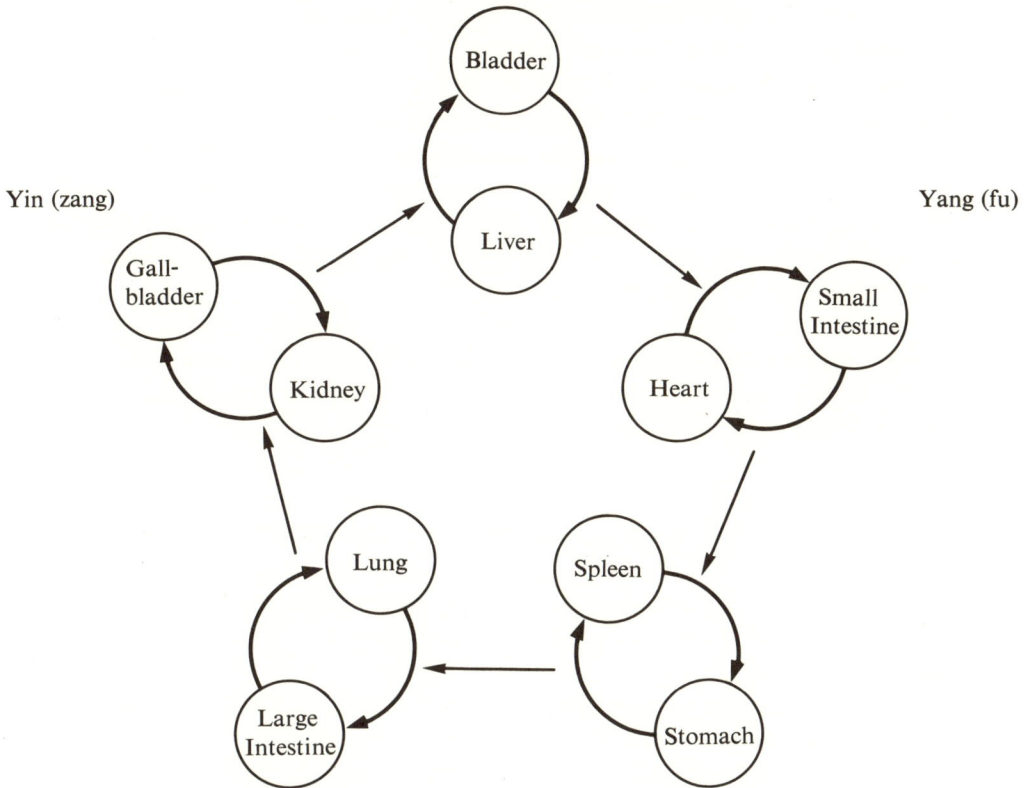

4. The Meridians (Energy Circulation System)

In Oriental medicine health is considered to be a result of the balanced and harmonious functioning of the six *zang* and six *fu* (internal organs). Disease is seen as a state in which the functions of these organs have been disturbed and the functional balance between the *zang-fu* is upset. As a means of maintaining smooth and balanced functioning of the six *zang* and six *fu*, pathways of energy circulation which connect every *zang* and *fu* to the body surface are said to exist. These routes of energy (*ki*) circulation are known as the meridians.

Meridian is the simple name for channel (vertical paths of circulation) and collateral (horizontal paths of circulation). There are main meridians and branch meridians, and internally the meridians connect to the *zang-fu* and superficially they travel within or close to the skin thus forming a complex network of energy circulation throughout the body. The meridians are pathways for the movement of what is known as *ki* and *ketsu* (*qi* and *xue*) in Oriental medicine. *Ki* and *ketsu* can be understood collectively as the vital energetic or functional components necessary for organic life.

The twelve meridians directly connected with the *zang-fu* are as follows: (1) lung meridian, (2) large intestine meridian, (3) stomach meridian, (4) spleen meridian, (5) heart meridian, (6) small intestine meridian, (7) bladder meridian, (8) kidney meridian, (9) pericardium meridian, (10) triple heater meridian, (11) gallbladder meridian, and (12) liver meridian. These meridians are also known as the twelve regular meridians. The energy circulation is said to start in the lung meridian and successively flow through each of the meridians and their associated *zang-fu* to complete the cycle by going through the liver meridian. After going through the liver meridian, the energy once more enters the lung meridian to repeat the same cycle of energy circulation through the body.

In addition to the twelve regular meridians, which comprise an energy circulation system directly associated with the *zang-fu*, there are eight extra meridians flowing through the body. The extra meridians serve to adjust any excesses or deficiencies in the energy flowing through the twelve regular meridians. The eight extra meridians are as follows: (1) conception vessel, (2) governor vessel, (3) *Yang Qiao* vessel, (4) *Yin Qiao* vessel, (5) *Yang Wei* vessel, (6) *Yin Wei* vessel, (7) *Dai* vessel, and (8) *Chong* vessel. Among these extra meridians the conception vessel, which is on the anterior median line of the body, and the governor vessel, which is on the posterior median line of the body, are especially important meridians. These two extra meridians added to the twelve regular meridians are called the fourteen major meridians.

In Oriental medicine, as already stated, the key to health is smooth and un-interrupted circulation of *ki* and *ketsu* (different forms of energy) through the meridians. Once there is some dysfunction in the organs or else if an external pathogenic factor invades the body, the circulation of *ki* and *ketsu* is impeded so that either the dysfunction of the *zang-fu* is reflected on the body surface or the invasion of the unhealthy environmental influence is relayed to the *zang-fu* by way of the meridians. The basic treatment principle in acupuncture is to accurately diagnose and treat any state of disruption in energy circulation.

It is necessary to explain *ki* and *ketsu*, which circulate through the meridians, in a little more detail. In Oriental medicine *ki* and *ketsu* are considered essential for carrying out various life processes. *Ki* is regarded to be a formless element some-what akin to a gas, and it appears in many Japanese words, such as air (*kūki*: empty *ki*) and weather (*tenki*: heaven's *ki*). More than just a gas, however, *ki* is understood as a form of energy which acts on matter to effect some change or carry out some function. *Ketsu*, on the other hand, refers to a liquid substance like our blood and body fluids, which is much more like physical matter and can actually be seen in our body. The "source *ki*" (*genki* in Japanese) received from one's parents prenatally causes the formation of *ketsu*, or blood and other fluid constituents of the body. *Ki* and *ketsu* work together to form our body and they are inextricably related. *Ki* and *ketsu* travel in the meridians together, but *ki* plays the main role. *Ki* is said to lead *ketsu* through the meridians. In this way *ki* and *ketsu* circulate throughout the body to carry out a multitude of life processes. The meridians (both the channels and collaterals) are thus a communication network for functional processes of the body and are an energetic system distinct from blood vessels and nerves.

5. Acupuncture Points (Tsubo)

Acupuncture points, which are commonly called *tsubo* in Japan, are key points along the energy pathways of the body known as meridians. The meridians do not remain consistent throughout whole body. In some places the meridians widen and in other places they become narrow. The size or thickness of meridians is thought to vary according to the location. The places on the meridian that are wider and where reactions appear on the skin surface are known as acupuncture points. The meridians connect the *zang-fu*, on the inside of the body, to the body surface. Acupuncture points are regarded as "gates" or openings by which the meridians communicate with the external environment.

As explained earlier, dysfunctions in the *zang-fu* are manifested at acupuncture points by transmission along the meridians, and otherwise, when external pathogenic factors afflict the body, the circulation of *ki* and *ketsu* along the meridians is disrupted by the unhealthy influence entering by way of the acupuncture points. Treating the meridians by stimulating the affected acupuncture points serves to alleviate the problem. Therefore the acupuncture points, in addition to being points at which one's condition can be diagnosed, are points at which treatment can be applied. In the case of abdominal pain, for example, the acupuncture points used to diagnose and to treat the problem will vary according to the location of the pain and which meridians are in the vicinity as well as whether it is a stomach condition or a liver condition.

This unique concept of disease in Oriental medicine is the reason an approach so different from Western medicine is used for diagnosis and treatment. Although the aim in Oriental medicine is basically the same as in Western medicine—to relieve the pain and suffering of patients—it emphasizes the subjective symptoms of every individual patient. More than identifying the exact type of disease, the thing needed to correct a physical problem is to determine what abnormalities the body is manifesting and to render a treatment according to the body's needs. The majority of physical problems are accompanied by a variety of abnormal reactions. These reactions include pain, numbness, tenderness, induration (knots), depressed areas, abnormally warm or cold areas, blemishes, freckles, and thin bands of tension. Treatment is provided on the acupuncture points in or around the area in which such reactions are felt. The overall physical condition may not be normalized just by one treatment. In some cases an acupuncture treatment causes a change in the location or nature of abnormal reactions. Wherever the reaction appears, if these manifestations are patiently dealt with one by one as they appear, the body will gradually return to a balanced condition and regain its original functional capacity in accordance with the laws of nature.

There are more than three hundred and sixty acupuncture points on the body. These are most commonly located in depressed spaces in the joints, creases in skin at joints, grooves between muscles, and clefts between muscle and bone, and otherwise in places where nerve trunks come close to the surface or in places where cutaneous nerves reach the skin through the muscles. In a sense these are all places in the body that are structurally more sensitive to physical stimulus than other areas.

Each meridian has a set of acupuncture points which more readily show the above mentioned physical reactions. These are the so-called command points, which are the acupuncture points on each meridian used most often in diagnosis and treatment. Every meridian has command points; these include the *Yuan* Source Point, *Xi* Cleft Point, *Luo* Connecting Point, Back *Shu* Point, and Front *Mu* Point. The table below lists the command points of the twelve regular meridians.

Table 4

Meridian	Yuan Point	Xi Point	Luo Point	Shu Point	Mu Point
Lung	LU-9	LU-6	LU-7	BL-13	LU-1
Large Intestine	LI-4	LI-7	LI-6	BL-25	ST-25
Stomach	ST-42	ST-34	ST-40	BL-21	CV-12
Spleen	SP-3	SP-8	SP-4	BL-19	LV-13
Heart	HT-7	HT-6	HT-5	BL-15	CV-14
Small Intestine	SI-4	SI-6	SI-7	BL-27	CV-4
Bladder	BL-64	BL-63	BL-58	BL-28	CV-3
Kidney	KI-3	KI-5	KI-4	BL-23	GB-25
Pericardium	PC-7	PC-4	PC-6	BL-14	CV-17
Triple Heater	TH-4	TH-7	TH-5	BL-22	CV-5
Gallbladder	GB-40	GB-36	GB-37	BL-19	GB-24
Liver	LV-3	LV-6	LV-5	BL-18	LV-14

Yuan Source Points
Among all the acupuncture points on a meridian, the most important one relating to that meridian is called the *Yuan* Source Point. If there is some problem in the internal organs, the pathology is always reflected in one of the *yuan* points. This fact is mentioned in the first chapter of the *Ling Shu*: "When there is disease in (one of) the five *zang*, a reaction appears at the twelve *yuan* points." Also it states, "When there is disease in the five *zang*, use the twelve *yuan* points." Thus the *yuan* points are valuable as points of diagnosis and they are also used directly for treatment.

Xi Cleft Points and Luo Connecting Points
Each meridian has a *xi* point and *luo* point. The character *xi* of the *Xi* Cleft Point means a groove or cleft between muscles and bone. In the classics, the *xi* points are identified as deep places between bone and muscle where *ki* and *ketsu* tend to collect. It is therefore a depression in muscles or between muscle and bones where a reaction appears. The *xi* points are considered to be points at which a reaction appears with acute problems, and these points are also useful for treating acute problems.

The *Luo* Connecting Point is said to be a point where a meridian branches (a collateral branches from a channel). The *luo* point is useful in modulating and regulating flow of *ki* and *ketsu* between the meridian's main trunk and its branch. The *luo* points are considered to be very useful in the treatment of chronic ailments.

Back Shu Points and Front Mu Points

The Back *Shu* Points are located on the back as the name implies, and each *shu* point is headed with the name of a *zang* or *fu*. The character *shu* of the Back *Shu* Points means a place where *ki* and *ketsu* pass through. Even though all the Back *Shu* Points are on the bladder meridian, they each show a reaction in response to problems in the corresponding *zang* or *fu*.

The Front *Mu* Points are located on the front of the body on the chest and abdomen. Most of the *mu* points, like the *shu* points, are found on a meridian other than the one they are associated with. Some *mu* points are located on the median line as a single point, and other *mu* points are located bilaterally on each side of the body as a pair of points. The character *mu* of the Front *Mu* Points means a place where *ki* and *ketsu* collect. Front *Mu* Points are very useful for diagnosis because they readily show a reaction of tenderness when there is some problem in their associated organ.

Chapter 2
Meridians and Acupuncture Points

1. The Circulation of Energy in the Meridians

The vital energy of the body known as *ki* circulates through the head, the trunk, the four limbs, and the viscera by way of the twelve meridians. The meridians are a network of interconnected channels which permeate the whole body. The energy flow begins in the *taiyin* lung meridian of the arm and goes to the *yangming* large intestine meridian of the arm and follows in sequence through the *yangming* stomach meridian of the leg, the *taiyin* spleen meridian of the leg, the *shaoyin* heart meridian of the arm, the *taiyang* small intestine meridian of the arm, the *taiyang* bladder meridian of the leg, the *shaoyin* kidney meridian of the leg, the *jueyin* pericardium meridian of the arm, the *shaoyang* triple heater meridian of the arm, the *shaoyang* gallbladder meridian of the leg, and the *jueyin* liver meridian of the leg (Fig. 4). After circulating through all twelve meridians, the energy returns to the *taiyin* lung meridian of the arm to repeat the above cycle again.

Fig. 4   The Twelve Meridians and Their Relationships

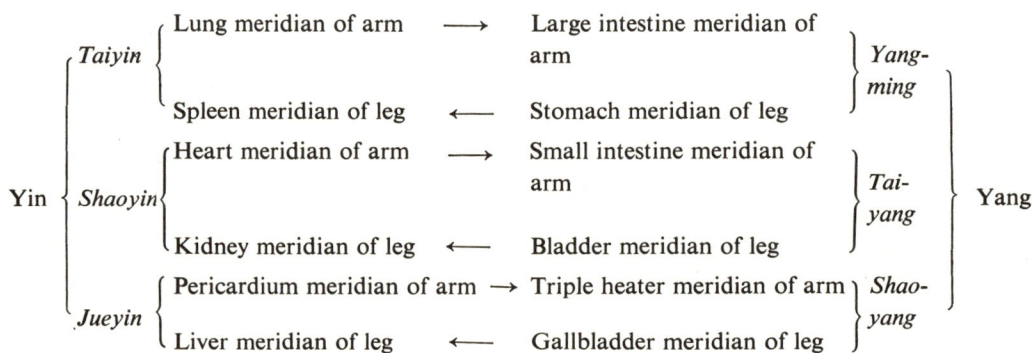

	Taiyin	Lung meridian of arm ⟶	Large intestine meridian of arm	*Yang-ming*
		Spleen meridian of leg ⟵	Stomach meridian of leg	
Yin	*Shaoyin*	Heart meridian of arm ⟶	Small intestine meridian of arm	*Tai-yang*	Yang
		Kidney meridian of leg ⟵	Bladder meridian of leg	
	Jueyin	Pericardium meridian of arm →	Triple heater meridian of arm	*Shao-yang*
		Liver meridian of leg ⟵	Gallbladder meridian of leg	

Vital energy flows in a single direction in each of the meridians and basically the energy travels upward in all yin meridians and downward in all yang meridians. This basic direction of energy flow in the meridians applies to a person standing up with both arms raised overhead. In this position the flow of energy in yin meridians goes from bottom to top, and from top to bottom in yang meridians. The meridians connect to each other either at the tips of the toes and fingers, or on the face or chest. In the case of the *shaoyin* heart meridian and the *taiyang* small intestine meridian, for example, the transfer of energy from one meridian into the other occurs at the tip of the little finger.

The internal branches of the twelve meridians, which connect the regular meridians to their corresponding organs (*zang* and *fu*), are significant because they establish the "interior and exterior relationship" of pairs of yin and yang meridians. Taking the yin-yang pair of the lung meridian and the large intestine meridian as an example, the lung meridian along with its primary association with the lung is also associated with the large intestine. Similarly the large intestine meridian is associated with the lung as well as the large intestine.

2. Symptoms Associated with the Meridians

When there is a disturbance in the energy circulation of any of the twelve meridians, a wide variety of associated symptoms appear. The name of the *zang* and *fu* which are also the name of the meridians, however, do not directly relate to the location of the pathological change in case a certain meridian is affected. A problem with the lung meridian, for example, does not necessarily mean that the lung is diseased. In Oriental medicine all the parts of the body that are involved in taking in the "*ki* of heaven" (air) and distributing it through the body (including the nose, pharynx, and bronchial tubes) are collectively referred to as the lung. A problem is considered to exist with the function of the lung as soon as there is some problem with taking in the "*ki* of heaven." In this case, the effect of the disturbance in lung *ki* (energy in the lung meridian) is conveyed along the lung meridian to produce certain signs on the body surface. Lung problems in particular tend to produce symptoms on the skin surface. When the disturbance becomes aggravated, pain most often occurs in the shoulders and upper back, and coughing and dryness of the mouth results. The disturbance in the circulation of lung *ki* also commonly leads to a problem in the large intestine, which is in a yin-yang (*zang-fu*) relationship with the lung.

Aside from the problems which can occur in one meridian or a pair of meridians, there are instances when the disruption in energy circulation spreads along the meridian system to produce a variety of different symptoms. For this reason, it is not always easy to attribute all the symptoms of a patient to specific meridians. Symptoms become especially difficult to classify according to the meridians when patients are old or when an illness reaches a chronic stage. Nevertheless, the area of the body in which each meridian runs basically correlates to the area where symptoms often appear when each meridian is affected. Therefore, the symptoms associated with each meridian (as recorded in the *Ling Shu*) will be listed for the sake of reference along with the description of the course of each meridian and its acupuncture points.

3. Location of Acupuncture Points

The location of acupuncture points were decided through the course of history by the accumulated experience of countless practitioners of Oriental medicine. Viewing the acupuncture points from a modern anatomical perspective, we find that in many cases they correspond to the location of major nerves or blood vessels and otherwise to parts of the body where viscerocutaneous reactions often appear.

Traditionally acupuncture points have been located by the use of proportional body measurements, which utilizes the traditional unit of *cun*. The cun used in proportional body measurements is a relative unit of distance derived by dividing a part of body into a number of equal segments. The exact length of the cun varies by the part of the body being measured as well as by the size of the person being measured. The number of cun, or segments of equal size, are used as a relative scale to measure various parts of the body and determine the location of acupuncture points. The length of each part of the body in cun has been designated in classical texts of acupuncture.

The proportional body measurements for the anterior aspect of the body are as follows:

> 9 cun between the lateral hairlines (ST-8–ST-8)
> 8 cun between the nipples
> 9 cun from the jugular notch to inferior border of the sternum
> 8 cun from the inferior border of the sternum to the umbilicus
> 5 cun from the umbilicus to superior border of the pubic symphysis
> 9 cun from the anterior axillary crease to the cubital skin fold
> 12 cun from the cubital skin fold to the skin fold of the wrist
> 19 cun from the superior margin of the trochanter to the inferior border of the lateral epicondyle
> 16 cun from the inferior border of the lateral epicondyle to the tip of the lateral malleolus

To use the proportional body measurements to locate acupuncture points, when locating points of the conception vessel on the lower abdomen for example, the distance between the superior border of the pubic symphysis and the umbilicus is divided into five equal segments (cun). The point CV-3, which is one cun above CV-2 (the superior border of the pubic symphysis), is located one-fifth the distance from CV-2 to CV-8 (the center of the umbilicus). This same principle of point location by proportional body measurements is applied to all other body parts as well.

In many instances it is much faster to locate a point by anatomical features than it is to divide parts of the body into equal segments and determine proportional distances. This is especially true for those points located next to bones and joints and points inside obvious depressions. Also sometimes it is not so practical to use proportional body measurements, since it is difficult to divide long body parts such as the thighs into many small segments. For this reason, through the ages practitioners have developed various shortcuts to expedite point location for clinical practice. The finger measurement is the simplest method which is used widely for acupuncture point location. In this method the width of the thumb at the interphalangeal joint is one cun. The width of the index, middle, and ring fingers at the distal interphalangeal joint is two cun. And the width of the four fingers (all fingers together except the thumb) across the proximal interphalangeal joint is three cun. The practitioner has to use his own fingers to find points on the patient, but he must first compare his fingers with the patient's fingers.

Methods of point location such as proportional body measurements, anatomical landmarks, and finger measurements allow a practitioner to find the general location of a particular acupuncture point. After deciding the approximate location of the point, the practitioner must determine the exact location by palpating cutaneous reactions or differences from the surrounding area. Even when the location of a point is correct according to a textbook, the point is not accurately located if no reaction or difference can be detected. It is inappropriate to insert a needle in a point based solely on textbook information. Acupuncture points, as part of an energy circulation system, are living phenomena in a constant state of flux. True acupuncture points move and change to reflect the functional condition of the body. Therefore, every practitioner must acquire the necessary skill and experience to accurately locate and appropriately choose the acupuncture points indicated for each patient.

4. The Fourteen Major Meridians and Their Acupuncture Points

Lung Meridian

Symptoms Associated with the Lung Meridian

Hotness in the face, oppression in chest, dryness in mouth, coughing, palpitations, shortness of breath, pain at the base of the neck, pain or numbness on the forearm in line with the thumb, hotness in the palms

---

The Path of the Lung Meridian

The lung meridian originates from the middle heater which corresponds to the point CV-12 on the body surface. The meridian descends internally to connect with the large intestine and then goes up again to travel around the bottom opening (pylorus) and top opening (cardia) of the stomach and pass through the diaphragm to enter the lungs. From the lungs the meridian goes up to the throat and comes down in the chest again to emerge on the body surface under the clavicle. The surface branch travels down the lateral side of the anterior aspect of the upper arm and passes through the cubital fossa to continue down the forearm

Fig. 5   Lung Meridian

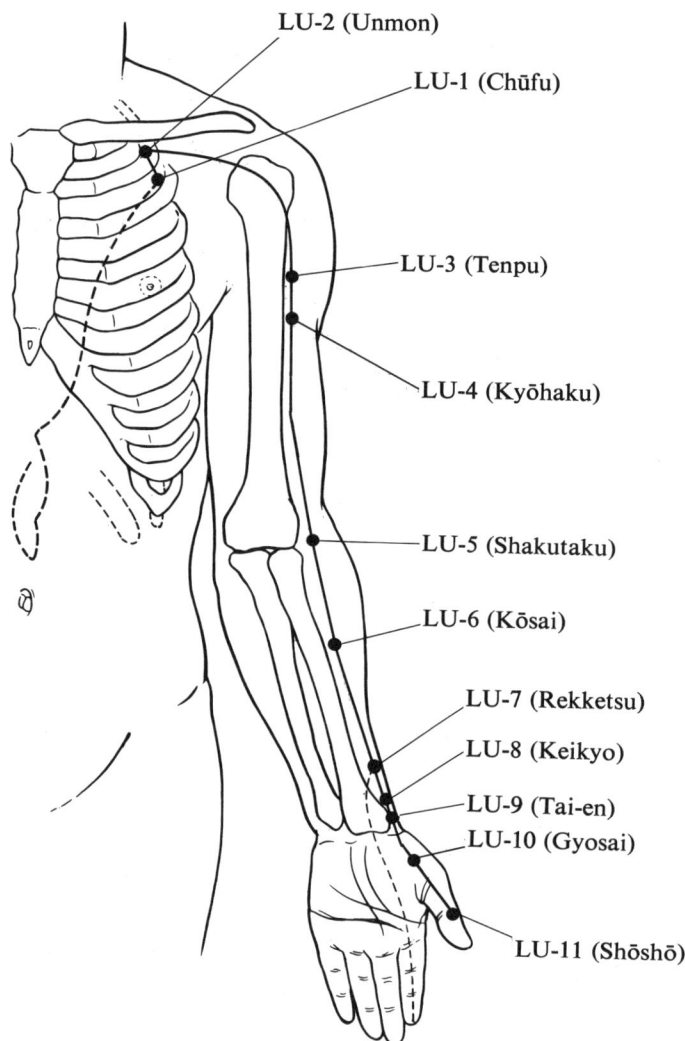

just medial to the styloid process of the radius. From there it passes down the lateral side of the first metacarpal to end up at the tip of the thumb. A branch of the lung meridian separates on the lower section of the forearm and goes to the tip of the index finger, where it connects with the large intestine meridian.

Acupuncture Points of the Lung Meridian

LU-1   Chūfu (Zhōngfǔ)—1 cun below LU-2
LU-2   Unmon (Yúnmén)—in depression of infraclavicular fossa 6 cun from median line
LU-3   Tenpu (Tiānfǔ)—on anterolateral aspect of upper arm 3 cun below the end of the axillary fold; on the lateral side of the biceps brachii
LU-4   Kyōhaku (Xiábái)—on upper arm 1 cun below LU-3

LU-5   Shakutaku (Chǐzé)—in the cubital skin fold on the radial side of the tendon of the biceps brachii

LU-6   Kōsai (Kǒngzuì)—on the anterolateral aspect of the forearm 3 cun below the cubital skin fold (LU-5)

LU-7   Rekketsu (Lièquē)—1.5 cun above the skin fold in the palmar aspect of the wrist just above the styloid process of the radius

LU-8   Keikyo (Jīngqú)—1 cun above LU-9 on the radial artery just medial to the styloid process of the radius

LU-9   Tai-en (Tàiyuān)—on the skin fold in the palmar aspect of the wrist; over the radial artery

LU-10   Gyosai (Yújì)—at midpoint of first metacarpal on the radial edge of the palm

LU-11   Shōshō (Shàoshāng)—on the radial side of the thumb, about 0.1 cun from the base of the thumbnail

Large Intestine Meridian

Symptoms Associated with the Large Intestine Meridian

Yellowish eyes, nasal discharge, epistaxis, toothache, dryness of mouth, swelling of throat and neck, pain from shoulder down to arm, pain and inability to use index finger

---

The Path of the Large Intestine Meridian

The large intestine meridian originates from the tip of the index finger and goes up the radial side of the index finger to pass between the heads of the first and second metacarpals. The meridian then goes up between the tendons of the thumb and continues up the radial side of the forearm to reach the lateral aspect of the elbow. It continues up the arm to the lateral edge of the shoulder joint and then goes to the point just above the first thoracic vertebra (GV-14), where the large intestine meridian communicates with the other yang meridians. An internal branch of the meridian descends through the supraclavicular fossa to connect with the lungs and passes through the diaphragm to enter the large intestine. The surface branch goes up the neck from the supraclavicular fossa and passes over the lower jaw and sends a branch into the lower teeth. The meridian then goes around the corner of the mouth and crosses over below the nose to end up on the other side at the base of the nose.

Acupuncture Points of the Large Intestine Meridian

LI-1   Shōyō (Shāngyáng)—on the radial side of the index finger about 0.1 cun from the base of the fingernail

LI-2   Jikan (Èrjiān)—on the radial aspect of the index finger; distal to the metacarpophalangeal joint

Fig. 6 Large Intestine Meridian

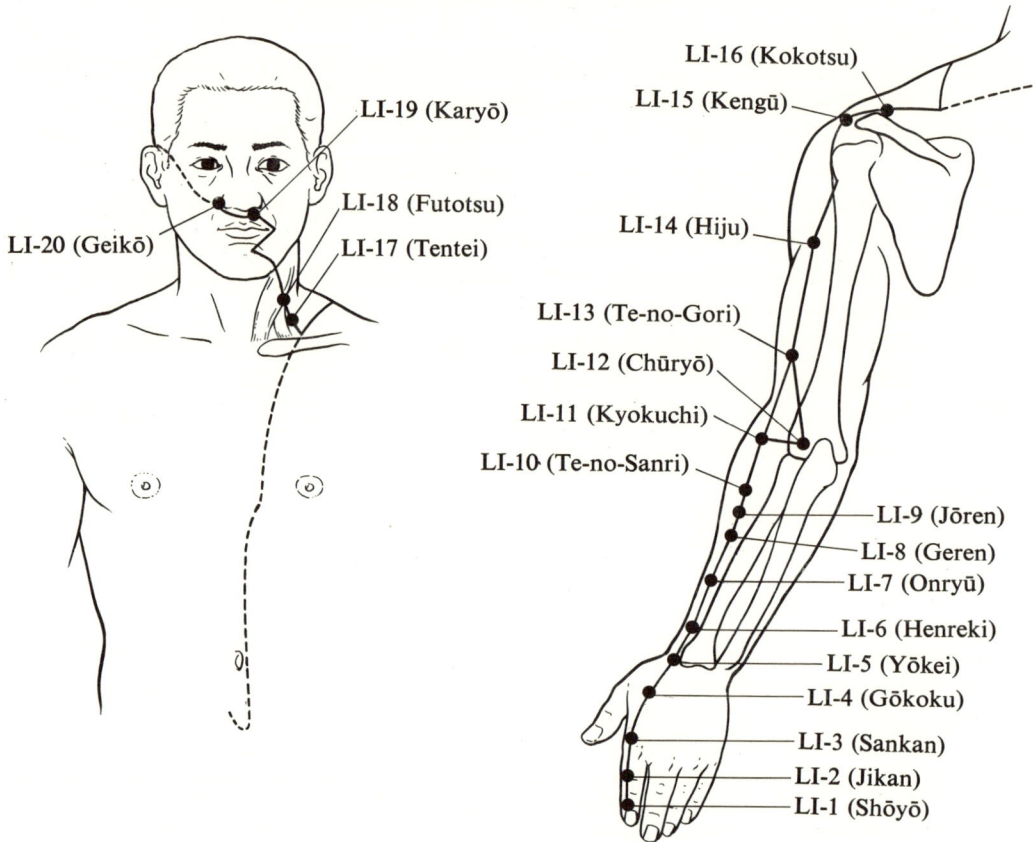

LI-19 (Karyō)

LI-18 (Futotsu)

LI-20 (Geikō)

LI-17 (Tentei)

LI-16 (Kokotsu)

LI-15 (Kengū)

LI-14 (Hiju)

LI-13 (Te-no-Gori)

LI-12 (Chūryō)

LI-11 (Kyokuchi)

LI-10 (Te-no-Sanri)

LI-9 (Jōren)

LI-8 (Geren)

LI-7 (Onryū)

LI-6 (Henreki)

LI-5 (Yōkei)

LI-4 (Gōkoku)

LI-3 (Sankan)

LI-2 (Jikan)

LI-1 (Shōyō)

LI-3   Sankan (Sānjiān)—on the radial aspect of the index finger proximal to the metacarpophalangeal joint

LI-4   Gōkoku (Hégǔ)—on the back of the hand distal to the bases of the first and second metacarpals

LI-5   Yōkei (Yángxī)—on the radial side of the wrist in the depression between the tendons of the extensor pollicis longus and the extensor pollicis brevis muscles

LI-6   Henreki (Piānlì)—on the radial side of the forearm 3 cun above LI-5

LI-7   Onryū (Wēnliū)—on the radial side of the forearm approximately halfway between LI-5 and LI-11

LI-8   Geren (Xiàlián)—on the radial side of the forearm 4 cun below LI-11

LI-9   Jōren (Shànglián)—on the radial side of the forearm 3 cun below LI-11

LI-10   Te-no-Sanri (Shŏu-Sānlĭ)—on the radial side of the forearm 2 cun below LI-11

LI-11   Kyokuchi (Qūchí)—in the depression at the lateral end of the cubital skin fold

LI-12   Chūryō (Zhŏuliáo)—on the lateral border of the humerus 1 cun above the lateral epicondyle

LI-13   Te-no-Gori (Shŏu-Wŭlĭ)—on the lateral border of the humerus; 3 cun above the lateral epicondyle

LI-14   Hiju (Bìnào)—lateral to the humerus on the lower border of the deltoid muscle

LI-15   Kengū (Jiānyú)—just inferior and anterior to the acromion in the anterior depression of the deltoid muscle

LI-16   Kokotsu (Jùgǔ)—just medial to the acromioclavicular joint

LI-17   Tentei (Tiāndǐng)—1 cun below LI-18 on the posterior border of the sternocleidomastoid muscle

LI-18   Futotsu (Fútū)—in the center of the sternocleidomastoid muscle at the level of the laryngeal prominence

LI-19   Karyō (Héliáo)—0.5 cun lateral to a point in the philtrum a third of the distance from the nose to the upper lip (GV-26)

LI-20   Geikō (Yíngxiāng)—in the nasolabial sulcus at the lateral margin of the nose

Stomach Meridian

Symptoms Associated with the Stomach Meridian

Pain in the forehead and the occipital area, dark complexion, constant yawning, epistaxis, sores and scabs around mouth, swelling of throat and neck, distension of abdomen, pain extending from the thigh down the shin to the third toe, tendency to sweat

---

The Path of the Stomach Meridian

The stomach meridian begins next to the base of the nose (LI-20) and goes up to meet the bladder meridian at the inner canthus (BL-1). From this point the meridian goes to the lower border of the orbit and begins its descent, traveling down beside the nose and sending an internal branch to the upper teeth. The meridian crosses over to the other side in the middle of the lower jaw (CV-24). It then branches and the ascending branch goes to the outside of the lower jaw (ST-5) and up to the mandibular angle (ST-6), curves up to pass in front of the ear (ST-7), and reaches a point at the corner of the hairline (ST-8). The descending branch goes over the lower jaw and down the anterior aspect of the neck. At the base of the neck, it curves laterally to go into the supraclavicular fossa. An internal branch goes down through the thorax and diaphragm to connect with the spleen and enter the stomach. The surface branch goes down the mammillary line over the nipple and passes beside the umbilicus to reach the inguinal region just lateral to the pubic hair. A portion of the internal branch from above exits the stomach through the lower opening (pylorus) and descends through the abdomen to rejoin the surface branch in the inguinal region. Then the meridian goes down the anterolateral aspect of the thigh and passes beside the knee, continues down just lateral to the tibia, and goes over the dorsum of the foot to reach the end of the second toe. A branch of the meridian separates at the midpoint of the lower leg (ST-40) and descends into the tip of the third toe on the lateral side. Another branch separates on the dorsum of the foot (ST-42) and goes to the tip of the big toe to connect with the spleen meridian.

Acupuncture Points of the Stomach Meridian

ST-1 Shōkyū (Chéngqì)—on the inferior ridge of the orbit directly below the pupil (looking straight ahead)

ST-2 Shihaku (Sìbái)—1 cun directly below the pupil in the infraorbital foramen

ST-3 Koryō (Jùliáo)—directly below the pupil at the level of the lower border of the nose

ST-4 Chisō (Dìcāng)—0.4 cun lateral to the corner of the mouth

ST-5 Daigei (Dàyíng)—on the lower border of the mandible about 1.3 cun anterior to ST-6

Fig. 7 Stomach Meridian

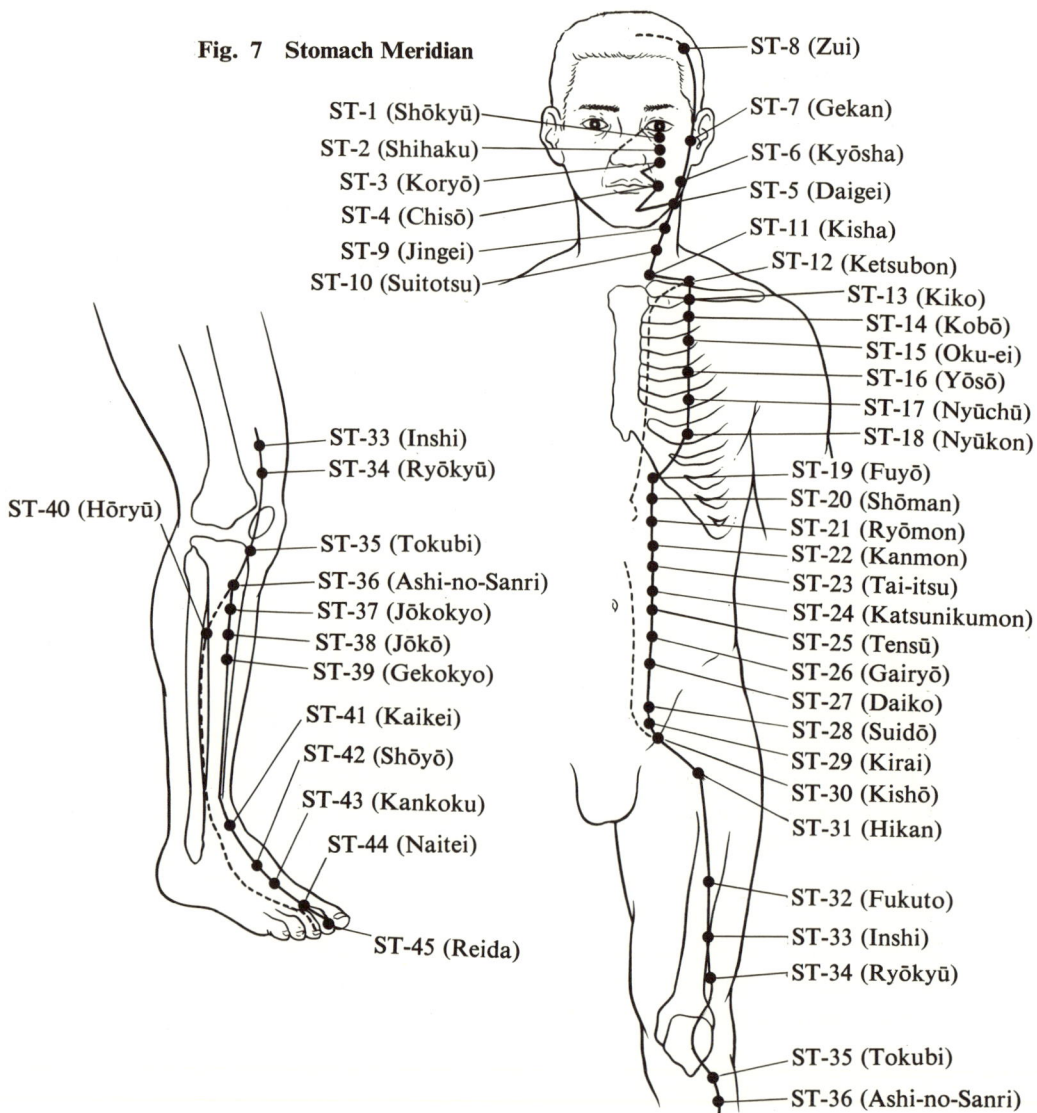

ST-8 (Zui)
ST-7 (Gekan)
ST-1 (Shōkyū)
ST-2 (Shihaku)
ST-6 (Kyōsha)
ST-3 (Koryō)
ST-5 (Daigei)
ST-4 (Chisō)
ST-11 (Kisha)
ST-9 (Jingei)
ST-12 (Ketsubon)
ST-10 (Suitotsu)
ST-13 (Kiko)
ST-14 (Kobō)
ST-15 (Oku-ei)
ST-16 (Yōsō)
ST-17 (Nyūchū)
ST-18 (Nyūkon)
ST-33 (Inshi)
ST-34 (Ryōkyū)
ST-19 (Fuyō)
ST-20 (Shōman)
ST-40 (Hōryū)
ST-21 (Ryōmon)
ST-22 (Kanmon)
ST-35 (Tokubi)
ST-23 (Tai-itsu)
ST-36 (Ashi-no-Sanri)
ST-24 (Katsunikumon)
ST-37 (Jōkokyo)
ST-25 (Tensū)
ST-38 (Jōkō)
ST-26 (Gairyō)
ST-39 (Gekokyo)
ST-27 (Daiko)
ST-41 (Kaikei)
ST-28 (Suidō)
ST-42 (Shōyō)
ST-29 (Kirai)
ST-43 (Kankoku)
ST-30 (Kishō)
ST-44 (Naitei)
ST-31 (Hikan)
ST-32 (Fukuto)
ST-45 (Reida)
ST-33 (Inshi)
ST-34 (Ryōkyū)
ST-35 (Tokubi)
ST-36 (Ashi-no-Sanri)

ST-6   Kyōsha (Jiáchē)—in the depression of the masseter muscle just anterior and superior to the mandibular angle

ST-7   Gekan (Xiàguān)—on the lower border of the zygomatic arch directly above ST-6

ST-8   Zui (Tóuwéi)—on the upper corner of the forehead at the lateral hairline

ST-9   Jingei (Rényíng)—at the level of the laryngeal prominence in the area over the common carotid artery

ST-10   Suitotsu (Shuǐtū)—1 cun below ST-9 on the anterior border of the sterno-cleidomastoid muscle

ST-11   Kisha (Qìshè)—on the superior border of the clavicle between the sternal and clavicular heads of the sternocleidomastoid muscle

ST-12   Ketsubon (Quēpén)—in the supraclavicular fossa on the mammillary line (4 cun from anterior median line)

ST-13   Kiko (Qìhù)—on the inferior border of the clavicle on the mammillary line (4 cun from anterior median line)

ST-14   Kobō (Kùfáng)—in the first intercostal space on the mammillary line (4 cun from anterior median line)

ST-15   Oku-ei (Wōyì)—in the second intercostal space on the mammillary line (4 cun from anterior median line)

ST-16   Yōsō (Yīngchuāng)—in the third intercostal space on the mammillary line (4 cun from anterior median line)

ST-17   Nyūchū (Rǔzhōng)—at the center of the nipple

ST-18   Nyūkon (Rǔgēn)—in the fifth intercostal space on the mammillary line (4 cun from anterior median line)

ST-19   Fuyō (Bùróng)—at the border of the costal arch 2 cun from the median line

ST-20   Shōman (Chéngmǎn)—1 cun below ST-19 and 2 cun from the median line

ST-21   Ryōmon (Liángmén)—2 cun below ST-19 and 2 cun from the median line

ST-22   Kanmon (Guānmén)—on a vertical line 2 cun from the median line; halfway between ST-19 and ST-25

ST-23   Tai-itsu (Tàiyǐ)—2 cun above ST-25 and 2 cun from the median line

ST-24   Katsunikumon (Huáròumén)—1 cun above ST-25 and 2 cun from the median line

ST-25   Tensū (Tiānshū)—2 cun from the median line at the level of the umbilicus

ST-26   Gairyō (Wàilíng)—1 cun below ST-25 and 2 cun from the median line

ST-27   Daiko (Dàjù)—2 cun below ST-25 and 2 cun from the median line

ST-28   Suidō (Shuǐdào)—2 cun above ST-30 and 2 cun from the median line

ST-29   Kirai (Gūilái)—1 cun above ST-30 and 2 cun from the median line

ST-30   Kishō (Qìchōng)—on superior border of pubic tubercle 2 cun from the median line; level with CV-2

ST-31   Hikan (Bìguān)—directly below the anterior superior iliac spine level with the lower border of the pubic bone

ST-32   Fukuto (Fútù)—on the thigh halfway between ST-31 and the lateral superior corner of the patella

ST-33   Inshi (Yīnshì)—3 cun above the lateral superior corner of the patella

ST-34   Ryōkyū (Liángqiū)—2 cun above the lateral superior corner of the patella

ST-35 Tokubi (Dúbí)—just inferior to the patella in the depression lateral to the patellar ligament

ST-36 Ashi-no-Sanri (Zú-Sānlǐ)—1 cun lateral to the inferior border of the tibial tuberosity

ST-37 Jōkokyo (Shàngjùxū)—1 cun lateral to tibia and 3 cun below ST-36; halfway between ST-36 and ST-39

ST-38 Jōkō (Tiáokǒu)—1 cun lateral to tibia and halfway between inferior border of patella and lateral malleolus; 1 cun above ST-39

ST-39 Gekokyo (Xiàjùxū)—1 cun lateral to tibia and 3 cun below ST-37

ST-40 Hōryū (Fēnglóng)—2 cun lateral to tibia halfway between inferior border of patella and lateral malleolus; 1 cun lateral to ST-38

ST-41 Kaikei (Jiěxī)—between the tendons of the extensor hallucis longus and extensor digitorum longus muscles, level with tip of lateral malleolus

ST-42 Shōyō (Chōngyáng)—on the dorsum of the foot 1.3 cun anterior to ST-41 where a pulse can be felt

ST-43 Kankoku (Xiàngǔ)—on the dorsum of the foot in the depression distal to the bases of the second and third metatarsals

ST-44 Naitei (Nèidíng)—above the web between the second and third toes just anterior to the heads of the metatarsals

ST-45 Reida (Lìduì)—on the lateral side of the second toe about 0.1 cun from the base of the toenail

Spleen Meridian

Symptoms Associated with the Spleen Meridian

Tightness of tongue, a stifling heavy sensation in the epigastrium or upper abdomen, nausea, constant belching, tightness in abdomen, difficulty in getting food down, diarrhea or constipation, scanty urination and occasional lack of urination, chilling of legs, swelling of thighs and knees on both sides when standing for long periods, jaundice, general sense of fatigue, insomnia

---

The Path of the Spleen Meridian

The spleen meridian begins at the tip of the big toe and goes along the border of the red and white skin on the medial side of the toe. It passes along the side of the metatarsophalangeal joint and the inferior border of the first metatarsal and then curves up just anterior to the medial malleolus. The meridian ascends the medial side of the leg on the posterior aspect of the tibia and intersects the liver meridian. It continues up the medial side of the knee and thigh and goes up to the inguinal region. An internal branch separates from the inguinal region and goes inside the abdomen to enter the spleen and connect with the stomach. The internal branch, after connecting to the stomach, continues upward through the diaphragm and communicates with the heart. The surface branch continues up the abdomen and goes up the side of the chest to end up directly below the axilla. From the chest

Fig. 8   Spleen Meridian

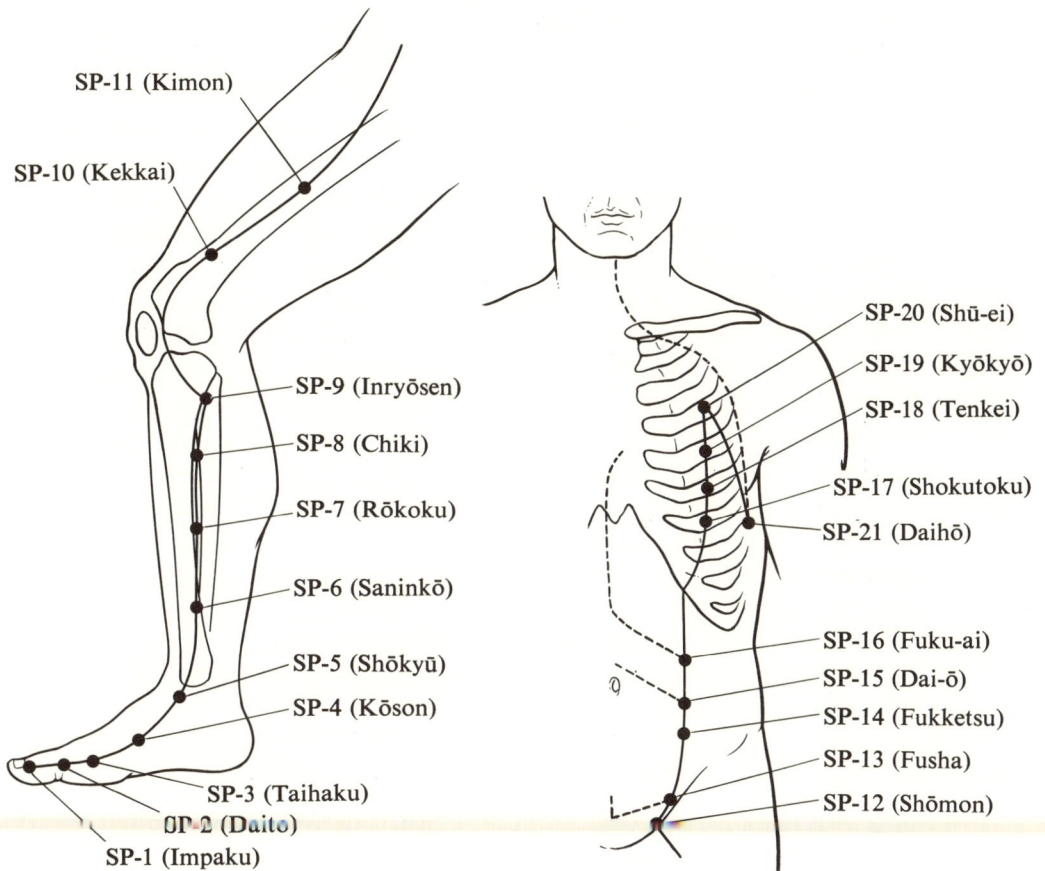

another branch goes inside to travel up the side of the trachea and reach the tongue.

Acupuncture Points of the Spleen Meridian

SP-1   Impaku (Yĭnbái)—on the medial side of the big toe about 0.1 cun from the base of the toenail

SP-2   Daito (Dàdū)—on the medial side of the big toe distal to the first metatarsophalangeal joint

SP-3   Taihaku (Tàibái)—on the medial side of the foot proximal to the first metatarsophalangeal joint

SP-4   Kōson (Gōngsūn)—1 cun posterior to SP-3

SP-5   Shōkyū (Shāngqiū)—in the depression anterior and inferior to the medial malleolus

SP-6   Saninkō (Sānyīnjiāo)—3 cun above the tip of the medial malleolus near the posterior border of the tibia

SP-7   Rōkoku (Lòugǔ)—3 cun above SP-6 on the posterior border of the tibia

SP-8   Chiki (Dìjī)—3 cun below SP-9 on the posterior border of the tibia; 5 cun below vertex of medial condyle

SP-9   Inryōsen (Yīnlíngqúan)—posterior to the tibia on the inferior border of the medial condyle

SP-10   Kekkai (Xuèhǎi)—2 cun superior to the medial superior corner of the patella

SP-11   Kimon (Jīmén)—6 cun above SP-10 on anteromedial aspect of thigh

SP-12   Shōmon (Chōngmén)—in the inguinal region level with the superior border of the pubic symphisis; 4 cun from the median line

SP-13   Fusha (Fǔshè)—1 cun above SP-12; 4 cun from the median line

SP-14   Fukketsu (Fùjié)—1.3 cun below SP-15; 4 cun from the median line

SP-15   Dai-ō (Dàhéng)—4 cun from the median line at the level of the umbilicus

SP-16   Fuku-ai (Fù'āi)—3 cun above SP-15; 4 cun from the median line

SP-17   Shokutoku (Shídòu)—in the fifth intercostal space on the anterolateral aspect; 6 cun from median line

SP-18   Tenkei (Tiānxī)—in the fourth intercostal space 6 cun from the median line; 2 cun lateral to the nipple

SP-19   Kyōkyō (Xiōngxiāng)—in the third intercostal space 6 cun from median line

SP-20   Shū-ei (Zhōuróng)—in the second intercostal space 6 cun from median line

SP-21   Daihō (Dàbāo)—6 cun directly below the center of the axilla; halfway between the axilla and tip of eleventh rib

Heart Meridian

Symptoms Associated with the Heart Meridian

Tendency for eyes to become yellowish, dry throat, pain in the epigastrium, occasional hotness and pain in the palms, pain, numbness, or a chilling sensation which extends from the upper arm past the elbow to the inside of the forearm on the ulnar side

---

The Path of the Heart Meridian

The heart meridian originates within the heart and is associated with the cardiovascular system. A descending branch goes through the diaphragm to connect with the small intestine. An ascending branch goes up along the trachea and connects to the back of the eye and the brain. The main branch of the meridian goes through the lungs and surfaces in the center of the axilla. It goes down the medial side of the arm to reach the pisiform bone and ends at the medial tip of the little finger, where it connects to the small intestine meridian.

Acupuncture Points of the Heart Meridian

HT-1   Kyokusen (Jíquán)—at the center of the axilla

Fig. 9   Heart Meridian

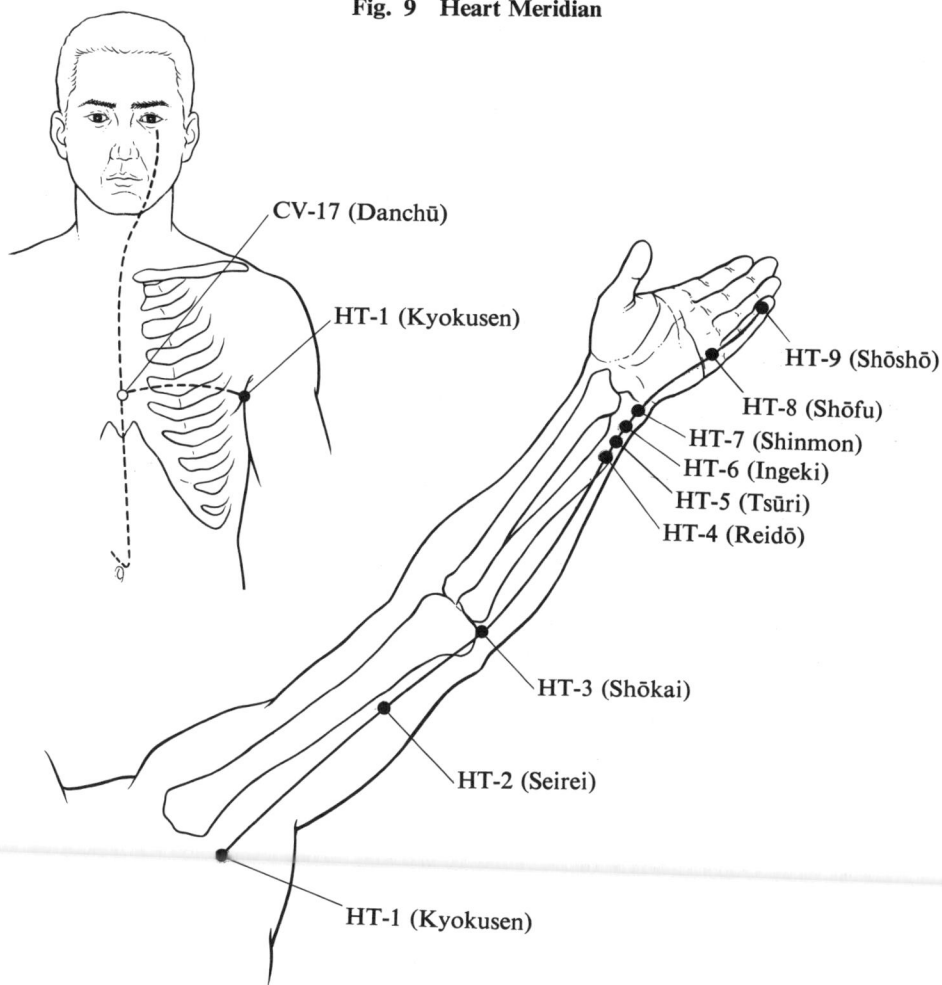

CV-17 (Danchū)

HT-1 (Kyokusen)

HT-9 (Shōshō)

HT-8 (Shōfu)

HT-7 (Shinmon)

HT-6 (Ingeki)

HT-5 (Tsūri)

HT-4 (Reidō)

HT-3 (Shōkai)

HT-2 (Seirei)

HT-1 (Kyokusen)

HT-2   Seirei (Qīnglíng)—3 cun above the medial epicondyle of the humerus, in depression medial to the biceps brachii muscle

HT-3   Shōkai (Shàohǎi)—at the medial end of the transverse cubital crease with elbow flexed

HT-4   Reidō (Língdào)—1.5 cun above HT-7, on the radial side of the tendon of the flexor carpi ulnaris muscle

HT-5   Tsūri (Tōnglǐ)—1 cun above HT-7, on the radial side of the tendon of the flexor carpi ulnaris muscle

HT-6   Ingeki (Yīnxì)—0.5 cun above HT-7, on the radial side of the tendon of the flexor carpi ulnaris muscle

HT-7   Shinmon (Shénmén)—in the palmar skin fold of the wrist on the radial side of the tendon of the flexor carpi ulnaris muscle

HT-8   Shōfu (Shàofǔ)—on the palm of the hand between the fourth and fifth metacarpals

HT-9   Shōshō (Shàochōng)—on the radial side of the little finger about 0.1 cun from the base of the fingernail

Small Intestine Meridian

Symptoms Associated with the Small Intestine Meridian

Yellowish eyes, loss of hearing, swelling of cheeks, sore throat, heaviness of head, pain or numbness from the top of shoulder and the scapulae extending down the upper arm beyond the elbow to the posteromedial aspect of the forearm

---

The Path of the Small Intestine Meridian

The small intestine meridian begins from the ulnar side of the little finger and goes up the medial aspect of the hand to the styloid process of the ulna. The meridian then goes up the posterior side of the ulna on the forearm and reaches the depression between the head of the ulna (olecranon) and the medial epicondyle. The meridian continues up the posteromedial aspect of the upper arm and passes over the shoulder joint to go up onto the scapula. The meridian then travels medially so that the right and left meridians connect just above the first thoracic vertebra (GV-14). From this point the meridian goes to the supraclavicular fossa and an internal branch enters the body to connect to the heart and continues through the diaphragm and stomach to enter the small intestine. The surface branch continues up the neck from the supraclavicular fossa and goes up onto the cheek. It then goes to the outer canthus and curves laterally over the zygomatic arch to end in the ear. A branch separates on the cheek to go up around the lower border of the orbit to the inner canthus to connect with the bladder meridian.

Acupuncture Points of the Small Intestine Meridian

SI-1 Shōtaku (Shàozé)—on the ulnar side of the little finger; about 0.1 cun from the base of the fingernail

SI-2 Zenkoku (Qiángǔ)—on the ulnar side of the hand in the depression distal to the metacarpophalangeal joint

SI-3 Gokei (Hòuxī)—on the ulnar side of the hand in the depression proximal to the metacarpophalangeal joint

SI-4 Wankotsu (Wànggǔ)—on the ulnar side of the wrist in the depression between the base of the fifth metacarpal and the triquetral bone

SI-5 Yōkoku (Yánggǔ)—on the ulnar side of the wrist in the depression proximal to the styloid process of the ulna

SI-6 Yōrō (Yánglǎo)—in the depression formed on the styloid process of the ulna when the wrist is turned

SI-7 Shisei (Zhīzhèng)—5 cun above the wrist on the radial border of the ulna

SI-8 Shōkai (Xiǎohǎi)—in the depression between the olecranon of the ulna and the medial epicondyle of the humerus

SI-9 Kentei (Jiānzhēn)—1 cun above the posterior end of the axillary skin fold

SI-10 Juyu (Nàoshū)—directly above SI-8 in the depression below the spine of the scapula

Fig. 10 Small Intestine Meridian

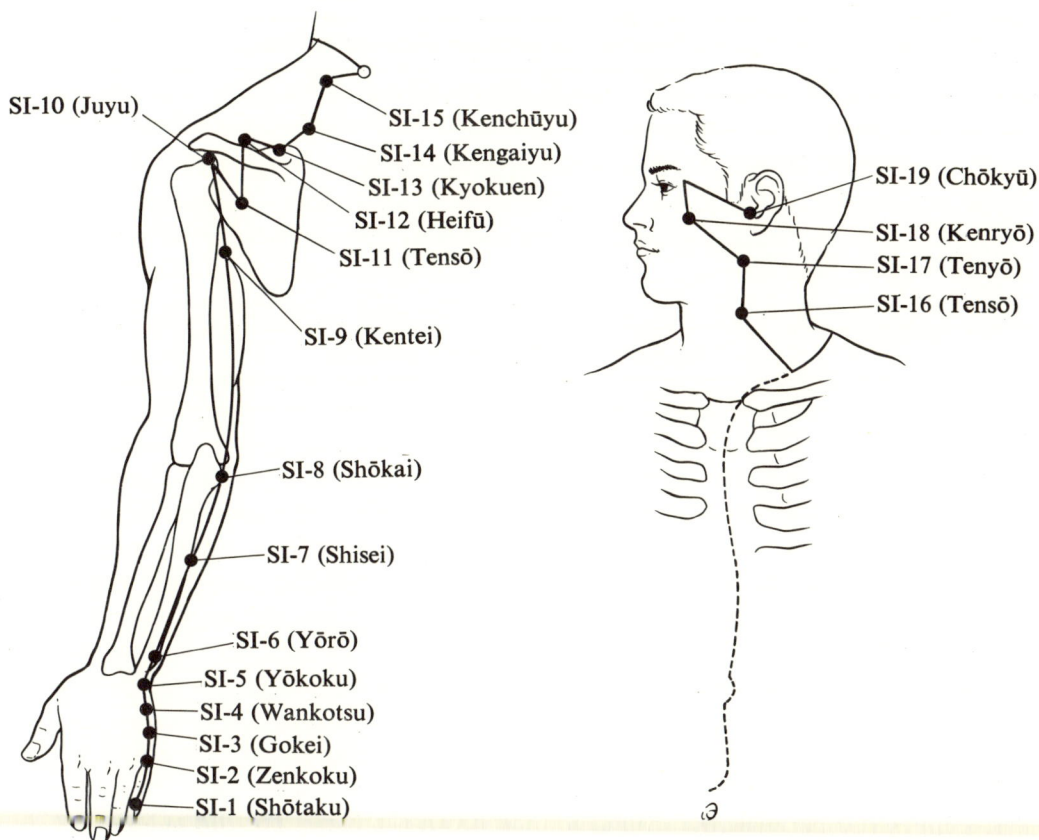

SI-10 (Juyu)

SI-15 (Kenchūyu)
SI-14 (Kengaiyu)
SI-13 (Kyokuen)
SI-12 (Heifū)
SI-11 (Tensō)

SI-9 (Kentei)

SI-8 (Shōkai)

SI-7 (Shisei)

SI-6 (Yōrō)
SI-5 (Yōkoku)
SI-4 (Wankotsu)
SI-3 (Gokei)
SI-2 (Zenkoku)
SI-1 (Shōtaku)

SI-19 (Chōkyū)
SI-18 (Kenryō)
SI-17 (Tenyō)
SI-16 (Tensō)

SI-11   Tensō (Tiānzōng)—1 cun below the midpoint of the inferior border of the scapular spine

SI-12   Heifū (Bǐngfēng)—1 cun above the midpoint of the superior border of the scapular spine

SI-13   Kyokuen (Qūyúan)—in the medial end of the depression above the scapular spine

SI-14   Kengaiyu (Jiānwàishū)—3 cun lateral to the point between the spinous processes of the first and second thoracic vertebrae (GV-13)

SI-15   Kenchūyu (Jiānzhōngshū)—2 cun lateral to the point between the spinous processes of the seventh cervical and first thoracic vertebrae (GV-14)

SI-16   Tensō (Tiānchuāng)—on the posterior border of the sternocleidomastoid muscle level with the laryngeal prominence

SI-17   Tenyō (Tiānróng)—on the anterior border of the sternocleidomastoid muscle level with the angle of the mandible

SI-18   Kenryō (Quánliáo)—on the lower border of the zygomatic bone directly below the outer canthus

SI-19   Chōkyū (Tīnggōng)—anterior to the tragus in the depression formed when mouth is opened

Bladder Meridian

Symptoms Associated with the Bladder Meridian

Pain which begins in the eyes and seems to shoot through to the occipital region, swelling in the scalp, nasal congestion, occasional epistaxis, tendency for eyes to water, pain in the occipital region, the interscapular area, along the spine, lower back, hips, in the hip joint, back of knees, calf muscles, lateral malleolus, and little toe, strong pain especially along the spine and in the lower back, sciatica, cramping of calf muscle, hemorrhoids

---

The Path of the Bladder Meridian

The bladder meridian begins at the inner canthus (inside corner of the eye) and goes up the forehead just next to the median line. The right and left sides of the meridian come together at the crown and a surface branch separates on either side and goes to the supra-auricular area. The meridian enters the cranium to circulate in the brain and then emerges posterior to the crown on either side of the median line to go down the back of the head. The meridian splits into two main branches in the occipital area. The medial branch goes down between the scapula and spine and descends along the spine. In the waist area the medial branch sends an internal branch which connects with the kidneys and enters the bladder. The medial branch continues downward next to the sacrum and over the buttocks to go down the center of the posterior aspect of the thigh and reaches the popliteal fossa. The lateral branch descends from the occipital area in line with the medial border of the scapula and parallels the medial branch down the back. This branch curves laterally on the buttocks to pass just behind the hip joint and travels down the posterolateral aspect of the thigh and rejoins the medial branch in the popliteal fossa. The bladder meridian continues down the back of the calf and curves laterally halfway down and passes just behind the lateral malleolus. Then it goes over the lateral aspect of the foot and the fifth metatarsal to end on the lateral side of the little toe.

Acupuncture Points of the Bladder Meridian

BL-1   Seimei (Jīngmíng)—0.1 cun medial to the inner canthus

BL-2   Sanchiku (Zǎnzhú)—on the medial tip of the eyebrow

BL-3   Bishō (Méichōng)—directly above BL-2 and 0.5 cun within the hairline; halfway between GV-24 and BL-4

BL-4   Kyokusa (Qūchāi)—1.5 cun lateral to the median line (GV-24); 0.5 cun within the hairline

BL-5   Gosho (Wǔchù)—1.5 cun lateral to the median line and 1 cun posterior to BL-4

BL-6   Shōkō (Chéngguāng)—1.5 cun lateral to the median line and 1.5 cun posterior to BL-5

Fig. 11 Bladder Meridian

BL-3 (Bishō)
BL-7 (Tsūten)
BL-6 (Shōkō)
BL-5 (Gosho)
BL-4 (Kyokusa)
BL-2 (Sanchiku)
BL-1 (Seimei)

BL-36 (Shōfu)

BL-37 (Inmon)
BL-38 (Fugeki)
BL-39 (Iyō)
BL-40 (Ichū)
BL-55 (Gōyō)
BL-56 (Shōkin)
BL-57 (Shōzan)
BL-58 (Hiyō)
BL-59 (Fuyō)

BL-8 (Rakkyaku)
BL-9 (Gyokuchin)
BL-10 (Tenchū)

BL-41 (Fubun)
BL-42 (Hakko)
BL-43 (Kōkō)
BL-44 (Shindō)
BL-45 (Iki)
BL-46 (Kakukan)
BL-47 (Konmon)
BL-48 (Yōkō)
BL-49 (Isha)
BL-50 (Isō)
BL-51 (Kōmon)
BL-52 (Shishitsu)
BL-27 (Shōchōyu)
BL-28 (Bōkōyu)
BL-53 (Kōkō)
BL-54 (Chippen)
BL-29 (Chūroyu)
BL-30 (Hakkanyu)

BL-11 (Daijo)
BL-12 (Fūmon)
BL-13 (Haiyu)
BL-14 (Ketsuinyu)
BL-15 (Shinyu)
BL-16 (Tokuyu)
BL-17 (Kakuyu)
BL-18 (Kanyu)
BL-19 (Tanyu)
BL-20 (Hiyu)
BL-21 (Iyu)
BL-22 (Sanshōyu)
BL-23 (Jinyu)
BL-24 (Kikaiyu)
BL-25 (Daichōyu)
BL-26 (Kangenyu)
BL-31 (Jōryō)
BL-32 (Jiryō)
BL-33 (Chūryō)
BL-34 (Geryō)
BL-35 (Eyō)

BL-59 (Fuyō)
BL-60 (Konron)
BL-61 (Bokushin)
BL-62 (Shinmyaku)
BL-63 (Kinmon)

BL-67 (Shi-in)
BL-66 (Ashi-no-Tsūkoku)
BL-65 (Sokkotsu)
BL-64 (Keikotsu)

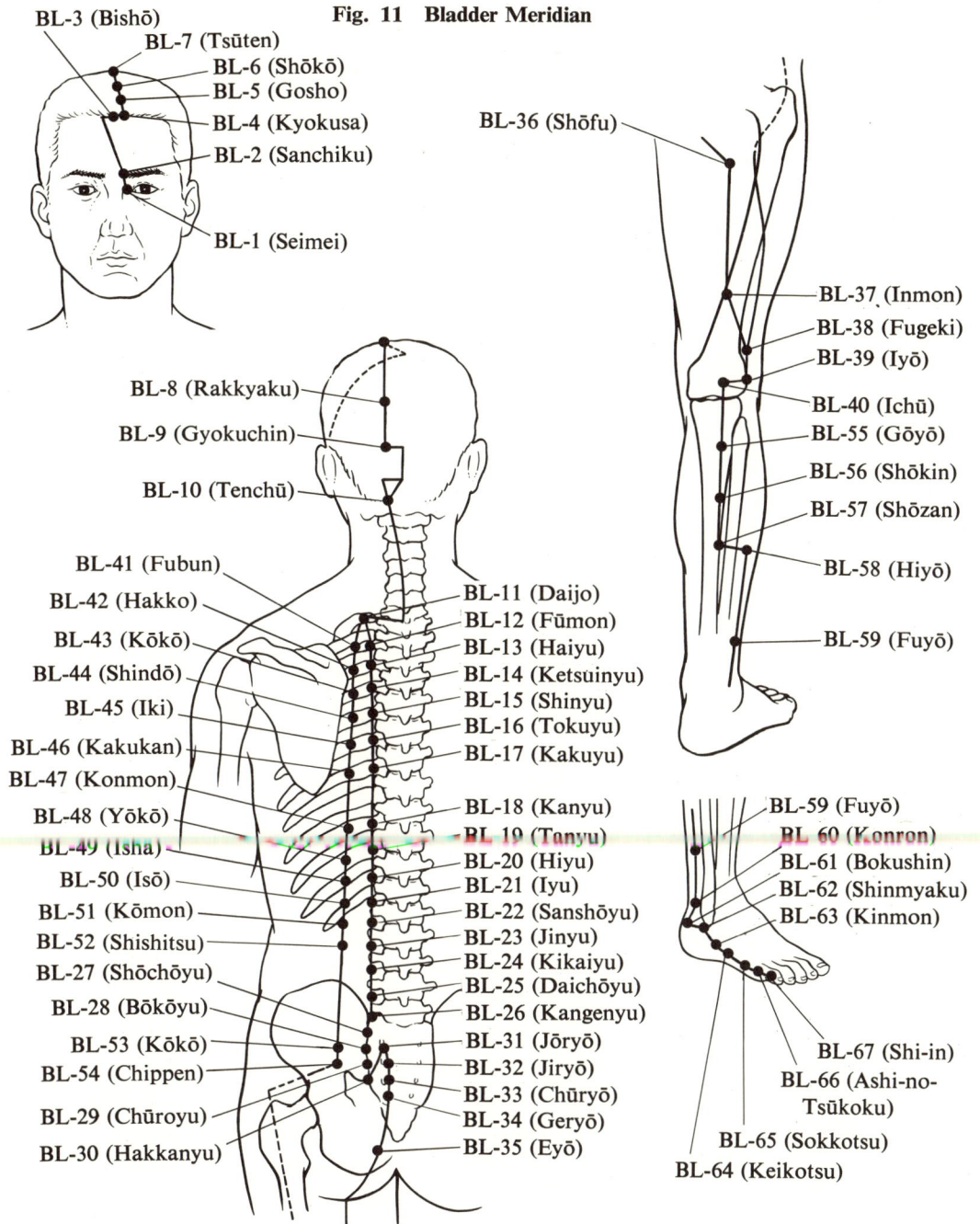

BL-7   Tsūten (Tōngtiān)—1.5 cun lateral to the median line and 1.5 cun posterior to BL-6; just to the front of GV-20

BL-8   Rakkyaku (Luòquè)—1.5 cun lateral to the median line and 1.5 cun posterior to BL-7; just to the back of GV-20

BL-9   Gyokuchin (Yùzhěn)—1.3 cun lateral to the median line and level with the superior border of the external occipital protuberance

BL-10   Tenchū (Tiānzhù)—1.3 cun lateral to the median line and 0.5 cun above the posterior hairline

BL-11   Daijo (Dàzhù)—1.5 cun lateral to the lower border of the spinous process of the first thoracic vertebra

BL-12   Fūmon (Fēngmén)—1.5 cun lateral to the lower border of the spinous process of the second thoracic vertebra

BL-13   Haiyu (Fèishū)—1.5 cun lateral to the lower border of the spinous process of the third thoracic vertebra

BL-14   Ketsuinyu (Juéyīnshū)—1.5 cun lateral to the lower border of the spinous process of the fourth thoracic vertebra

BL-15   Shinyu (Xīnshū)—1.5 cun lateral to the lower border of the spinous process of the fifth thoracic vertebra

BL-16   Tokuyu (Dūshū)—1.5 cun lateral to the lower border of the spinous process of the sixth thoracic vertebra

BL-17   Kakuyu (Géshū)—1.5 cun lateral to the lower border of the spinous process of the seventh thoracic vertebra

BL-18   Kanyu (Gānshū)—1.5 cun lateral to the lower border of the spinous process of the ninth thoracic vertebra

BL-19   Tanyu (Dǎnshū)—1.5 cun lateral to the lower border of the spinous process of the tenth throracic vertebra

BL-20   Hiyu (Píshū)—1.5 cun lateral to the lower border of the spinous process of the eleventh thoracic vertebra

BL-21   Iyu (Wèishū)—1.5 cun lateral to the lower border of the spinous process of the twelfth thoracic vertebra

BL-22   Sanshōyu (Sānjiāoshū)—1.5 cun lateral to the lower border of the spinous process of the first lumbar vertebra

BL-23   Jinyu (Shènshū)—1.5 cun lateral to the lower border of the spinous process of the second lumbar vertebra

BL-24   Kikaiyu (Qìhǎishū)—1.5 cun lateral to the lower border of the spinous process of the third lumbar vertebra

BL-25   Daichōyu (Dàchángshū)—1.5 cun lateral to the lower border of the spinous process of the fourth lumbar vertebra

BL-26   Kangenyu (Guānyuǎnshū)—1.5 cun lateral to the lower border of the spinous process of the fifth lumbar vertebra

BL-27   Shōchōyu (Xiǎochángshū)—1.5 cun lateral to the median sacral crest on the medial border of the posterior superior iliac spine; adjacent to BL-31

BL-28   Bōkōyu (Pángguāngshū)—1.5 cun lateral to the median sacral crest level with the inferior border of the posterior superior iliac spine; adjacent to BL-32

BL-29   Chūroyu (Zhōnglǔshū)—1.5 cun lateral to the median sacral crest; adjacent to BL-23 and halfway between BL-28 and BL-30

BL-30   Hakkanyu (Báihuánshū)—1.5 cun lateral to the center of the sacral hiatus (GV-2); adjacent to BL-34

BL-31   Jōryō (Shàngliáo)—about halfway between the posterior superior iliac spine and the median sacral crest; over the first posterior sacral foramen

BL-32   Jiryō (Cìliáo)—about halfway between the lower border of the posterior

superior iliac spine and the median sacral crest; over the second posterior
sacral foramen

BL-33 Chūryō (Zhōngliáo)—about halfway between BL-32 and BL-34; over the
third posterior sacral foramen

BL-34 Geryō (Xiàliáo)—about halfway between the median sacral crest and
BL-30; over the fourth posterior sacral foramen

BL-35 Eyō (Huìyáng)—0.5 cun lateral to the inferior tip of the coccyx (GV-1)

BL-36 Shōfu (Chéngfú)—at the midpoint of the gluteal fold

BL-37 Inmon (Yīnmén)—6 cun below BL-36 in the middle of the posterior
aspect of the thigh

BL-38 Fúgekì (Fúxì)—on the medial side of the tendon of the biceps femoris
muscle and 1 cun above the lateral end of the transverse crease of the
popliteal fossa (BL-39)

BL-39 Iyō (Wěiyáng)—on the medial side of the tendon of the biceps femoris
muscle at the lateral end of the transverse crease of the popliteal fossa

BL-40 Ichū (Wěizhōng)—at the midpoint of the transverse crease of the popliteal
fossa

BL-41 Fubun (Fùfēn)—3 cun lateral to the lower border of the spinous process
of the second thoracic vertebra

BL-42 Hakko (Pòhù)—3 cun lateral to the lower border of the spinous process
of the third thoracic vertebra

BL-43 Kōkō (Gaōhuāng)—3 cun lateral to the lower border of the spinous
process of the fourth thoracic vertebra

BL-44 Shindō (Shéntáng)—3 cun lateral to the lower border of the spinous
process of the fifth thoracic vertebra

BL-45 Iki (Yìxǐ)—3 cun lateral to the lower border of the spinous process of the
sixth thoracic vertebra

BL-46 Kakukan (Géguān)—3 cun lateral to the lower border of the spinous
process of the seventh thoracic vertebra

BL-47 Konmon (Húnmén)—3 cun lateral to the lower border of the spinous
process of the ninth thoracic vertebra

BL-48 Yōkō (Yánggāng)—3 cun lateral to the lower border of the spinous
process of the tenth thoracic vertebra

BL-49 Isha (Yìshè)—3 cun lateral to the lower border of the spinous process of
the eleventh thoracic vertebra

BL-50 Isō (Wèicāng)—3 cun lateral to the lower border of the spinous process
of the twelfth thoracic vertebra

BL-51 Kōmon (Huāngmén)—3 cun lateral to the lower border of the spinous
process of the first lumbar vertebra

BL-52 Shishitsu (Zhìshì)—3 cun lateral to the lower border of the spinous
process of the second lumbar vertebra

BL-53 Hōkō (Baōhuāng)—3 cun lateral to the median sacral crest and level with
the inferior border of the posterior superior iliac spine

BL-54 Chippen (Zhìbiān)—3 cun lateral to the center of the sacral hiatus
(GV-2); lateral to BL-30

BL-55 Gōyō (Héyáng)—3 cun below the midpoint of the popliteal crease (BL-40) at the point where the medial and lateral heads of the gastrocnemius muscle meet

BL-56   Shōkin (Chéngjīn)—in the center of the gastrocnemius muscle; halfway between BL-55 and BL-57

BL-57   Shōzan (Chéngshān)—at the origin of the Achilles tendon where the medial and lateral head of the gastrocnemius muscle separate

BL-58   Hiyō (Fēiyáng)—on the inferior border of the lateral head of the gastrocnemius muscle about 1 cun inferior and lateral to BL-57

BL-59   Fuyō (Fūyáng)—3 cun directly above BL-60

BL-60   Konron (Kūnlún)—in the depression between the lateral malleolus and the Achilles tendon

BL-61   Bokushin (Púshēn)—about 1.5 cun below BL-60 in the depression on the lateral side of the calcaneus

BL-62   Shinmyaku (Shēnmài)—in the depression about 1 cun below the apex of the lateral malleolus

BL-63   Kinmon (Jīnmén)—in the depression halfway between BL-62 and BL-64

BL-64   Keikotsu (Jīnggǔ)—on the lateral side of the foot just posterior and inferior to the tuberosity of the fifth metatarsal

BL-65   Sokkotsu (Shùgǔ)—on the lateral side of the foot posterior and inferior to the head of the fifth metatarsal

BL-66   Ashi-no-Tsūkoku (Zú-Tōnggǔ)—on the side of the little toe in the depression anterior and inferior to the fifth metatarsophalangeal joint

BL-67   Shi-in (Zhìyīn)—on the lateral side of the little toe, about 0.1 cun from the base of the toenail

Kidney Meridian

Symptoms Associated with the Kidney Meridian

Dark complexion without luster, hotness in mouth and dry tongue, swelling and soreness in throat, shortness of breath, frequent choking, dizziness on standing, hemoptysis, lack of appetite even on an empty stomach, lack of strength in lower abdomen, tendency toward diarrhea and weight loss, pain or chilling sensation down the back, in the hips, and on the inside of the thighs and lower legs, hotness and pain in soles

---

The Path of the Kidney Meridian

The kidney meridian begins at the bottom of the little toe and travels diagonally on the sole of the foot to cross over a point just anterior to its center (KI-1). The meridian continues across onto the arch of the foot and passes under the tuberosity of the navicular bone and goes up behind the medial malleolus. Here it curves downward to make a loop over the medial aspect of the calcaneus and then begins to travel up the medial aspect of the gastrocnemius muscle. The kidney meridian goes up the medial edge of the popliteal fossa and continues to ascend the medial aspect of the thigh to reach the tip of the coccyx. After this the meridian

Fig. 12 Kidney Meridian

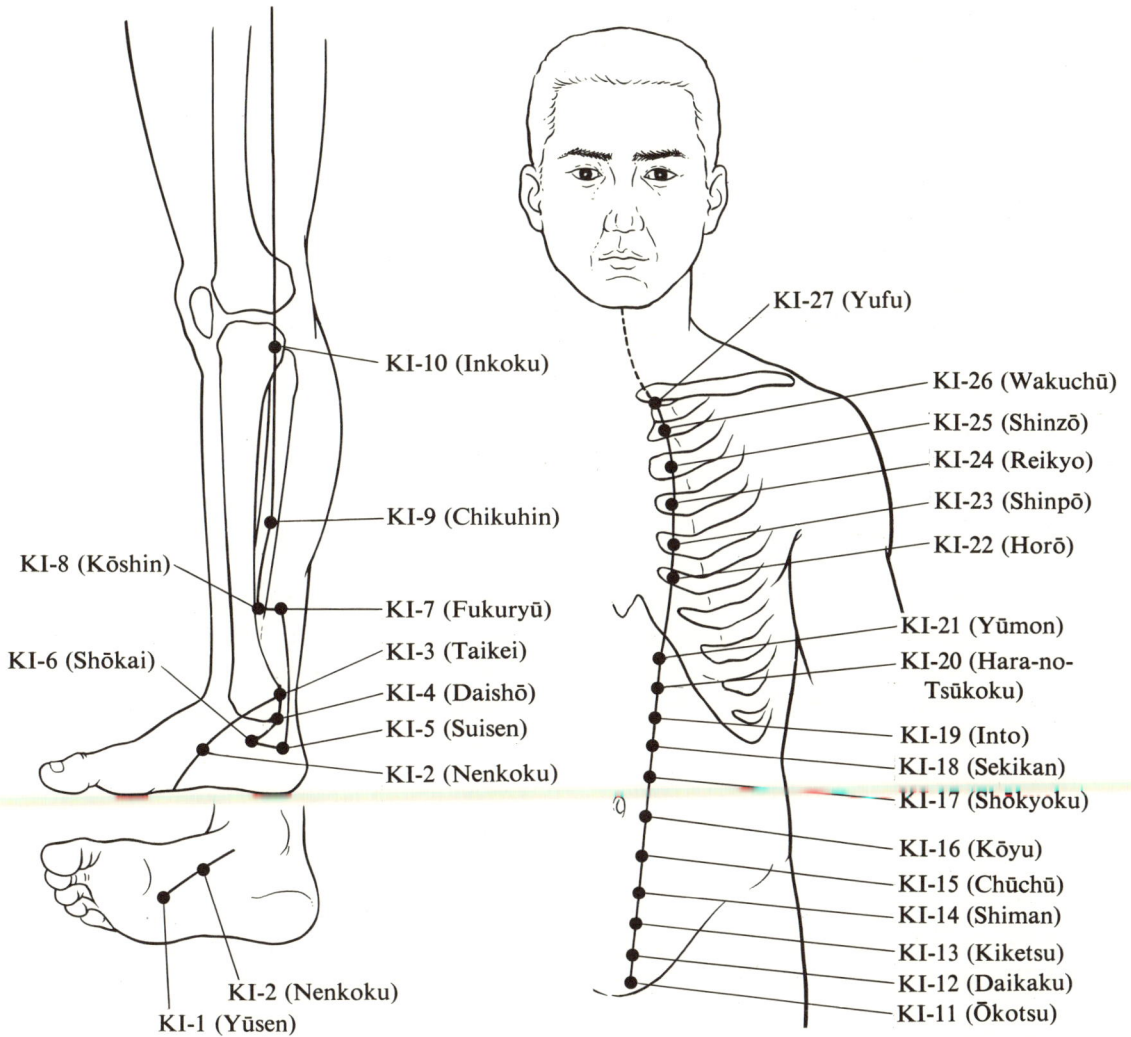

KI-27 (Yufu)

KI-26 (Wakuchū)

KI-25 (Shinzō)

KI-24 (Reikyo)

KI-23 (Shinpō)

KI-22 (Horō)

KI-21 (Yūmon)

KI-20 (Hara-no-Tsūkoku)

KI-19 (Into)

KI-18 (Sekikan)

KI-17 (Shōkyoku)

KI-16 (Kōyu)

KI-15 (Chūchū)

KI-14 (Shiman)

KI-13 (Kiketsu)

KI-12 (Daikaku)

KI-11 (Ōkotsu)

KI-10 (Inkoku)

KI-9 (Chikuhin)

KI-8 (Kōshin)

KI-7 (Fukuryū)

KI-6 (Shōkai)

KI-3 (Taikei)

KI-4 (Daishō)

KI-5 (Suisen)

KI-2 (Nenkoku)

KI-2 (Nenkoku)

KI-1 (Yūsen)

travels internally up the lower spine and enters the kidneys and connects with the bladder. Then the meridian returns to the surface of the body on the abdomen just above the pubic bone and travels up over the abdomen and chest to end up just below the clavicle. An internal branch separates inside the kidneys and passess through the liver and diaphragm and enters the lungs. From the lungs one branch goes up the throat to reach the base of the tongue and another branch enters the heart to connect with the pericardium meridian.

Acupuncture Points of the Kidney Meridian

KI-1   Yūsen (Yǒngquán)—on the sole of the foot in the depression posterior to the second metatarsophalangeal joint

KI-2   Nenkoku (Rángǔ)—just above the arch of the foot, just anterior and inferior to lower border of navicular bone

KI-3   Taikei (Tàixī)—in the depression between the medial malleolus and the Achilles tendon in the area of the dorsal tibial artery

KI-4   Daishō (Dàzhōng)—0.5 cun below KI-3 on the superior border of the calcaneus

KI-5   Suisen (Shuǐquán)—1 cun below KI-3 in the depression on the medial side of the calcaneus

KI-6   Shōkai (Zhàohǎi)—in the depression about 1 cun below the apex of the medial malleolus

KI-7   Fukuryū (Fùliū)—2 cun above the tip of the medial malleolus on the medial border of the Achilles tendon

KI-8   Kōshin (Jiāoxìn)—just anterior to KI-7 on the posterior border of the tibia

KI-9   Chikuhin (Zhùbīn)—5 cun above the tip of the medial malleolus, on the medial border of the Achilles tendon

KI-10   Inkoku (Yīngǔ)—on the medial side of the popliteal fossa between the tendons of the semitendinosus and the semimembranosus muscles

KI-11   Ōkotsu (Hénggǔ)—on the superior border of the pubic symphysis 0.5 cun from the median line

KI-12   Daikaku (Dàhè)—1 cun above KI-11 and 0.5 cun from the median line

KI-13   Kiketsu (Qìxúe)—2 cun above KI-11 and 0.5 cun from the median line

KI-14   Shiman (Sìmǎn)—2 cun below KI-16 and 0.5 cun from the median line

KI-15   Chūchū (Zhōngzhù)—1 cun below KI-16 and 0.5 cun from the median line

KI-16   Kōyu (Huāngshū)—at the level of the umbilicus 0.5 cun from the median line

KI-17   Shōkyoku (Shōngqū)—2 cun above KI-16 and 0.5 cun from the median line

KI-18   Sekikan (Shíguān)—3 cun above KI-16 and 0.5 cun from the median line

KI-19   Into (Yīndū)—1 cun above KI-18 and 0.5 cun from the median line

KI-20   Hara-no-Tsūkoku (Fù-Tōnggǔ)—2 cun above KI-18 and 0.5 cun from the median line

KI-21   Yūmon (Yōumén)—3 cun above KI-18 and 0.5 cun from the median line

KI-22   Horō (Bùláng)—in the fifth intercostal space 2 cun from the median line

KI-23   Shinpō (Shénfēng)—in the fourth intercostal space 2 cun from the median line

KI-24   Reikyo (Língxū)—in the third intercostal space 2 cun from the median line

KI-25   Shinzō (Shéncáng)—in the second intercostal space 2 cun from the median line

KI-26   Wakuchū (Yùzhōng)—in the first intercostal space 2 cun from the median line

KI-27   Yufu (Shūfǔ)—at the inferior border of the clavicle 2 cun from the median line

Pericardium Meridian

Symptoms Associated with the Pericardium Meridian

Hotness in face causing flushed complexion, palpitations, yellowish eyes, pain and occasional numbness in the chest and sides, pain and numbness on the palmar aspect of the upper and lower arms, hotness in the palms

---
The Path of the Pericardium Meridian

The pericardium meridian originates inside the chest at the pericardium and descends through the diaphragm to connect with the upper, middle, and lower sections of the triple heater. Another branch of the meridian goes anteriorly in the chest from the pericardium and surfaces just lateral to the nipple. Then it goes upward to the axillary region and travels down the anterior aspect of the arm

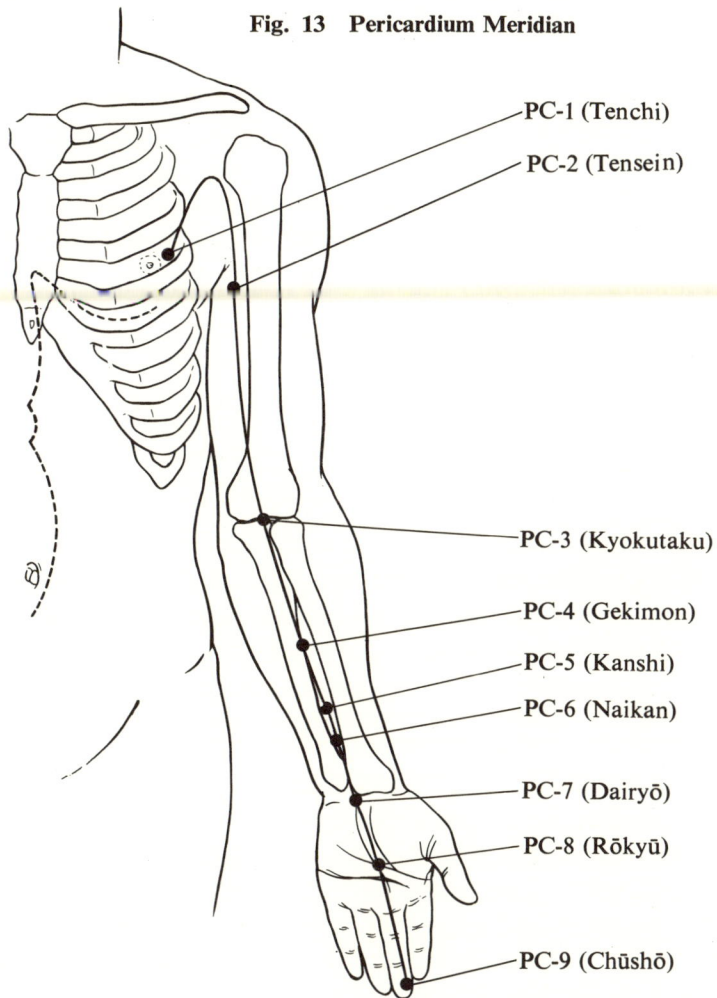

Fig. 13   Pericardium Meridian

PC-1 (Tenchi)

PC-2 (Tensein)

PC-3 (Kyokutaku)

PC-4 (Gekimon)

PC-5 (Kanshi)

PC-6 (Naikan)

PC-7 (Dairyō)

PC-8 (Rōkyū)

PC-9 (Chūshō)

between the lung and heart meridians. It passes on the medial side of the tendon of the biceps brachii muscle in the cubital fossa and continues down the center of the anterior aspect of the forearm. The pericardium meridian goes down the center of the palm and ends at the tip of the middle finger.

Acupuncture Points of the Pericardium Meridian

PC-1 Tenchi (Tiānchí)—1 cun lateral to the nipple in the fourth intercostal space

PC-2 Tensen (Tiānquán)—2 cun below the anterior end of the axillary skin fold between the long and short heads of the biceps brachii muscle

PC-3 Kyokutaku (Qūzé)—in the cubital skin fold on the ulnar side of the tendon of the biceps brachii muscle

PC-4 Gekimon (Xìmén)—on the forearm 5 cun above the transverse crease of the wrist between the tendons of the palmaris longus and flexor carpi radialis muscles

PC-5 Kanshi (Jiānshǐ)—on the forearm 3 cun above the transverse crease of the wrist between the tendons of the palmaris longus and flexor carpi radialis muscles

PC-6 Naikan (Nèiguān)—on the forearm 2 cun above the transverse crease of the wrist between the tendons of the palmaris longus and flexor carpi radialis muscles

PC-7 Dairyō (Dàlíng)—in the center of the transverse crease of the wrist between the tendons of the palmaris longus and flexor carpi radialis muscles

PC-8 Rōkyū (Láogōng)—in the palmar crease of the hand between the second and third metacarpals

PC-9 Chūshō (Zhōngchōng)—on the radial side of the middle finger about 0.1 cun from the base of the fingernail

Triple Heater Meridian

Symptoms Associated with the Triple Heater Meridian

Poor hearing, pain in the outer corner of the eyes and the cheeks, swelling of throat, tendency to sweat excessively, pain which extends from the back of the jaw to the neck and from the back of the shoulder down the back of the arm on the radial side

---

The Path of the Triple Heater Meridian

The triple heater meridian begins at the tip of the ring finger and goes up the back of the hand between the fourth and fifth metatarsals to reach the wrist. It continues up the posterior aspect of the forearm between the radius and ulna and goes over the elbow to travel up the posterior aspect of the upper arm and reach the back of the shoulder. The triple heater meridian intersects the gallbladder meridian as it crosses over to the front of the shoulder and then goes down to the supraclavicular fossa, where it enters into the thoracic cavity. This internal branch

Fig. 14   Triple Heater Meridian

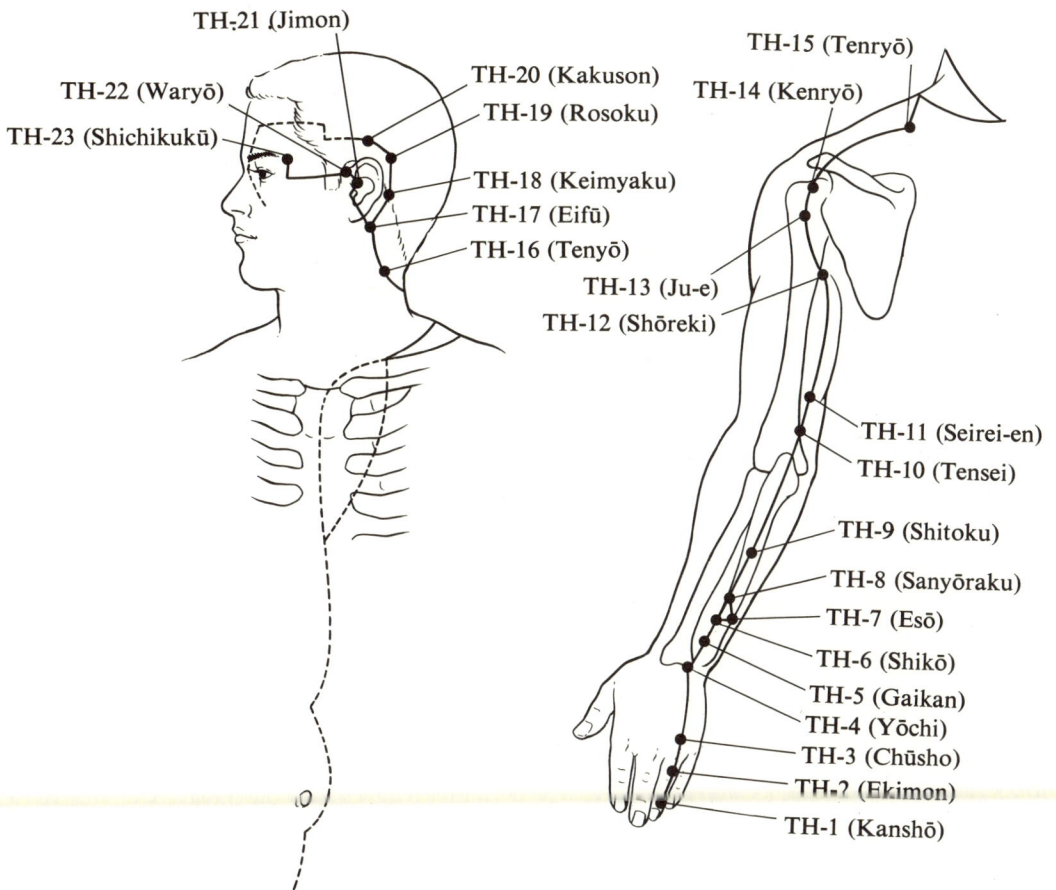

descends between the lungs to a point posterior to CV-17 and connects with the pericardium. One branch which descends through the diaphragm joins the three parts of the triple heater. Another branch travels back up to the supraclavicular fossa and, after going to a point at the posterior base of the neck (GV-14), emerges on the skin surface to go up the side of the neck to the retroauricular region. This branch continues up around the ear and then goes down over the temporal and zygomatic areas to the infraorbital region. Another branch arising from the retro-auricular region goes through the ear and surfaces once again in front of the ear. This branch passes over a point on the zygomatic arch (GB-3) and goes to the outer canthus, where it connects to the gallbladder meridian.

Acupuncture Points of the Triple Heater Meridian

TH-1   Kanshō (Gūnāchōng)—on the ulnar side of the ring finger about 0.1 cun from the base of the fingernail

TH-2   Ekimon (Yèmén)—on the back of the hand above the web between the ring finger and little finger, just distal to the metacarpophalangeal joints

TH-3   Chūsho (Zhōngzhǔ)—on the back of the hand between the fourth and fifth metacarpals, proximal to the metacarpophalangeal joints

TH-4 Yōchi (Yángchí)—on the back of the wrist directly above the ring finger between the tendons of the extensor digitorum communis and the extensor digitorum minimi muscles

TH-5 Gaikan (Wàiguān)—2 cun above TH-4 in the center of the arm between the radius and ulna

TH-6 Shikō (Zhīgōu)—3 cun above TH-4 in the center of the arm between the radius and ulna

TH-7 Esō (Huìzōng)—3 cun above TH-4 on the radial border of the ulna

TH-8 Sanyōraku (Sānyángluò)—4 cun above TH-4 in the center of the arm between the radius and ulna

TH-9 Shitoku (Sìdú)—5 cun below the tip of the olecranon between the radius and ulna

TH-10 Tensei (Tiānjǐng)—in the depression 1 cun above the tip of the olecranon

TH-11 Seirei-en (Qīnglěngyuān)—2 cun above the tip of the olecranon

TH-12 Shōreki (Xiāoluò)—halfway between TH-11 and TH-13

TH-13 Ju-e (Nàohuì)—on the lower border of the deltoid muscle 3 cun below TH-14

TH-14 Kenryō (Jiānliáo)—in the depression inferior to the lateral extremity of the acromion

TH-15 Tenryō (Tiānliáo)—just above the superior angle of the scapula

TH-16 Tenyō (Tiānyǒu)—on the posterior border of the sternocleidomastoid muscle level with the mandibular angle

TH-17 Eifū (Yìfēng)—under the earlobe in the depression between the mandible and the mastoid process

TH-18 Keimyaku (Qìmài)—one-third the distance from TH-17 to TH-20 on a curved line just under the rim of the auricle; in a depression on the mastoid process

TH-19 Rosoku (Lúxī)—two-thirds the distance from TH-17 to TH-20 on a curved line just under the rim of the auricle; in a depression superior to the mastoid process

TH-20 Kakuson (Jiǎosūn)—on the hairline directly above the apex of the auricle

TH-21 Jimon (Ěrmén)—just in front of the ear in the depression anterior to the supratragic tubercle

TH-22 Waryō (Héliáo)—just anterior and superior to TH-21 on the posterior border of the hairline over the temporal artery

TH-23 Shichikukū (Sīzhúkōng)—in the depression at the lateral tip of the eyebrow

Gallbladder Meridian

Symptoms Associated with the Gallbladder Meridian

Headaches, lack of luster in face and skin, migraine headaches with pain extending to the outer corner of the eyes and the base of the neck, bitter taste in mouth, scrofula around ears and on neck, pain in the epigastrium and axilla extending to the sides, hotness in outer edge of foot, pain in the fourth toe, occasional spells of

Fig. 15 Gallbladder Meridian

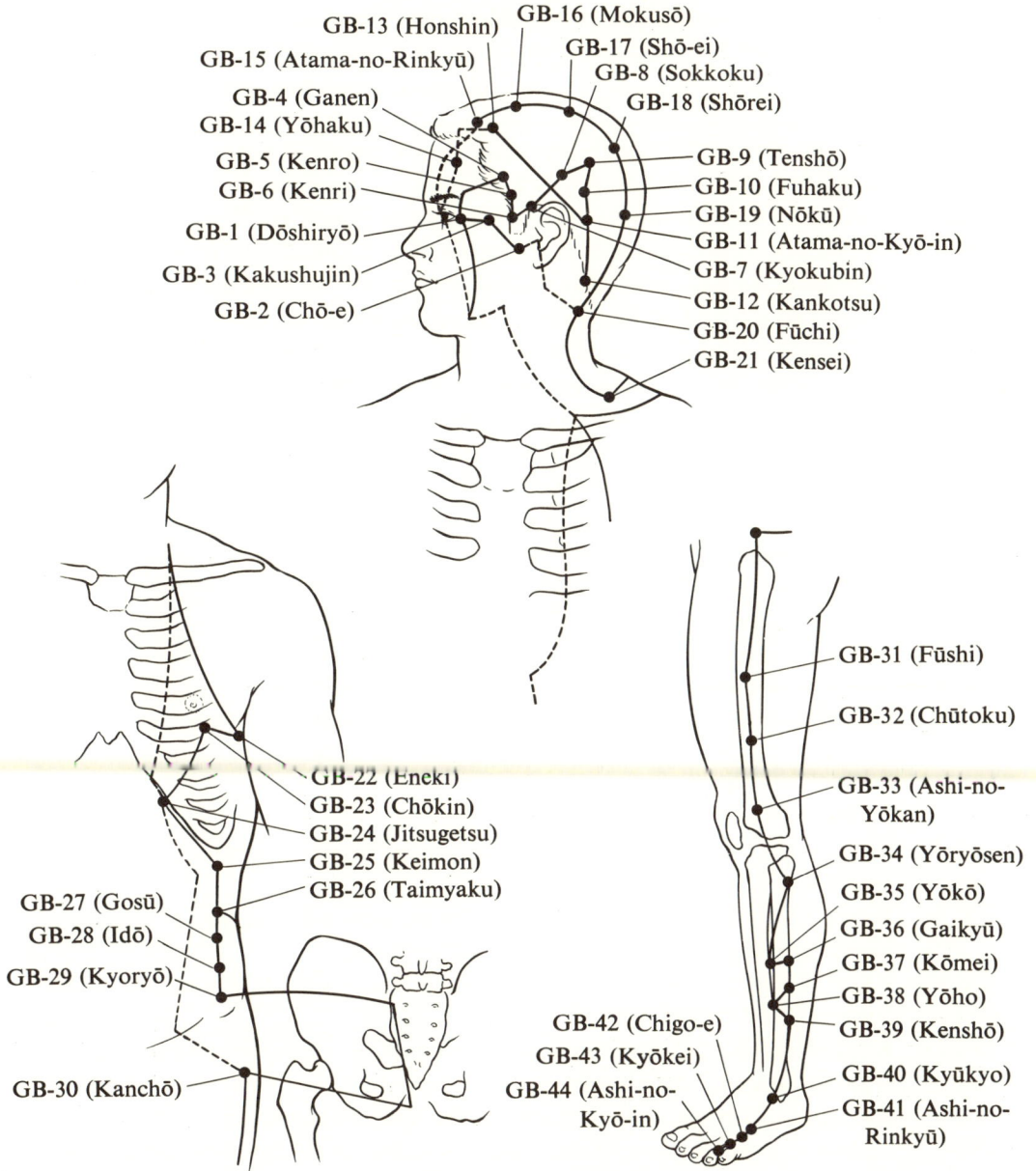

GB-13 (Honshin)   GB-16 (Mokusō)
GB-15 (Atama-no-Rinkyū)   GB-17 (Shō-ei)
   GB-8 (Sokkoku)
GB-4 (Ganen)   GB-18 (Shōrei)
GB-14 (Yōhaku)
GB-5 (Kenro)   GB-9 (Tenshō)
GB-6 (Kenri)   GB-10 (Fuhaku)
   GB-19 (Nōkū)
GB-1 (Dōshiryō)   GB-11 (Atama-no-Kyō-in)
GB-3 (Kakushujin)   GB-7 (Kyokubin)
GB-2 (Chō-e)   GB-12 (Kankotsu)
   GB-20 (Fūchi)
   GB-21 (Kensei)

GB-22 (Eneki)   GB-31 (Fūshi)
GB-23 (Chōkin)   GB-32 (Chūtoku)
GB-24 (Jitsugetsu)
GB-25 (Keimon)   GB-33 (Ashi-no-Yōkan)
GB-26 (Taimyaku)
GB-27 (Gosū)   GB-34 (Yōryōsen)
GB-28 (Idō)   GB-35 (Yōkō)
GB-29 (Kyoryō)   GB-36 (Gaikyū)
   GB-37 (Kōmei)
   GB-38 (Yōho)
GB-42 (Chigo-e)   GB-39 (Kenshō)
GB-43 (Kyōkei)   GB-40 (Kyūkyo)
GB-44 (Ashi-no-Kyō-in)   GB-41 (Ashi-no-Rinkyū)
GB-30 (Kanchō)

chilling, feverishness, and sweating, pain and symptoms appearing on the side of body such as the flank region, the hip joints, the outside of the knees and lower legs, and lateral malleoli

---

The Path of the Gallbladder Meridian

The gallbladder meridian begins at a point next to the outer canthus, from which one branch goes up the temporal region to the corner of the anterior hairline. It continues down along the lateral hairline and goes down around the ear to the back of the mastoid process. An internal branch separates from this point to pass through the ear and return to the point next to the outer canthus. Another internal branch of the gallbladder meridian goes down from the outer canthus to ST-5 on the mandible and joins a branch of the triple heater meridian. From this point the branch goes upward and then curves downward to go over the cheek. It passes over ST-6 on the mandibular angle and goes down the neck to the supraclavicular fossa. Here it penetrates into the thoracic cavity and passes down through the diaphragm to connect with the liver and enter the gallbladder. This internal branch continues down the abdomen from the hypochondriac region to the inguinal region and reaches the hip joint. The surface branch of the meridian from the back of the mastoid process goes down to GV-14, at the posterior base of the neck, and then it goes forward over the shoulder into the supraclavicular fossa. From here it goes down the front of the shoulder to the axilla and descends the side of the body to reach the hip joint, where it rejoins the internal branch. The gallbladder meridian then passes down the side of the thigh and knee and passes just in front of the head of the fibula. The meridian continues down the side of the lower leg and passes in front of the lateral malleolus to go anteriorly on the dorsum of the foot to the tip of the fourth toe. Another branch separates on the dorsum of the foot to reach the lateral tip of the big toe and connect with the liver meridian.

Acupuncture Points of the Gallbladder Meridian

GB-1   Dōshiryō (Tóngzǐliáo)—0.5 cun lateral to the outer canthus

GB-2   Chō-e (Tīnghuì)—in the depression anterior to the intertragic notch

GB-3   Kakushujin (Shàngguān)—in the depression above the zygomatic arch on anterior side of temporal hairline

GB-4   Ganen (Hànyàn)—one-fourth the distance from the corner of the anterior hairline (ST-8) to GB-7

GB-5   Kenro (Xuánlú)—halfway between the corner of the anterior hairline (ST-8) and GB-7

GB-6   Kenri (Xuánlí)—one-fourth the distance from GB-7 to the corner of the anterior hairline (ST-8)

GB-7   Kyokubin (Qūbìn)—on the anterior side of the temporal hairline level with the apex of the auricle

GB-8   Sokkoku (Shuáigǔ)—1.5 cun above the apex of the auricle

GB-9   Tenshō (Tiānchōng)—posterior and superior to the apex of the auricle; 0.5 cun posterior to GB-8

GB-10   Fuhaku (Fúbái)—one-third the distance from GB-9 to GB-12; about 1 cun posterior to the apex of the auricle

GB-11   Atama-no-Kyō-in (Toū-Qiàoyīn)—posterior and superior to the mastoid process; one-third the distance from GB-12 to GB-9

GB-12   Kankotsu (Wángǔ)—in the depression posterior to the inferior aspect of the mastoid process

GB-13   Honshin (Běnshén)—on the anterior hairline about 1 cun medial to the corner of the hairline (ST-8)

GB-14 Yōhaku (Yángbái)—1 cun above the eyebrow; directly above the pupil when looking straight ahead

GB-15 Atama-no-Rinkyū (Tóu-Línqì)—halfway between the median line (GV-24) and the corner of the anterior hairline (ST-8); 0.5 cun behind the hairline

GB-16 Mokusō (Mùchuāng)—1.0 cun posterior to GB-15 and 2.25 cun lateral to the median line

GB-17 Shō-ei (Zhèngyíng)—1.0 cun posterior to GB-15 and 2.25 cun lateral to the median line

GB-18 Shōrei (Chénglíng)—halfway between GB-17 and GB-19 and 2.25 cun from the median line

GB-19 Nōkū (Nǎokōng)—directly above GB-20 level with the superior border of the external occipital protuberance

GB-20 Fūchi (Fēngchí)—at inferior border of the occiput in the depression between the insertions of the trapezius and sternocleidomastoid muscles

GB-21 Kensei (Jiānjǐng)—on the shoulder halfway between the spinous process of the seventh cervical vertebra and the acromion

GB-22 Eneki (Yuānyè)—3 cun straight below the center of the axilla at the level of the nipple

GB-23 Chōkin (Zhéjīn)—1 cun anterior to GB-22 at the level of the nipple

GB-24 Jitsugetsu (Rìyuè)—in the seventh intercostal space on the mammillary line (4 cun from anterior median line)

GB-25 Keimon (Jīngmén)—on the lower border of the tip of the twelfth rib

GB-26 Taimyaku (Dàimài)—directly below the tip of the eleventh rib at the level of the umbilicus

GB-27 Gosū (Wǔshū)—on the anterior end of iliac crest just above the anterior superior iliac spine; 3 cun below the level of the umbilicus

GB-28 Idō (Wéidào)—just medial to the inferior border of the anterior superior iliac spine; 0.5 cun below GB-27

GB-29 Kyoryō (Jūliáo)—halfway between the anterior superior iliac spine and the greater trochanter

GB-30 Kanchō (Huántiào)—in the depression above the superior border of the greater trochanter

GB-31 Fūshi (Fēngshì)—on the side of the thigh about 2.5 cun below the midpoint between the greater trochanter and the lateral epicondyle of the femur; about 7 cun above the inferior border of the lateral epicondyle of the femur

GB-32 Chūtoku (Zhōngdú)—2 cun below GB-31; about one-fourth the way from the inferior border of the lateral epicondyle of the femur to the superior border of the greater trochanter

GB-33 Ashi-no-Yōkan (Xī-Yángguān)—in the depression anterior to the ilio-tibital tract just above the lateral epicondyle of the femur

GB-34 Yōryōsen (Yánglíngquán)—directly anterior and inferior to the head of the fibula

GB-35 Yōkō (Yàngjiào)—on the posterior border of the fibula 7 cun above the tip of the lateral malleolus; about 1 cun below the midpoint between the tip of the lateral malleolus and the inferior border of the lateral epicondyle of the femur

GB-36 Gaikyū (Wàiqiū)—on the anterior border of the fibula level with GB-36

GB-37 Kōmei (Guāngmíng)—on the posterior border of the fibula 5 cun above the tip of the lateral malleolus; about one-third of the way from the lateral malleolus to the inferior border of the lateral epicondyle of the femur

GB-38 Yōho (Yángfǔ)—on the anterior border of the fibula 4 cun above the tip of the lateral malleolus

GB-39 Kenshō (Xuánzhōng)—3 cun above the tip of the lateral malleolus in the depression between the posterior border of the fibula and the peroneus longus and brevis muscles

GB-40 Kyūkyo (Qiūxū)—in the depression anterior and inferior to the lateral malleolus

GB-41 Ashi-no-Rinkyū (Zú-Línqì)—on the dorsum of the foot in the depression between the fourth and fifth metatarsals; posterior to the tendon of the extensor digiti minimi muscle

GB-42 Chigo-e (Dìwǔhuì)—on the dorsum of the foot in the depression just proximal to the bases of the fourth and fifth metatarsals

GB-43 Kyōkei (Xiáxī)—above the web between the fourth and fifth toes just anterior to the head of the metatarsals

GB-44 Ashi-no-Kyō-in (Zú-Qiàoyīn)—on the lateral side of the fourth toe about 0.1 cun from the base of the toenail

Liver Meridian

Symptoms Associated with the Liver Meridian

Dingy complexion, dry throat, feeling of congestion in chest, nausea, tendency toward diarrhea, low back pain, occasional chilling or feverishness, pain extending down to the big toe, difficulty in urinating at nighttime, pain in the inguinal region and genitals for men, swelling of scrotum, distention of lower abdomen for women

---

The Path of the Liver Meridian

The liver meridian begins at the lateral tip of the big toe and goes proximally across the dorsum of the foot to pass in front of the medial malleolus. It continues up the medial aspect of the lower leg and crosses the spleen meridian about eight cun above the malleolus. The meridian then goes up the medial side of the knee and the thigh and then goes inside the pubic region to connect with the external genitalia. The main branch continues up the side of the abdomen next to the stomach meridian. At a point below the rib cage (LV-13) the meridian goes inward to connect to the gallbladder and enter the liver. One branch of the meridian travels upward from the hypochondriac region to pass through the diaphragm and reach the lateral thoracic region. It continues up the back of the throat and comes out through the maxillary fossa and connects with the eyes and goes over the

Fig. 16 Liver Meridian

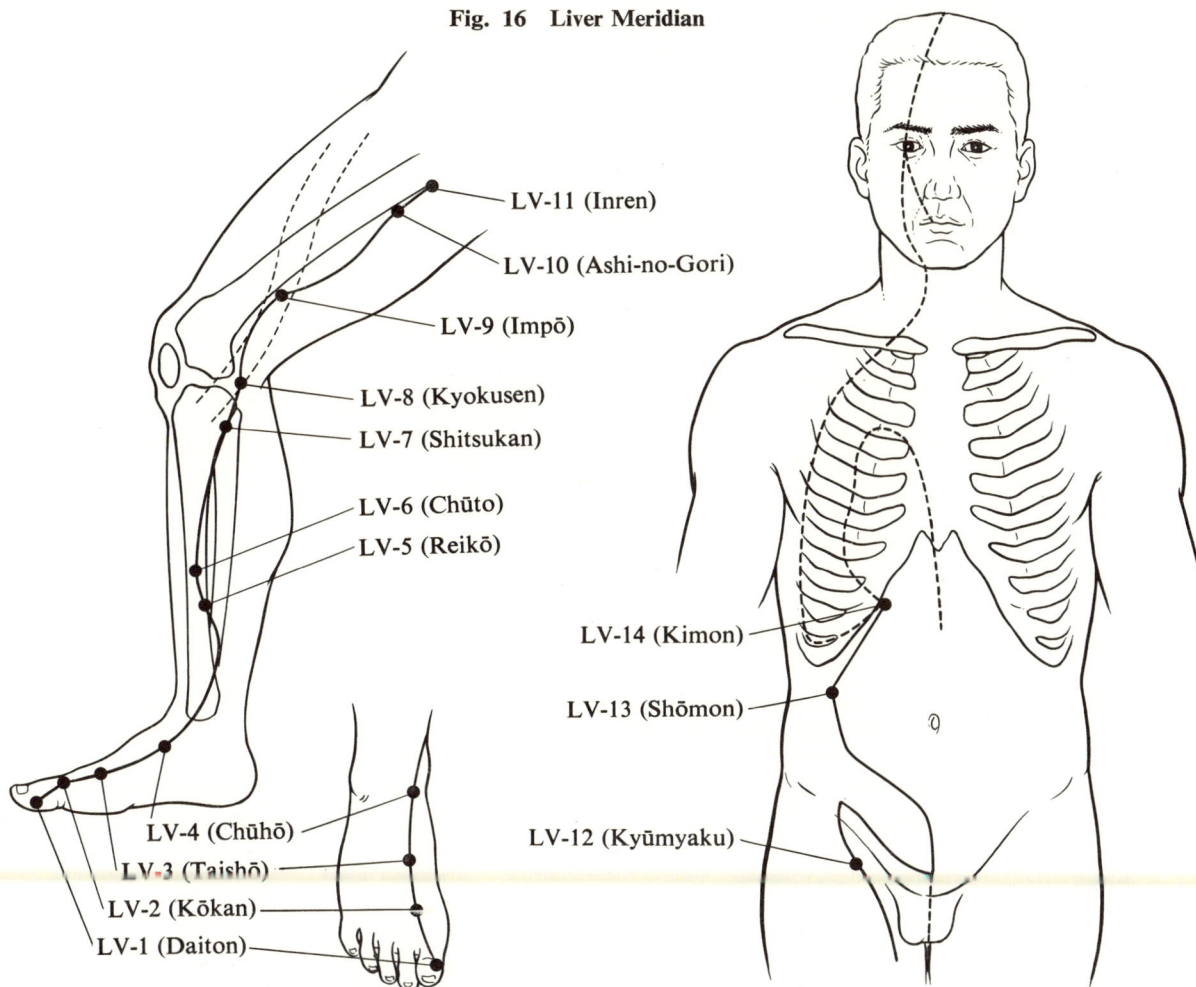

LV-11 (Inren)
LV-10 (Ashi-no-Gori)
LV-9 (Impō)
LV-8 (Kyokusen)
LV-7 (Shitsukan)
LV-6 (Chūto)
LV-5 (Reikō)
LV-14 (Kimon)
LV-13 (Shōmon)
LV-4 (Chūhō)
LV-12 (Kyūmyaku)
LV-3 (Taishō)
LV-2 (Kōkan)
LV-1 (Daiton)

forehead to reach the vertex of the head and thus the liver meridian connects with the governor vessel. Another branch arising from inside the liver goes through the diaphragm and enters the lungs.

Acupuncture Points of the Liver Meridian

LV-1 Daiton (Dàdūn)—on the lateral side of the big toe, about 0.1 cun from the base of the toenail

LV-2 Kōkan (Xíngjiān)—above the web between the first and second toes just anterior to the head of the metatarsals

LV-3 Taishō (Tàichōng)—in the depression between the first and second metatarsals posterior to the metatarsophalangeal joints

LV-4 Chūhō (Zhōngfēng)—level with the tip of the medial malleolus in the depression on the medial side of the tendon of the tibialis anterior muscle

LV-5 Reikō (Lígōu)—on the medial aspect of the tibia 5 cun above the tip of the medial malleolus

LV-6 Chūto (Zhōngdū)—on the medial aspect of the tibia 7 cun above the tip of

the medial malleolus; 0.5 cun above midpoint between the medial malleolus and the medial condyle

LV-7   Shitsukan (Xīguān)—on the inferior border of the medial condyle; about
halfway between LV-8 and SP-9

LV-8   Kyokusen (Qūquán)—in the depression between the upper border of the
medial epicondyle of the femur and the tendon of the semimembranosus
muscle

LV-9   Impō (Yīnbāo)—on the border of the vastus medialis muscle 4 cun above
LV-8

LV-10   Ashi-no-Gori (Zú-Wŭlĭ)—on the medial aspect of the thigh 3 cun below
ST-30

LV-11   Inren (Yīnlián)—on the medial aspect of the thigh 2 cun below ST-30

LV-12   Kyūmyaku (Jímài)—in the inguinal region 2.5 cun lateral to the midpoint
of the inferior border of the pubic symphysis; over the femoral artery

LV-13   Shōmon (Zhāngmén)—on the lower border of the tip of the eleventh rib

LV-14   Kimon (Qīmén)—in the sixth intercostal space on the mammillary line
(4 cun from anterior median line)

Governor Vessel

Symptoms Associated with the Governor Vessel

Symptoms accompanying diseases in the cranium as well as in the reproductive,
digestive, and respiratory systems; a pain thrusting up from the lower abdomen to
the epigastrium, strong pain when bending forward or backward, hotness in the
head, sharp pain, dry and sore throat

The Path of the Governor Vessel

The governor vessel originates in the pelvic cavity and an internal branch ascends
inside the abdomen to connect with the kidneys. The surface branch emerges at
the perineum and goes to the tip of the coccyx, from where it ascends the spinal
column all the way to the occiput. The six yang meridians converge at GV-14, just
to the top of the spinous process of the first thoracic vertebra, and thus the
governor vessel modulates the energy in all the yang meridians. An internal branch
of the governor vessel separates at GV-16, on the posterior median line just under
the occiput, to enter the brain. The surface branch continues up the back of the
head and goes over the vertex and down the center of the forehead. This branch
goes over the tip of the nose and onto the upper lip and then enters the mouth to
end in the center of the upper gum.

Acupuncture Points of the Governor Vessel

GV-1   Chōkyō (Chángqiáng)—at the tip of the coccyx
GV-2   Yōyu (Yāoshū)—at the center of the sacral hiatus

Fig. 17   Governor Vessel

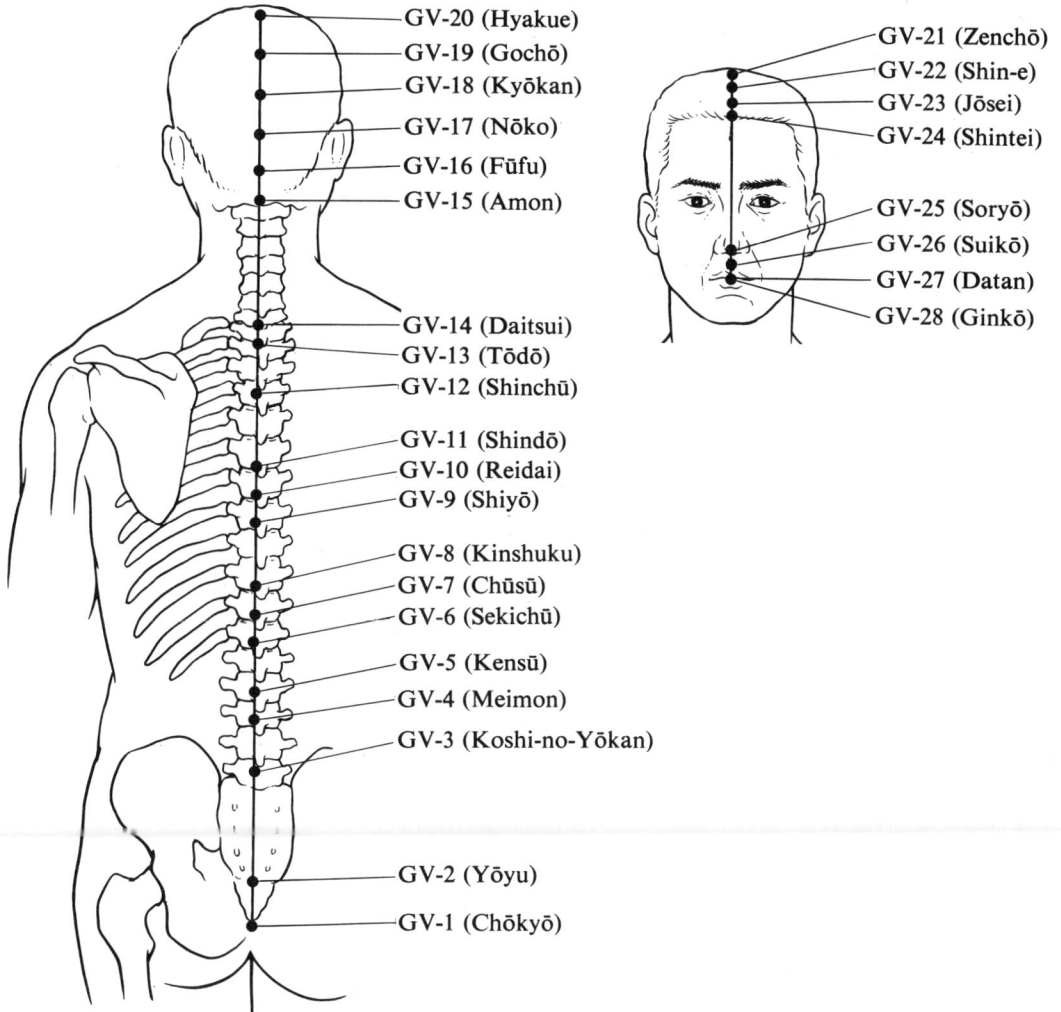

- GV-20 (Hyakue)
- GV-19 (Gochō)
- GV-18 (Kyōkan)
- GV-17 (Nōko)
- GV-16 (Fūfu)
- GV-15 (Amon)
- GV-21 (Zenchō)
- GV-22 (Shin-e)
- GV-23 (Jōsei)
- GV-24 (Shintei)
- GV-25 (Soryō)
- GV-26 (Suikō)
- GV-27 (Datan)
- GV-28 (Ginkō)
- GV-14 (Daitsui)
- GV-13 (Tōdō)
- GV-12 (Shinchū)
- GV-11 (Shindō)
- GV-10 (Reidai)
- GV-9 (Shiyō)
- GV-8 (Kinshuku)
- GV-7 (Chūsū)
- GV-6 (Sekichū)
- GV-5 (Kensū)
- GV-4 (Meimon)
- GV-3 (Koshi-no-Yōkan)
- GV-2 (Yōyu)
- GV-1 (Chōkyō)

GV-3   Koshi-no-Yōkan (Yāo-Yángguān)—below the spinous process of the fourth lumbar vertebra

GV-4   Meimon (Mìngmén)—below the spinous process of the second lumbar vertebra

GV-5   Kensū (Xuánshū)—below the spinous process of the first lumbar vertebra

GV-6   Sekichū (Jǐzhōng)—below the spinous process of the eleventh thoracic vertebra

GV-7   Chūsū (Zhōngshū)—below the spinous process of the tenth thoracic vertebra

GV-8   Kinshuku (Jīnsuō)—below the spinous process of the ninth thoracic vertebra

GV-9   Shiyō (Zhìyáng)—below the spinous process of the seventh thoracic vertebra

GV-10   Reidai (Língtái)—below the spinous process of the sixth thoracic vertebra

GV-11 Shindō (Shéndào)—below the spinous process of the fifth thoracic vertebra

GV-12 Shinchū (Shēnzhù)—below the spinous process of the third thoracic vertebra

GV-13 Tōdō (Táodào)—below the spinous process of the first thoracic vertebra

GV-14 Daitsui (Dàzhuī)—below the spinous process of the seventh cervical vertebra

GV-15 Amon (Yǎmén)—on the median line in the back of the neck, 0.5 cun above the posterior hairline

GV-16 Fūfu (Fēngfǔ)—on the median line in the back of the neck, about 1 cun below the external occipital protuberance

GV-17 Nōko (Nǎohù)—on the superior border of the external occipital protuberance

GV-18 Kyōkan (Qiángjiān)—one-third the distance from GV-17 to GV-20

GV-19 Gochō (Hòudǐng)—one-third the distance from GV-20 to GV-17

GV-20 Hyakue (Bǎihuì)—in the small depression over the saggital suture at the midpoint of the line connecting the apexes of the ears

GV-21 Zenchō (Qiándǐng)—on the anterior median line about 1.5 cun in front of GV-20

GV-22 Shin-e (Xìnhuì)—on the anterior median line about 3.0 cun in front of GV-20

GV-23 Jōsei (Shàngxīng)—on the anterior median line about 1 cun above the frontal hairline

GV-24 Shintei (Shéntíng)—on the anterior median line at the level of the frontal hairline

GV-25 Soryō (Sùliáo)—at the tip of the nose in the depression between the nasal cartilage

GV-26 Suikō (Rénzhōng)—below the nose just above the midpoint of the philtrum

GV-27 Datan (Duìduān)—at the center of the upper lip on the border of the skin and the mucous membrane

GV-28 Ginkō (Yínjiāo)—on the superior frenulum

Conception Vessel

Symptoms Associated with the Conception Vessel

Disease of the reproductive organs, gynecological problems, symptoms accompanying disease of the excretory and digestive systems as well as that of heart disease; primary symptoms include hard masses in abdomen, extreme tightness in abdomen from the umbilicus down to the pubic bone, and accumulation of intestinal gas

---

The Path of the Conception Vessel

The conception vessel originates in the pelvic cavity and descends to emerge at the perineum. It passes through the pubic region and goes up the abdomen on the

Fig. 18   Conception Vessel

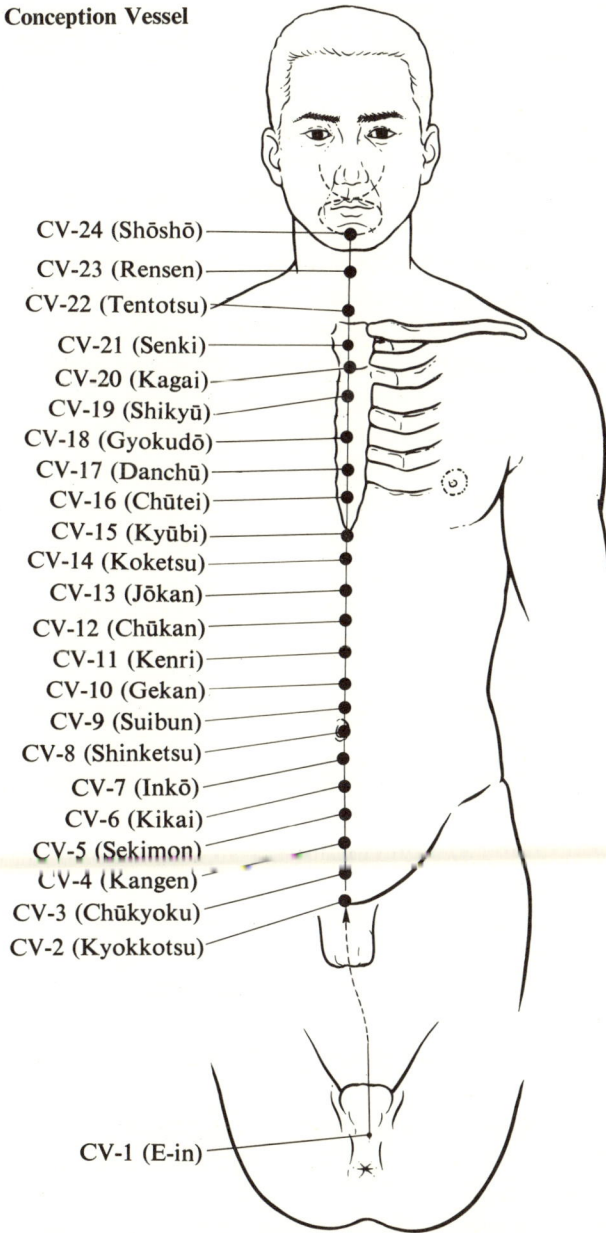

CV-24 (Shōshō)
CV-23 (Rensen)
CV-22 (Tentotsu)
CV-21 (Senki)
CV-20 (Kagai)
CV-19 (Shikyū)
CV-18 (Gyokudō)
CV-17 (Danchū)
CV-16 (Chūtei)
CV-15 (Kyūbi)
CV-14 (Koketsu)
CV-13 (Jōkan)
CV-12 (Chūkan)
CV-11 (Kenri)
CV-10 (Gekan)
CV-9 (Suibun)
CV-8 (Shinketsu)
CV-7 (Inkō)
CV-6 (Kikai)
CV-5 (Sekimon)
CV-4 (Kangen)
CV-3 (Chūkyoku)
CV-2 (Kyokkotsu)

CV-1 (E-in)

anterior median line. Below the umbilicus around CV-4, three yin meridians of the legs connect to the conception vessel and thus this meridian serves to modulate the energy in the yin meridians of the lower extremities. The conception vessel continues up the center of the abdomen and over the midline of the sternum and the throat to a point above the laryngeal prominence. It then goes up the center of the lower jaw and penetrates deeper just below the lip and splits into two branches, which encircle the mouth and cross over each other above the upper lip and go upward to reach the eyes.

Acupuncture Points of the Conception Vessel

CV-1   E-in (Hùiyīn)—at the center of the perineum

CV-2   Kyokkotsu (Qūgǔ)—at the superior border of the pubic symphysis on the anterior median line

CV-3   Chūkyoku (Zhōngjí)—on median line 1 cun above CV-2

CV-4   Kangen (Guānyuán)—on median line 2 cun above CV-2

CV-5   Sekimon (Shímén)—on the median line 2 cun below the umbilicus

CV-6   Kikai (Qìhǎi)—on the median line 1.5 cun below the umbilicus

CV-7   Inkō (Yīnjiāo)—on the median line 1.0 cun below the umbilicus

CV-8   Shinketsu (Shénquè)—in the center of the umbilicus

CV-9   Suibun (Shǔifēn)—on the median line 1.0 cun above the umbilicus

CV-10   Gekan (Xìawǎn)—on the median line 2.0 cun above the umbilicus

CV-11   Kenri (Jiànlǐ)—on the median line 3.0 cun above the umbilicus

CV-12   Chūkan (Zhōngwǎn)—on the median line halfway between the umbilicus and the inferior border of the sternal body; 4.0 cun above the umbilicus

CV-13   Jōkan (Shàngwǎn)—on the median line 1.0 cun above CV-12

CV-14   Koketsu (Jùquè)—on the median line 2.0 cun above CV-12

CV-15   Kyūbi (Jiūwěi)—on the median line about 3.0 cun above CV-12 at the tip of the xyphoid process

CV-16   Chūtei (Zhōngtíng)—on the midline of the sternum at the level of the fifth intercostal space

CV-17   Danchū (Shānzhōng)—on the midline of the sternum at the level of the fourth intercostal space (between the nipples)

CV-18   Gyokudō (Yùtáng)—on the midline of the sternum at the level of the third intercostal space

CV-19   Shikyū (Zǐgōng)—on the midline of the sternum at the level of the second intercostal space

CV-20   Kagai (Huágài)—on the midline of the sternum at the level of the first intercostal space

CV-21   Senki (Xuánjī)—on the midline of the sternum halfway between CV-20 and CV-22

CV-22   Tentotsu (Tiāntū)—in the center of the jugular fossa

CV-23   Rensen (Liánquán)—on the anterior median line at the superior border of the hyoid bone

CV-24   Shōshō (Chéngjiāng)—in the center of the lower jaw in the deepest part of the mentolabial furrow

Chapter 3
The Scientific Rationale for
Acupuncture Therapy

1. A Modern Perspective on Meridians and Acupuncture Points

The concept of meridians and acupuncture points is the basis of acupuncture therapy. The concept of meridians is based on Chinese philosophical principles and it is a system of vertical correlations of reactive points on the body discovered and systematized through the experience accumulated by many generations of Chinese medical workers from ancient times. Acupuncture points are reactive points along the path of meridians, and they are also the points most receptive to stimulation.

The meridians are a functional bands on or closer to the body surface where reactions tend to appear and acupuncture points are the reactive points on the meridians. When there is some abnormality in the body, the meridians and acupuncture points reveal the condition of the internal organs on the body surface. These reactions are not confined to the surface of the skin, but are instead regarded as a three dimensional phenomena involving subcutaneous tissues. Research has been conducted from various angles since the beginning of this century to study the physiological effects of acupuncture stimulation and to elucidate the physical basis of meridians and acupuncture points. Despite this fact, to this day no attempt to analyze and organize all the findings and scientific theories regarding acupuncture has been adequate and comprehensive enough to gain unanimous acceptance.

For this reason, today there are a variety of viewpoints regarding the significance of meridians and acupuncture points, and a number of theories are advocated. One theory is that the meridians are basically nerve reflexes, or a system of reflexes which connect the internal organs with the body surface. Another theory adopts the model of an energy circulation system as spoken of in the classical texts and postulates another circulation system for body fluids independent of the circulatory system and the nervous system. Another theory relates the meridians to blood vessels and lymphatic vessels. Yet another theory equates the meridians to the peripheral nerves.

Amidst all the disagreement over the matter, the theory which seems most plausible from the standpoint of clinical practice is the first theory of nerve reflexes based on a modern medical viewpoint. The meridians and acupuncture points will therefore be discussed below in terms of this perspective.

(1) Viscerocutaneous Reflex

When there is some abnormality in the internal organs or other deep tissues, the abnormality is reflected in the skin and muscles controlled by the nerves of the same spinal segment, and various changes can be detected on the surface. This is known as the viscerocutaneous reflex. In this reflex, impulses from the sensory nerves in the affected internal organs or deep tissues are transmitted afferently to the central nervous system, which produces reflexive changes close to the body surface. The changes caused by the viscerocutaneous reflex actually result as a combination of the viscerosensory reflex, visceromotor reflex, and visceroautonomic reflex. The viscerosensory reflex is a mechanism by which any abnormal impulse going into the spinal cord from internal organs causes hypersensitivity in the skin in the areas corresponding to the spinal nerves on the same level as the affected reflex center. This makes mild stimulation of the skin, which is normally painless, cause pain or numbness. This reaction occurs especially on the surface of the skin, in subcutaneous connective tissues, and in superficial muscles because these tissues have an abundance of sensory nerve endings.

The visceromotor reflex is a mechanism by which sensory impulses received by the central nervous system from internal organs are reflected as motor responses in the superficial muscle groups at the level of the same spinal nerves. Such a motor response generally appears as hard spots or masses in the muscles and as tension or muscular contracture over a certain body part. This is the localized muscular tension and "stiffness" associated with fatigue and chronic disorders. This results from a type of defensive reaction occurring with abnormalities of the internal organs in which receptivity to adverse stimulation is reduced. This reaction initially begins as hard spots or masses, but after the abnormal impulses from the internal organs reaches a certain level, it turns into broad bands of muscular tension.

The visceroautonomic reflex is the reflexive changes occurring in the sweat glands, sebaceous glands, arrectores pilorum muscles, and subcutaneous capillary networks. The reflexive change in the sweat glands leads to sweating, and that in the sebaceous glands causes oily hair and skin. A reflexive effect on the arrectores pilorum muscles causes goose bumps to form on the skin. The vascular reflex in the skin leads either to abnormal coolness or heating of the skin surface.

(2) Cutaneovisceral Reflex

When certain points on the body surface are stimulated, impulses are transmitted to the spinal cord, and this produces a reflexive effect on an internal organ which is controlled by the spinal nerve on the same level. The following changes are apt to occur in the internal organs by this reaction:

Motor response—increased peristalsis or contraction
Sensory response—greater sensitivity to adverse stimuli
Autonomic response—constriction of arterioles

Fig. 19 The Spinal Cord   **Fig. 20 Spinal Dermatomes**

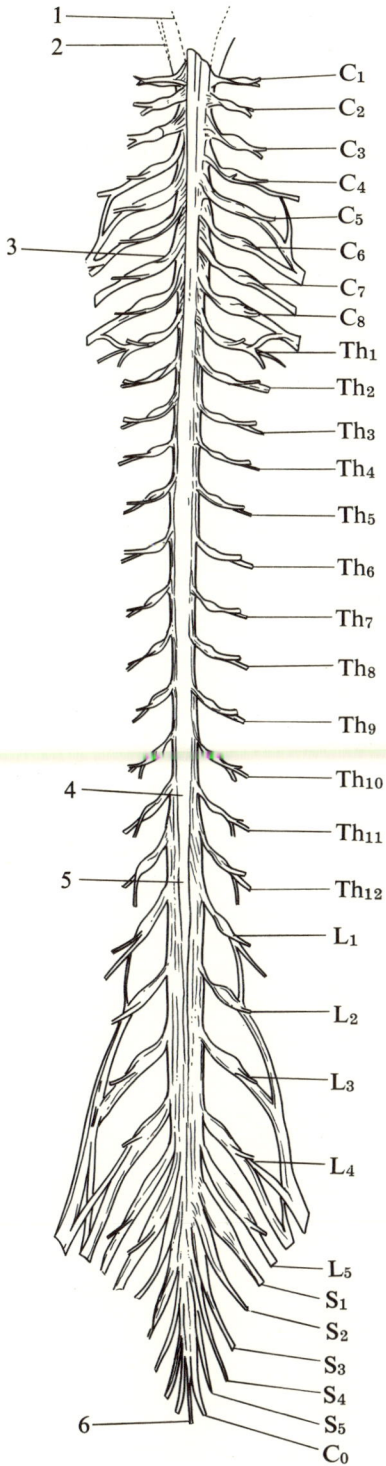

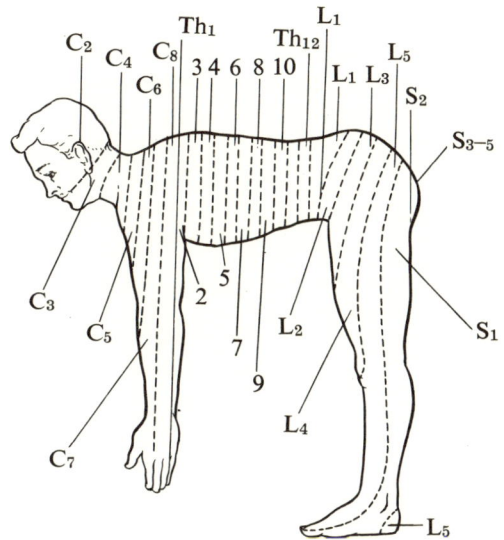

1. Medula oblongata
2. Accesory nerve
3. Cervical plexus
4. Brachial plexus
5. Lumbar plexus
6. Medullary conus (end of spinal cord)
7. Sacral plexus
8. Cauda equina
9. Terminal filum

C_1–C_8: First cervical nerve to eighth cervical nerve
Th_1–Th_{12}: First thoracic nerve to twelfth thoracic nerve
L_1–L_5: First lumbar nerve to fifth lumbar nerve
S_1–S_5: First sacral nerve to fifth sacral nerve
Co: Coccygeal nerve

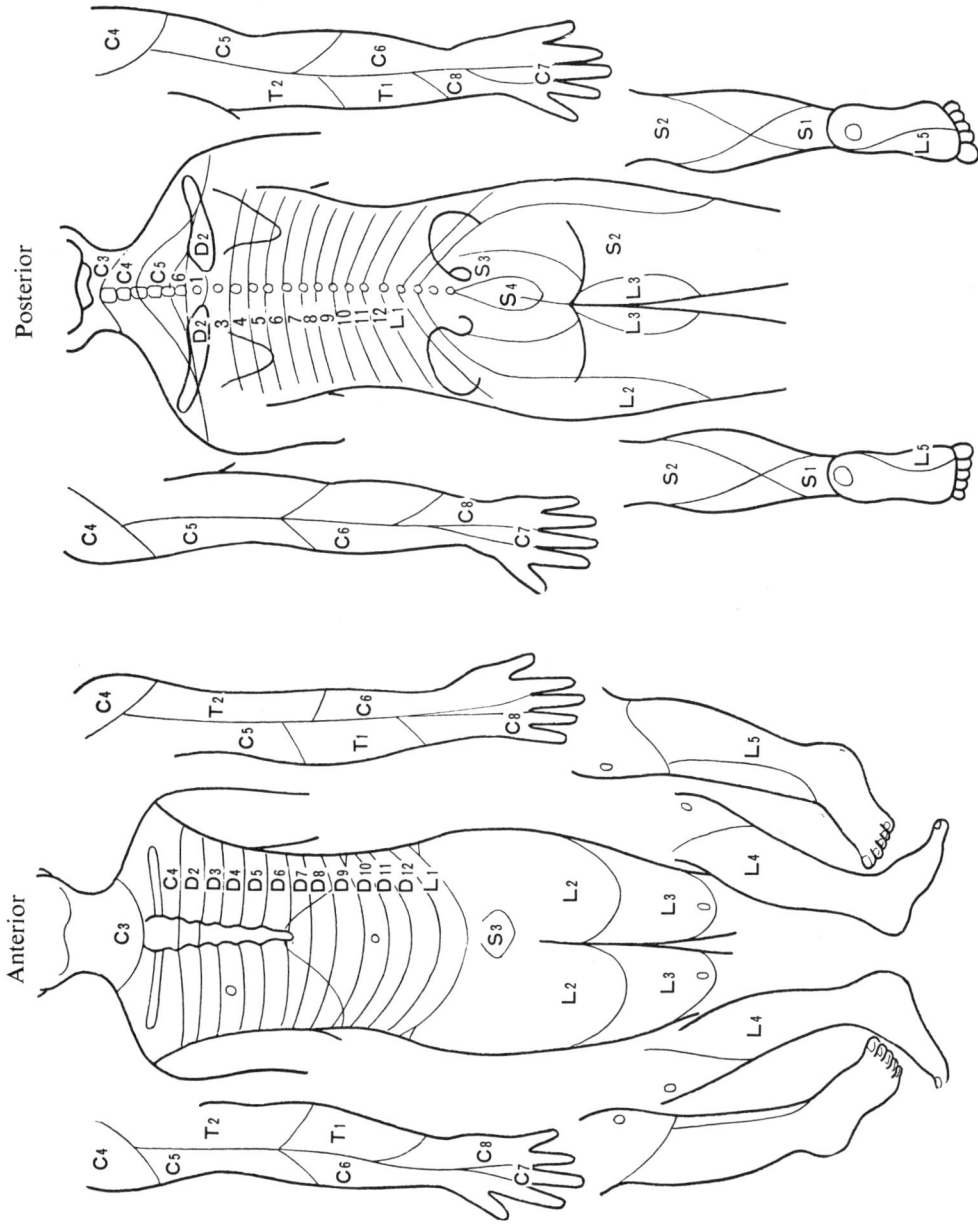

Fig. 21 Sensory Dermatomes (viscerosensory reflex)

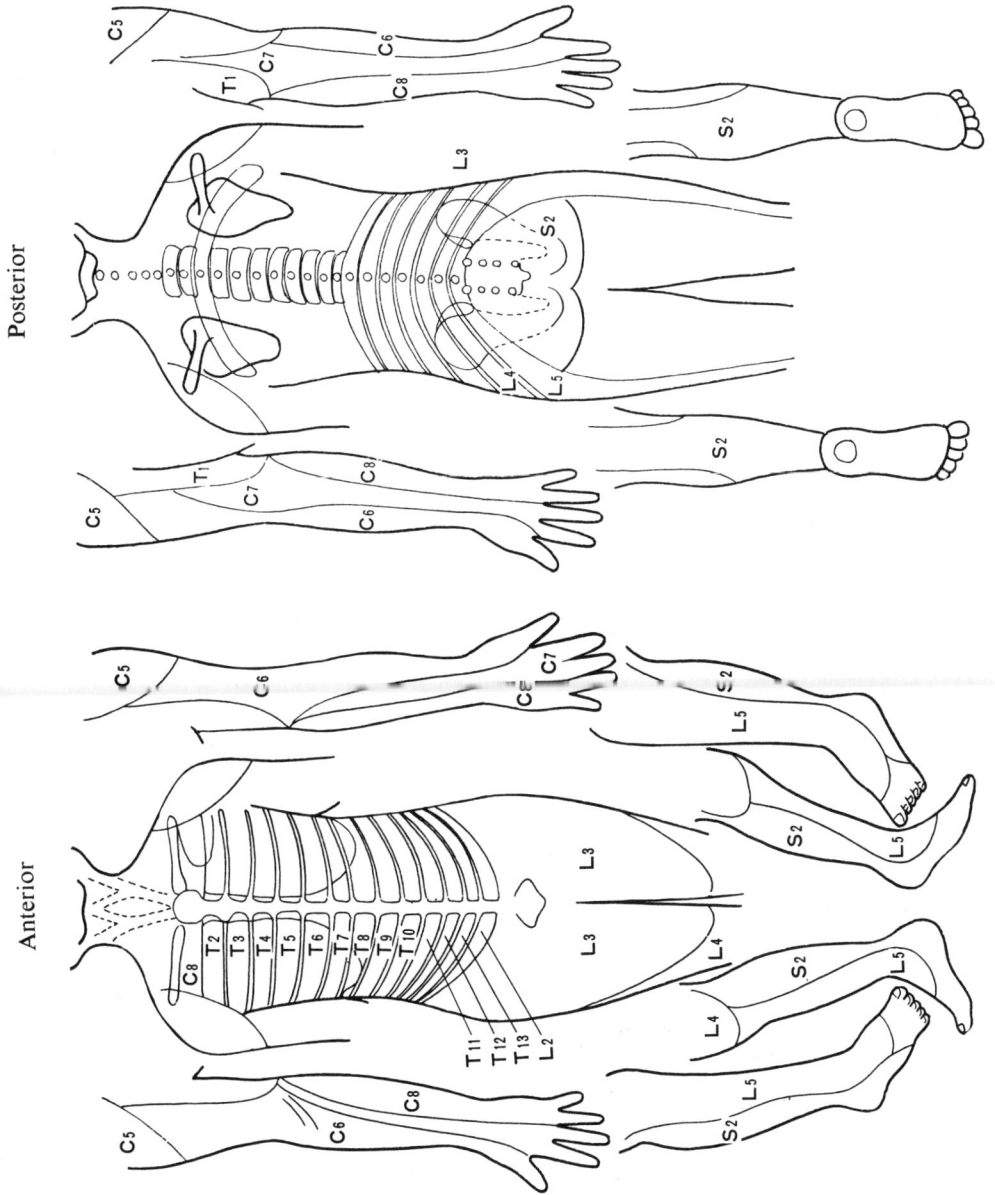

Fig. 22 Myotomes (visceromotor reflex)

It is no overstatement to say that the clinical effects of acupuncture therapy, which is an attempt to regulate the function of the internal organs by applying the appropriate stimulation to the skin, are derived primarily from the cutaneovisceral reflex. Among all the above mentioned reflexive effects, the viscerosensory reflex occurs in relation to the spinal dermatomes, the visceromotor reflex occurs in relation to the myotomes, and the visceroautonomic reflex occurs in relation to sympathetic dermatomes.

The spinal dermatomes refer to the skin segments supplied with a single pair of spinal nerves. The spinal nerves include the first to the eighth cervical nerves, the first to the twelfth thoracic nerves, the first to the fifth lumbar nerves, and the first to the fifth sacral nerves (Fig. 19). The dermatomes line up in a very orderly fashion when a person assumes a posture like that of a four-legged animal (Fig. 20). In the figure showing sensory dermatomes the boundary between the dermatomes is very clearly drawn as a line (Fig. 21), but in reality the borderline between dermatomes is not at all distinct and it is typical for dermatomes to overlap in quite a complex manner.

The myotomes refer to muscle segments controlled by a single pair of spinal nerves. Myotomes were discovered based on the premise that muscles were supplied with spinal nerves in the same way as skin. Although this premise is correct, the arrangement of myotome segments is far more complex than dermatomes since many of the motor nerves extend a long way down the trunk and the upper and lower limbs from spinal nerve plexes to create a great deal of overlap and juxtaposition. Furthermore, the muscle fibers of a particular muscle are grouped together according to a common function and the motor nerve fibers supplying a long muscle often come from spinal nerves originating from different levels of the spinal cord (Fig. 22).

Another aspect which complicates the location of myotomes is that the sensory fibers associated with the deep sensation present in muscles, tendons, and joints merge with motor fibers to form fascicles, or nerve bundles, which supply the muscle fibers. This explains the presence of the deep sensation of tenderness, or pressure sensitivity, along with localized muscular tension. In the clinical work of acupuncture one commonly finds tenderness, or pressure sensitivity, appearing together with localized muscular tension (hard spots). Nevertheless, it is usually hard to determine exactly what spinal nerve a particular tense spot in a superficial muscle is associated with. This is especially true on the back over the trapezius, latissimus dorsi, and the serratus anterior muscles.

The autonomic nervous system consists of sympathetic and parasympathetic components and the visceroautonomic reflex is associated with the sympathetic system. The paravertebral ganglia are the reflex center for sympathetic nerves and they exist next to each one of the spinal nerves from the level of the first thoracic vertebra down to that of the second lumbar vertebra. Since both the sympathetic and sensory nerves originate from the same spinal nerves in the trunk, the sympathetic dermatomes largely correspond with the sensory dermatomes. On the neck and four limbs, however, the sympathetic and sensory dermstomes are not so closely related because the distribution of these nerves differs in the peripheral

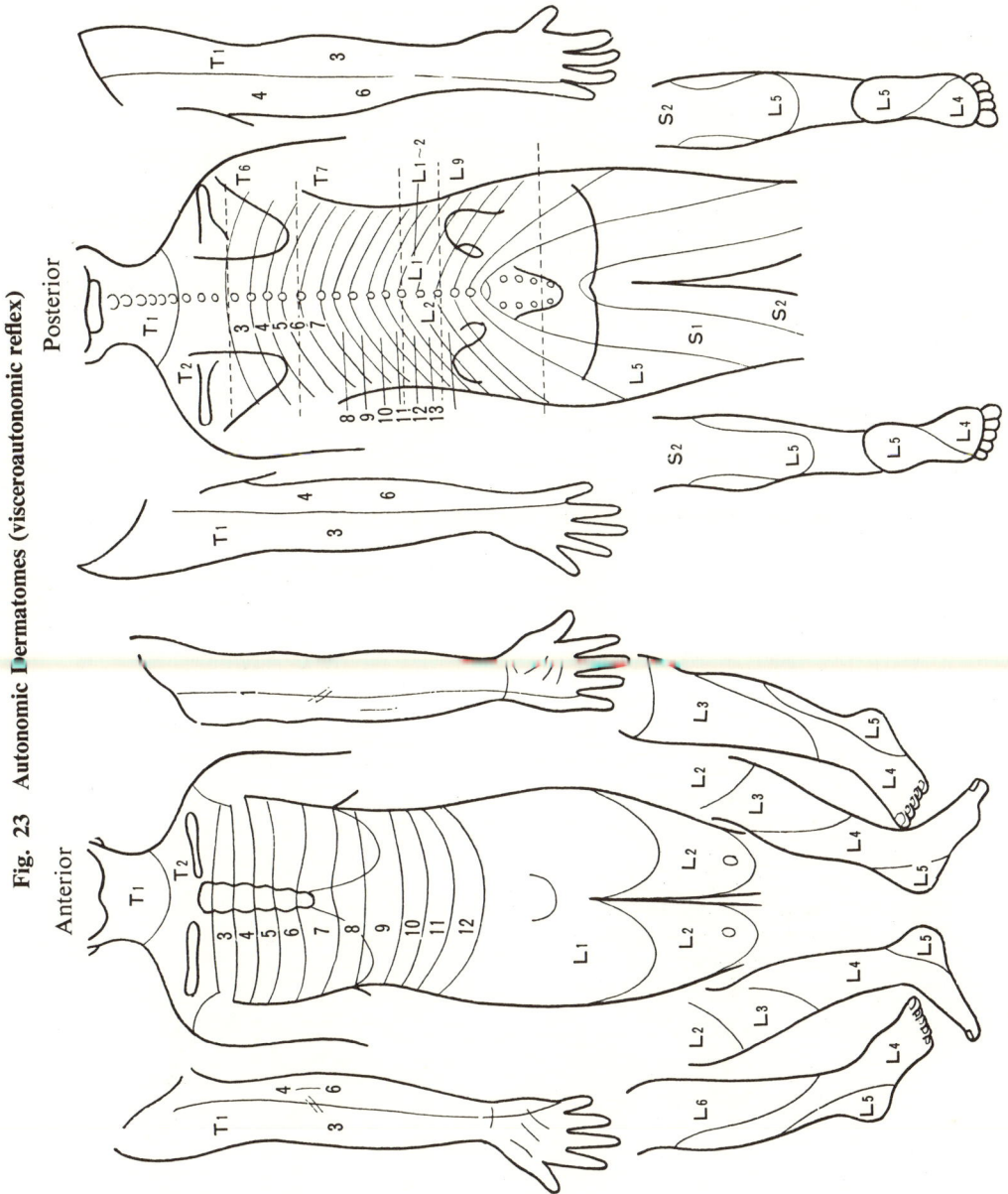

Fig. 23   Autonomic Dermatomes (visceroautonomic reflex)

anatomy. The figure for the autonomic dermatomes shows those skin segments on which there is some consistency (Fig. 23).

The Front *Mu* Points and Back *Shu* Points are some of the most important points in acupuncture, and the relationship between these special points and sensory dermatomes are shown in Fig. 24. It can be seen from this figure that the Front *Mu* Points and Back *Shu* Points have a clear relationship with the spinal dermatomes. Front *Mu* Points and Back *Shu* Points belonging to the same meridian are used diagnostically to correlate the yin (anterior) and yang (posterior) aspects of the torso. The meridians comprise a system of vertical correlations, but they also relate to the dermatomes and myotomes which are for the large part a system of horizontal correlations.

Many complex physiological functions are carried out by means of the nervous system and the musculoskeletal system. One of these functions is to produce many different types of reactions on specific points of the body by a reflex mechanism whenever there is some abnormality in internal organs and tissues. Among these reactions close to the body surface, those of pain and numbness are associated with the viscerosensory reflex. Those of localized muscular tension and tenderness are associated with the visceromotor reflex. Those of chilling and overheating are related to the cutaneovascular reflex. And changes in the appearance of skin such as

Fig. 24 Front *Mu* and Back *Shu* Points and Sensory Dermatomes

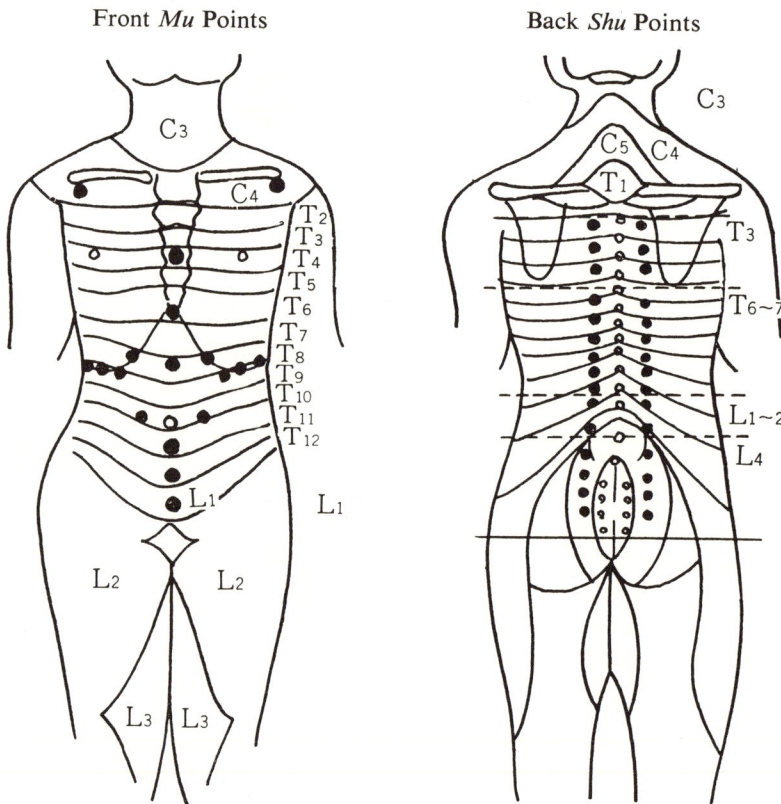

Front *Mu* Points   Back *Shu* Points

dark spots, blemishes, freckles, and pimples are related to the visceroautonomic reflex. Changes in the skin's electrical properties (e.g., lower resistivity around acupuncture points or differences in electrical potential between acupuncture points and other areas) are also associated with the visceroautonomic reflex.

The various changes which occur at acupuncture points as a result of the viscerocutaneous reflex are a response to signals recieved from the internal organs. Acupuncture or tsubo therapy, which apply various types of stimulation on the skin, can be regarded as a way of utilizing the cutaneovisceral reflex to send impulses to the internal organs to correct their abnormal state.

2. Physiological Mechanisms at Work in Acupuncture

(1) The Synergistic Workings of the Body

The phenomenon of life in our body can be divided into the animal functions of sensation and motor activity and the vegetable functions of growth, nourishment, and reproduction. In the process of life these various functions never operate independently by themselves. Each function works in conjunction with all the other functions and maintains an intricate balance to contribute to the total process of life. In all organisms each and every physical part and process is integrated to actualize one whole life process. Furthermore all the functions necessary for life, in all their complexity, are in continuous operation without rest and without letup. This process of life can be called a synergistic action. An organism can therefore be understood as a dynamic whole operating synergistically to maintain itself.

We human beings, as individual organisms, are highly integrated life systems with all parts of our body working together as one for the purpose of maintaining life. Furthermore, the activity of our body is intimately connected with our external environment. Obviously our lives are totally dependent on air, water, and heat originating from the sun. The instinct of self-preservation can be regarded as being one and the same as that for adapting to one's environment. The influences, or various stimuli, from our environment not only affect the receptors or the localized area receiving the influence but affect all parts of the body to a greater or lesser extent. The reaction of our body to external stimulus is likewise a combination of the reactions of various parts of our body. Our response to external stimulus is for the large part an unconscious process.

Acupuncture therapy applies this principle of synergistic action of the organism. Specific points on the body are stimulated to prompt an appropriate physiological response which brings about a therapeutic effect by correcting imbalances and bringing about functional and structural integration. Naturally acupuncture stimulation produces many complex reactions, both physical and psychological, that are integrated by the body to produce a concerted response which works to normalize its functional condition. This effect of acupuncture treatments is utilized widely not only to treat various physical conditions but also for prevention and the continued improvement of health.

(2) The Homeostatic Mechanism of the Body

The word homeostasis comes from the Greek words *homeo*, which means same and *stasis*, which means standing. Homeostasis is a biological action of maintaining a certain physiological equilibrium. Observing the totality of physiological mechanisms of the body, it is clear that activity in one aspect of the body to a greater or lesser extent causes a corresponding action in other parts. The activity of each organ or tissue always occurs in relation to the body as a whole. Also the body is constantly being influenced by the environment it is in, and it modulates its activity to adapt to any changes in the environment.

The physiological activity of the body in response to both internal and external factors is complex and varied, but in general all activity occurs in a way which best enables an individual to accommodate changes and survive. One of the key mechanisms of the body for ensuring its own survival can be called the automatic balancing mechanisms of homeostasis. For example, if for some reason the venous return from the systemic circulation increases to the right atrium, the increase in blood pressure at the vena cava and right atrium causes the Bainbridge reflex*, which increases the heart rate. This then increases the rate of blood flow to the ventricles, which automatically increase their stroke volume so that optimal circulation is maintained. Otherwise, when the blood volume in the arteries rises to cause an increase in vascular resistance, a reflex mechanism increases the output pressure of the left ventricle to maintain a normal blood flow rate. In both the above cases, there is an adjusting mechanism which prevents an overreaction in one part of the body from leading to a life threatening situation for the body as a whole.

The body also has a defensive homeostatic mechanism for changes in temperatures in the external environment. When the air temperature increases, the blood vessels near the skin dilate and sweating increases to give off excess body heat. Conversely when temperatures outside go down, the blood vessels near the skin surface constrict and body heat is conserved and internally metabolic activity increases to produce more heat. In this way the body is constantly reacting in various ways to changes in external temperature to maintain a constant temperature.

Mechanisms for maintaining physiological equilibrium exist in many aspects of organic function, and Walter Cannon named this principle homeostasis. The nervous system (especially the autonomic nervous system) and the endocrine system are most intimately related to homeostasis. The sympathico-adrenal activity occurring when an individual is suddenly confronted with imminent danger or harm was also explained as a kind of homeostatic mechanism by Cannon. The

---

* Bainbridge reflex—a reflex in which the heart rate accelerates due to the distention of the right atrium and vena cava with an increase in blood volume.

principle of homeostasis also provides powerful grounds for explaining the therapeutic mechanism of acupuncture.

It is clear that our body has a great variety of homeostatic mechanisms and is capable of protecting itself from changes in the environment. Changes in the external environment, or external stimuli, are recieved by the skin and other sensory organs, which then play a role in modifying internal conditions to adapt to the environment. Vision and hearing are the most advanced receptors of external stimuli by which animals are capable of a variety of complex adaptive responses through the mediation of the cerebrum. Skin, on the other hand, is the most primitive and largest receptor of stimulus which covers the entire body. The skin responds to external stimulus largely by way of the autonomic nervous system which is associated with the regulation of basic physiological factors essential for survival.

Sensitivity to temperature and pain, among all the stimuli which affect skin, is the most important for survival. For this reason the response of the autonomic nervous system, especially the sympathetic nerves, is great when heat or pain is felt. The stimulation of heat receptors by moxibustion or various other forms of heat therapy utilize this mechanism. The stimulation of pain and pressure receptors of the skin is the effect utilized in acupressure and acupuncture therapy. The aim in acupuncture and related physiotherapies is to elicit a corrective physiological response by the stimulation of specific points on the skin surface.

(3) The Stress Theory

The stress theory advanced by Dr. Hans Selye was a radical break away from the mainstream of Western medical thought, which emphasized the pathophysiology of individual organs and tissues. This new theory of stress gave credence to the more holistic concept of diseases in Oriental medicine.

In his clinical work Dr. Selye noticed a high incidence of cases with the common symptoms of fever, general fatigue, loss of appetite, and headache in which there was no traceable cause. He began animal experiments to determine the cause and discovered that applying psychologically and physiologically stressful stimulus lead to hypertrophy of the adrenal glands, atrophy of the thymus gland, and peptic ulcers. Dr. Selye's work proved that aside from those factors conventionally understood in medicine as being specific causes of pathology (e.g., arthritis due to infection by germs) mechanical, chemical, and psychological stimulus can also cause similar pathological changes.

Dr. Selye applied a variety of adverse stimuli to laboratory animals and found that the basic physiological reaction was the same in every case. He named the reaction of the body to adverse stimuli stress, and the stimuli creating a pathological change stressors. Dr. Selye named the group of typical physiological changes in reaction to the stressors the general adaptation syndrome. He divided the general adaptation syndrome into three stages. The first stage is the so-called alarm period when body temperature, blood pressure, and blood sugar rise or fall in response to the presence of a stressor. The second stage is called the reaction period when the resistance of the body to the stressor increases and the pulse rate, blood pressure, and blood sugar increase. When the stressor acts strongly or persists for a long time, the body enters the third stage called the fatigue period. In this final stage there is a decline in the pulse rate and blood pressure, and resistance to the stressor decreases and edema appears. If the stressor continues to act powerfully on the body and exceeds the body's limit of adaptation, it eventually leads to death.

In some cases, when the body is under the influence of one stressor, it has a higher than normal resistance to another stressor. This happens in the first stage of reaction to stress during the alarm response period and is called cross-resistance. In the second and third period of the general adaptation syndrome, however, the body loses almost all of its resistance to other stressors and no longer responds. This is thought to be due to the exhaustion of energy in reaction to the primary stressor. This is called cross-susceptibility. These concepts of cross-resistance and cross-susceptibility are useful in explaining the therapeutic effects of acupuncture and moxibustion, which in one sense are applications of artificial stressors. There is one theory that acupuncture is effective in treating diseases because it creates cross-resistance in the body and that moxibustion is effective as a treatment because it induces cross-susceptibility. There are actually a number of scientific studies on acupuncture which examine the effects of acupuncture as a stressor. Acupuncture is generally accepted as being a form of therapy applying a controlled amount of stimulation, in varying degrees from mild to strong, to enhance the body's ability to cope with stress.

(4) The Principle of Cybernetics

Cybernetics is a principle developed in 1947 by a mathematician named Norbert Wiener. It is a principle which compares the human nervous system to computers and views the mind and body in terms of cross-communication and servomechanisms. This principle evolved out of a technological need in the postwar period because the products manufactured by machines needed to be checked by human beings even though dramatic increases in production had been achieved since the industrial revolution. There still was a need to compensate for the shortcomings of mechanized production. A machine simply performs the tasks given to it and cannot take responsibility for the results.

A production system where only the designated work is performed without confirmation of the results was termed an open cycle. All animals including human beings differ from such open cycle systems in that they consciously or unconsciously confirm their performance. That is, animals all have feedback systems. In the case of human beings, for example, when we write something, in addition to signals from our brain to move our hand, our eyes look at the outcome. Messages from our eyes reach the area of our brain where the impulses to write are originating and thus we confirm whether the writing is being done satisfactorily. If there is a discrepancy, our brain sends corrective signals to write in the way intended. The signals returning to our brain from our eyes are known as feedback signals. In contrast to the open cycle of simple mechanical production, in living organisms there are always automatic adjustment systems at work, and such organic systems are called closed cycles.

Our bodies maintain homeostasis by feedback mechanisms like the one just mentioned. Designing machines with feedback systems based on cybernetics, which enabled complex quality control operations to be performed automatically, brought remarkable advancements in the industrial sector. Viewing the biological implications of cybernetics, the muscular activity of the body provides another good example of a feedback mechanism. Motor nerves, which extend from the spine to the skeletal muscles, are composed of thick fibers and thin fibers. When the motor nerve is stimulated, the thick fibers cause a muscular contraction by sending impulses to the muscle spindles and the thin fibers serve to regulate the sensitivity of these muscle spindles to nervous impulses. Thus, when the muscle spindles are under pressure due to muscular activity, this is transmitted back as an impulse by the sensory nerves to provide feedback. By this the central nervous system senses the condition of muscular contraction and regulates the muscular activity accordingly. Such muscular activity is regulated not only by the sensitivity of muscle spindles but also by other feedback mechanisms such as skin sensations and vision to make up a multifaceted self-regulation system. One of the primary characteristics of a living organism is the presence of such complex regulating mechanisms. Biological feedback mechanisms maintain organic systems and make it possible for life to exist.

If acupuncture were to be viewed in terms of the principle of feedback in cybernetics, its effects could be explained as follows. Even though the actual amount of stimulation may be quite small, acupuncture stimulation creates an afferent impulse which travels from the muscles to the central nervous system and intervenes in the biological feedback mechanism and serves to normalize its operation.

(5) Reilly Phenomenon

The Reilly phenomenon is something discovered by a group of scientists led by Dr. J. Reilly of France who investigated the reasons no animal except the human being could contract typhoid fever. Through their research and experimentation they found that the reason typhoid fever could not be caused in other animals was not due to any antibody produced by the animals but rather due to a kind of cellular response in animals which prevented the spread of the disease. They came to this conclusion because they succeeded for the first time in creating infections in other animals with the typhoid bacillus by direct inoculation of the mesenteric glands. These scientists further investigated the reason inoculation of the mesenteric glands had caused infections on the intestinal wall, and they came to the conclusion that stimulation of autonomic nerve fibers was the primary anatomical factor causing the infection to occur elsewhere.

In other words, it became clear that initially the irritation of the autonomic nerves caused reactive symptoms that were pathological changes in vasomotor properties and that eventually this functional change led to histological changes. Furthermore, it was discovered that such pathology could be produced not only by inoculation with bacilli but also by various toxins and chemicals such as nicotine, lead, nickel, and arsenic as well as by nonspecific physical stimuli such as pinching with tweezers and applying an electrical potential. It was ascertained that the reason a wide variety of pathological changes result from the reactive symptoms caused by stimulation affecting the autonomic nerves is due to differences in the amount and duration of the stimulation.

Viewed from the perspective of the Reilly phenomenon, acupuncture may be regarded as a form of therapy in which light stimulation is applied to the autonomic nerves to thus produce mild reactive symptoms. Acupuncture can therefore be viewed as a form of counter-irritation which elicits a natural response in the body that works to correct any pathological change.

3. The Mechanims of Pain and the Analgesic Effect of Acupuncture

(1) Theories on the Mechanism of Pain

Many theories have been proposed since the olden days regarding pain sensation and the physiological basis of how pain is felt. There are two theories on pain that are widely subscribed to today. One is known as the specialization theory, which holds that the receptors and nerves which transmit pain sensations are specialized structures. This theory is based purely on anatomical findings. The other theory is called the patterning theory, which holds that pain is felt when the brain detects a certain pattern, regardless of which nerves transmit the stimuli. Actually neither of these theories offer a complete explanation of the varied and complex phenomena called pain. In any case, the specialization theory, which is the more widely accepted pain theory among the two, will be explained below in some detail.

According to the specialization theory the receptors of pain are free nerve endings, and the pain impulse reaches the brain by two pathways. The first pathway is the new spinothalamic tract. When a pain impulse follows this course, first it travels along a sensory nerve to reach the spinal cord by the posterior root of the spinal nerve. The impulse then crosses over to the other side of the spinal cord and ascends the anterolateral portion of the spinal cord to go through the thalamus and reach the sensory area of the cerebral cortex. This pathway is considered to be useful in sensing the location and intensity of the pain, and it is thought to transmit mostly sharp pain sensations. The second pathway is the old spinothalamic tract. This pathway is embryologically older than the new spinothalamic tract, and it travels up the spinal cord just medial to the new spinothalamic tract. It goes through the thalamus and reaches a wider area of the cerebral cortex than does the new spinothalamic tract. This pathway is considered to transmit dull pain sensations, and also it is held to play a role in the general discomfort, emotional reactions, and the psychological aspect of pain.

Another part of the specialization theory is the differentiation of various types of nerve fibers which transmit pain. Two types of nerve fibers, A delta fibers and C fibers, are held to transmit pain sensations. Both of these fibers are relatively thin fibers among nerve fibers. The A delta fiber has a thickness of four to eight microns and conducts impulses at a fast speed of about fifty meters per second. This fiber transmits sharp pain. The C fiber has a thickness of one to three microns and its conducting speed is slow at two to four meters per second. This fiber transmits dull pain sensations. Both of these fibers, in addition to transmitting pain, transmit sensations of heat. The new spinothalamic tract is said to contain mostly A delta fibers, while the old spinothalamic tract in comparison is said to have more C fibers. If we were to bang our shin against a low table for example, we usually feel a sharp pain right at that instant and later this becomes a dull throbbing pain. It can be assumed that the initial sharp sensation is carried by A delta fibers and that the subsequent dull sensation is carried by C fibers.

(2) The Gate Control Theory

The gate control theory is a new theory regarding pain which was proposed by Dr. Ronald Melzack and Dr. Patrik Wall. According to this theory, when some painful stimulus is applied to the skin, not only do the nerve fibers for pain transmission, such as the A delta and C fibers, transmit pain but thicker nerve fibers, such as A beta fibers, which are associated with the sensation of touch, also transmit the painful stimulus. All the impulses transmitted by these nerve fibers go to the spinal cord. In the gate control theory it is suggested that there is a gate at the point where these nerve fibers enter the spinal cord. This gate opens and closes according to the situation. There is no physical structure resembling a gate which actually opens and closes. The gate is a neurochemical one, and the opening of the gate occurs when the pain sensation is enhanced at the entrance to the spinal cord and the closing occurs when the pain sensation is inhibited. When the gate is open, pain impulses are able to enter the spinal cord and reach the brain by way of the spinothalamic tract.

It is suggested in this theory that stimulation of A delta and C fibers (the thin nerve fibers which transmit pain) serves to open the gate, while stimulation of A beta fibers (the thick nerve fibers which transmit the sensation of touch) serves to close the gate. The neurochemical gate is caused to close not only by the stimulation of the thick nerve fibers originating in the skin but also by nervous impulses coming from the brain which travel down the spinal cord. This phenomenon is called descending inhibition. This phenomenon is indispensable for explaining the analgesic effects of morphine and of acupuncture.

(3) The Mechanism in the Analgesic Effect of Morphine

It is common knowledge that even small amounts of morphine have a pain killing effect, but how morphine works was a mystery until recently. Experiments such as the following were performed to study the operating mechanism of morphine.

In an experiment on cats, an electrode was implanted in the nerve cells in the posterior horn of the spinal cord, where the impulses from the sciatic nerve travel. In this way the electrical activity of these nerve cells were monitored. When painful stimulus was applied on the sciatic nerve, the electrical activity in the nerve cells naturally increased. Next the animals were given injections of morphine and the same stimulus was applied. In this case the electrical activity in the nerve cells was reduced drastically. The larger the amount of morphine injected, the greater the reduction of such electrical activity became. It was discovered, however, that severing the spinal cord above the area where the electrode was implanted brought a change in the electrical activity when painful stimulus was applied. The decrease in electrical activity occurring with injections of morphine was reduced substantially with the spinal cord severed. The conclusion drawn from this experiment was that the electrical activity of the nerve cells in the posterior horn which transmitted pain was inhibited by morphine and also that descending inhibition from the brain played a major role in this effect of morphine. This was proven because severing the descending nervous pathway from the brain drastically undermined the effect of morphine in reducing electrical activity in affected nerve cells.

Based on such experiments the effects of morphine are now considered to be a result of its inhibiting effect on the activity of nerve cells in the posterior horn which transmit pain. The mode of morphine's inhibition on these nerve cells is two fold—a direct inhibition of the nerve cells and descending inhibition. There are many neurological studies which confirm the above conclusion. It is important to get a clear grasp of the neurological mechanism of morphine in order to understand the analgesic effects of acupuncture.

(4) Morphine-like Substances in the Brain

When a specimen of the spermatic cord (vas deferens) of a guinea pig is electrically stimulated, it contracts, but when the specimen is placed in a solution of morphine and then electrically stimulated, it contracts less. It was found that placing a specimen of spermatic cord in cerebrospinal fluid extracted from the brain also caused the contraction under electrical stimulation to decrease. From this finding, it was assumed that there were substances in the brain which had similar effects as morphine, and since that time a great deal of research has been done to identify these substances. As a result enkephalins and endorphins were discovered to be the morphinelike substances in the brain and their chemical composition has been clarified. Further, scientists succeeded in synthesizing these compounds and have confirmed that injecting these into the ventricles of the brain produces an analgesic effect.

Both enkephalins and endorphins are chains of amino acids. Enkephalins are a chain of five amino acids, while endorphins are a more complex compound, beta-endorphins being a chain of thirty-one amino acids. The analgesic effect of enkephalins is short-lived compared to beta-endorphins because enkephalins are more readily broken down by enzymes. It is thought that these morphinelike substances in the brain work by binding to morphine receptors in the brain. Another factor which makes these substances similar to morphine is that the administration of naloxone, a morphine antagonist which counteracts the effects of morphine, also inhibits the effects of these substances.

(5) The Analgesic Effect Produced by Electrical Stimulation of Specific Areas of the Brain

It has been known for over a decade that electrical stimulation of the central nervous system produces an analgesic effect. This phenomenon is termed stimulation produced analgesia (SPA). The types of stimulation which produce such an effect and the neurological mechanisms involved will be discussed below in detail because SPA is closely related to the analgesic effect of acupuncture.

In 1969 Dr. D. V. Reinold reported that he succeeded in performing abdominal surgery on rats painlessly by electrical stimulation of the periaqueductal gray matter in their midbrain. Sometime later Dr. J. C. Liebeskind and his associates performed some experiments on cats and confirmed that the areas of the brain in which electrical stimulation produced an analgesic effect were in the periphery of the aqueduct of the midbrain in the vicinity of the dorsal raphe nuclei. They further verified that electrical stimulation of this area of the midbrain reduced the electrical activity in the nerve cells in the posterior horn involved in pain transmission during the application of painful stimulus.

Subsequently it was confirmed by other researchers that an analgesic effect could be produced in monkeys and human subjects by electrical stimulation. It was further found that the area of the brain in which electrical stimulation caused an analgesic effect was not limited to the periaqueductal gray matter but extended over a wide area of the gray matter from the third and fourth ventricles.

As to the mechanism of the analgesic effect produced by electrical stimulation of the central gray matter of the midbrain, it is quite clear that SPA causes descending inhibition on the nerve cells of the posterior horn which transmit pain. The relationship of SPA to increases in morphinelike substances, however, is not so clear. The results vary according to the study, and some researchers report increases while others report no increase.

Otherwise it has been reported that electrical stimulation of the dorsal raphe nuclei and the major raphe nuclei, which are lower on the brain stem compared to the central gray matter of the midbrain, also produces an analgesic effect. These nuclei have nerve fibers which extend from the central gray matter of the midbrain. The direct stimulation of these nuclei inhibits the response of nerve cells in the posterior horn to pain, which in effect is descending inhibition. The descending inhibition caused by stimulation of the central gray matter of the midbrain can also be seen as being conveyed by way of these nuclei.

In China investigators conducting SPA experiments with rabbits found that electrical stimulation on the head of the caudate nucleus also produces an analgesic effect. In this study it is also reported that there was an increase in acetylcholine and morphinelike substances in the animals' brain and that the analgesic effect was counteracted by the morphine antagonist naloxone. Currently in China, based on the above findings, SPA is applied for pain control in cancer patients.

Dr. D. Bowsher, a neurophysiologist, explains the analgesic effect produced by the electrical stimulation of certain areas of the central nervous system as well as the mechanism of descending inhibition in the following way:

Fig. 25   The Path of the Old and New Spinothalamic Tracts

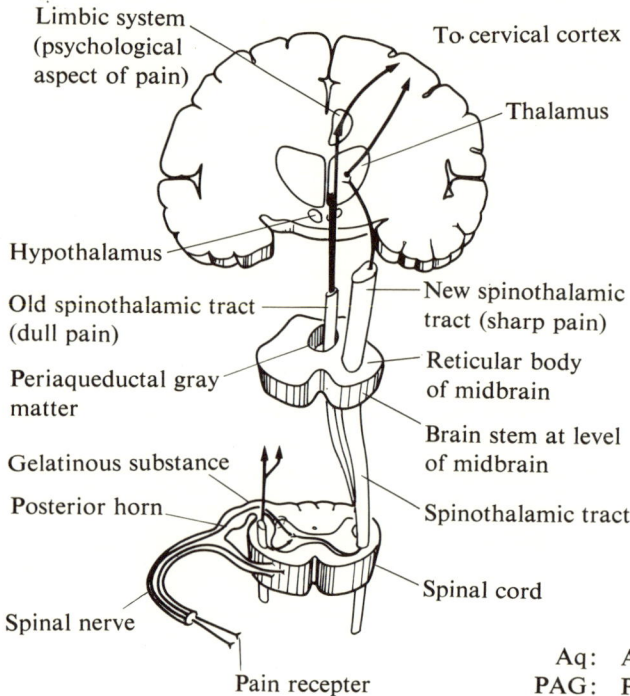

Fig. 26   Mechanism of Analgestic Effect Caused by Stimulation of the Periaqueductal Gray Matter

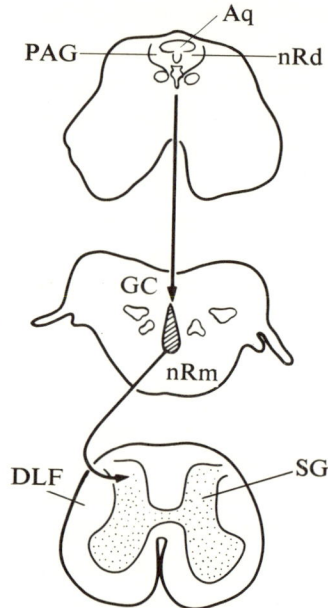

Aq: Aqueduct of midbrain
PAG: Periaqueductal gray matter
nRd: Nuclei raphe dorsalis (dorsal raphe nuclei)
GC: Giant cell
nRm: Nuclei raphe magnus (major raphe nuclei)
DLF: Dorsal longitudinal fasciculus
SG: Substantia gelatinosa (gelatinous substance)

The electrical stimulation first reaches the enkephalin neuron in the periaqueductal gray matter and next goes to the dorsal raphe nuclei. This impulse then goes to the major raphe nuclei and the giant cell in the lower brain stem, which in turn transmits the impulse via the dorsal longitudinal fasciculus to the neurons of the enkephalin receptors, which are found in the gelatinous substance of the posterior horn. This impulse acts to inhibit the activity of the nerve cells in the posterior horn which are associated with the transmission of pain.

Some of the neurotransmitters which are involved in the transmission of nervous impulses initiated by electrical stimulation of the central nervous system are enkephalin, serotonin, and noradrenalin.

(6) The Mechanism of the Analgesic Effect of Acupuncture

There are several explanations as to why acupuncture has an analgesic effect, and some of the most plausible ones are listed below.

When the area of pain and the site of needle insertion for the analgesic effect is on the same dermatome, it is possible to explain the effect by the gate control theory. It is said that acupuncture stimulation is transmitted by A beta fibers, and if this is true, it means the insertion of a needle stimulates the thick nerve fibers which acts to close the neurological gate of pain transmission. This would produce the effect of reducing sensitivity to pain in that area.

The electrical nerve block effect also accounts for some of the analgesic effect of acupuncture. It is a well-known fact in physiology that inserting a needle into a nerve trunk and applying electrical stimulation blocks the transmission of nervous impulses including that of pain. Therefore an analgesic effect can be obtained when a needle is inserted into a nerve which supplies the painful area or an area about to be operated on and electrical stimulation is applied. This principle is most often applied in surgical procedures utilizing acupuncture anesthesia.

Stimulation produced analgesia (SPA) is another phenomenon with close parallels to acupuncture analgesia. The nuclei in the central nervous system associated with SPA have just been discussed, but apparently acupuncture stimulation has an affect on some of these nuclei. It has been confirmed that inserting needles in the acupuncture points LI-4 and ST-36 on human subjects induces electrical potentials at the head of the caudate nucleus. Also it was found that among the neurons of this nucleus, those receptive to acetylcholine show the greatest electrical response with acupuncture stimulation. Another study with cats found that inserting needles in locations corresponding to LI-4 increases electrical activity in the raphe nuclei of the midbrain.

Further, an experiment was conducted to determine the exact site of the induced potentials in SPA by applying acupuncture stimulation in the ears of rabbits. Induced potentials were found to occur in localized areas of the posterior portion of the periaqueductal gray matter and in the central neuron of the thalamus as well as in the septum pellucidum (septal nuclei), cingulum, and hippocampus. These are all structures along the pathway of pain transmission leading from the periaqueductal gray matter through the medial forebrain bundle to the limbic system (the old spinothalamic tract).

These are some of the known effects of acupuncture on the nuclei associated with SPA, and from this it is obvious that there is some relationship between SPA and the analgesic effect of acupuncture. Further, many studies have shown that acupuncture causes an increase in the morphinelike substances in the brain. Also it has been shown that the analgesic effects of acupuncture are counteracted by naloxone, the morphine antagonist. In addition, since rendering a nerve block procedure above the area of acupuncture stimulation reduces the effects of acupuncture analgesia, descending inhibition seems to be a factor in much the same way as in SPA.

The neurological mechanism of pain and the reasons for the analgesic effect of acupuncture have been explained in some detail above. Nevertheless, many difficult questions remain concerning the mechanism of acupuncture analgesia. Although an overview of recent research has been presented, much remains to be explained about the effects of acupuncture. It is expected that further research will shed light on the mechanisms of acupuncture which are as of yet poorly understood.

Chapter 4
The Equipment and Techniques of Acupuncture and Moxibustion

1. The Tools of Acupuncture and Moxibustion

(1) The History of Acupuncture Needles

The use of acupuncture needles in China preceded the development of iron and steel technology. The most primitive form of acupuncture needles is recorded in Chinese classics as being the *bianshi*. These "needles" were slivers of flint stones used to drain abscesses. In primitive times needles were also fashioned out of bone and bamboo, but once metal working technology arrived, gold, silver, and bronze became the preferred materials for acupuncture needles. Recent excavations into Han Dynasty tombs has yielded fine examples of gold needles used in ancient times. The development of iron and steel technology during the Han Dynasty enabled the production of thin acupuncture needles which closely resemble those used today.

In the first chapter of the *Ling Shu*, which is part of the *Huangdi Nei Jing* (*The Yellow Emperor's Classic of Internal Medicine*), nine types of needles and their uses are described in detail. This record implies that acupuncture was traditionally prac-

Fig. 27   The Nine Traditional Needles

A—Dazhen: large needle
B—Chanqzhen: long needle
C—Haozhen: filliform needle
D—Yuanlizhen: sharp round needle
E—Pizhen: swordlike needle
F—Fengshen: three-edged needle
G—Chizhen: blunt needle
H—Yuanzhen: round-headed needle
I—Chanzhen: arrow-headed needle

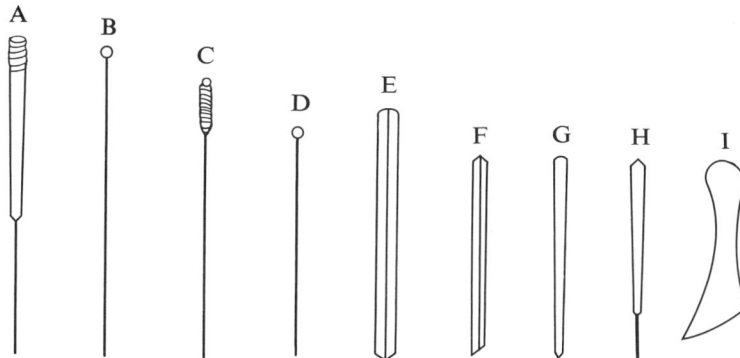

ticed with nine types of needles. Some of these "needles" more closely resemble scalpels used for surgery. Among the nine traditional needles, the *haozhen*, or filiform needle, was the most often employed in acupuncture treatments. *Hao* means hair and *zhen* means needle so *haozhen* means a hair-thin needle.

(2) Japanese Acupuncture Needles

The acupuncture needles used today can be largely classified into three types: needles for external stimulation, needles for insertion, and needles for bleeding. Needles for external stimulation are for stimulating the skin surface without puncturing, and most pediatric needles belong in this category. Needles for insertion are those used to penetrate the skin either superficially or deeply to reach underlying tissues. Needles for bleeding are those instruments used to pierce superficial veins and cause a limited amount of bleeding. Today the three-edged needle is the most widely used needle for bleeding. Needles for insertion are the type of acupuncture needle used the most often today, and among them the thinnest variety —the filiform needles—accounts for the vast majority of needles used in acupuncture. When people speak of acupuncture needles, it is almost certain that they are referring to filiform needles.

Japanese acupuncture needles originally were very similar to Chinese needles in their construction, but they underwent various modifications in the course of history to become very thin and better suited for use with insertion tubes. The

Fig. 28   The Japanese Filiform Needle

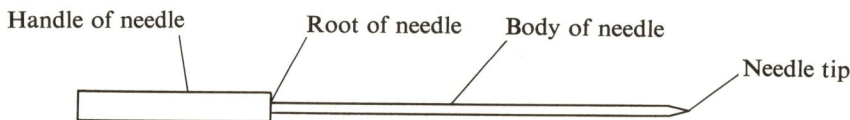

Handle of needle   Root of needle   Body of needle

Needle tip

Table 5

Thickness of Needles			Length of Needles (needle body)	
0	gauge	0.14 mm diameter	1 cun needle	30 mm
1	gauge	0.16 mm diameter	1.3 cun needle	40 mm
2	gauge	0.18 mm diameter	1.6 cun needle	50 mm
3	gauge	0.20 mm diameter	2 cun needle	60 mm
4	gauge	0.22 mm diameter	2.5 cun needle	80 mm
5	gauge	0.24 mm diameter	3 cun needle	100 mm
6	gauge	0.26 mm diameter (Chinese 32 gauge)		
7	gauge	0.28 mm diameter		
8	gauge	0.30 mm diameter		
9	gauge	0.32 mm diameter (Chinese 30 gauge)		
10	gauge	0.34 mm diameter		

needle shown in Fig. 28 is the standard Japanese filiform needle which is usually used with an insertion tube.

The standard acupuncture needle consists of a handle and the needle body. The needle tip is shaped like the end of a pine needle and is sharpened to a fine point to facilitate the insertion. The Japanese filiform needle in standard use (with an average thickness of 3 gauge) is much thinner than the Chinese variety so Japanese filiform needles are more deserving of the name "hair-thin needle." The Japanese filiform needle does come in a variety of thicknesses and lengths as shown in Table 5.

Japanese acupuncture needles are made of gold, silver, steel, imitation platinum, and stainless steel. Each material has its advantages and disadvantages as listed below. The most widely used Japanese acupuncture needles are silver needles and stainless steel needles. Silver needles are used by many acupuncturists because it provides milder stimulation. Stainless steel needles are by far the most popular because they are easier to insert and they hold up to repeated autoclaving. Furthermore stainless steel needles almost never break.

Table 6

Material	Advantages	Disadvantages
Gold	soft and pliant minimal damage to tissue does not corrode	expensive breakage possible hard to insert
Silver	soft and pliant minimal damage to tissue relatively inexpensive	corrodes to dark color breakage possible hard to insert
Steel	easy to insert inexpensive	corrodes easily breakage possible easier to damage tissue
Imitation platinum	easy to insert very little corrosion inexpensive	easier to damage tissue breakage possible
Stainless steel	easy to insert breakage rare does not corrode	easier to damage tissue

(3) Insertion Tubes

Insertion tubes are used to insert thin Japanese needles. Insertion tubes make it easier to insert needles painlessly. The vast majority of acupuncturists in Japan use insertion tubes to insert filiform needles since insertion tubes enable a quick and smooth beginning to needle insertion. The length of the insertion tube is three to five millimeters shorter than the total length of the needle (handle and body of

Fig. 29   Various Insertion Tubes

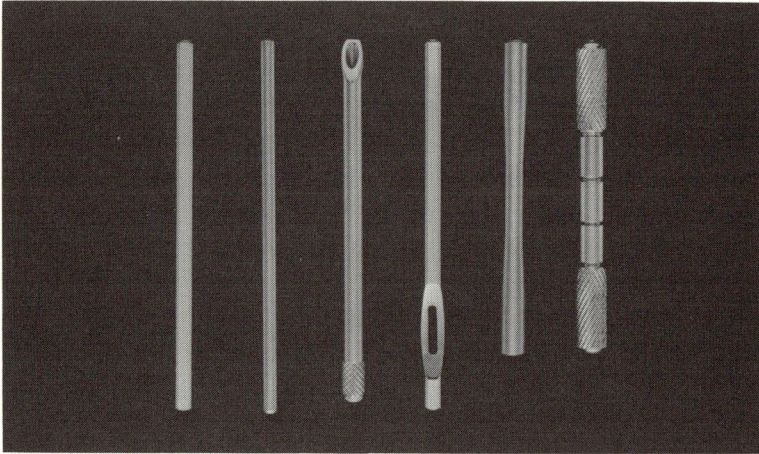

needle). Insertion tubes come in a variety of sizes and shapes, but the common cross-sectional shapes are round, hexagonal, and octagonal (Fig. 29). Insertion tubes are made of either chrome plated brass or stainless steel.

(4) The Production of Moxa and Its Qualities

Moxibustion is the application of heat stimulation by the combustion of moxa on or near the skin. Moxa is a refined product of the leaves of the Chinese wormwood plant (*Artemesia vulgaris*). To produce moxa the mature wormwood plant is cut and dried in the sun. Next all the thick stems are removed and the plant is stored for several months to a year. After that the plant is thoroughly dried in an oven at a low temperature. Then it is shredded and placed in sifters to remove all the unnecessary matter to yield a soft downy material with a light yellow color.

   Moxa is produced in several qualities from fine to coarse, and generally it is divided into two categories of use. The fine or high quality moxa is used for direct moxibustion; the coarse or low quality moxa is used for indirect moxibustion. The combustion temperature of high quality moxa is lower than that of low

Table 7:   Features of High Quality Moxa and Low Quality Moxa

	High Quality	*Low Quality*
Age	old	new
Texture	soft	hard
Fibers	thin and long	thick and coarse
Impurities	none	some remaining
Color	light yellow	grayish brown
Moisture	low	high
Combustion	fast	slow
Stimulation	small	large

quality moxa. Also the temperature gradient of high quality moxa during combustion is said to describe a sine curve, and this gradient is held to be most suitable for direct heat stimulation on the skin. The coarse moxa used for indirect moxibustion burns hotter than fine moxa, and even though it may sometimes be used directly on the skin, it is removed as soon as the heat becomes too much to bear. The low quality moxa is usually applied over some heat buffer or is otherwise held a short distance from the skin. Some practitioners, in applying direct moxibustion, use fine moxa with lower combustion temperatures for reinforcing deficiencies (tonification) and use coarse moxa for dispersing excesses (dispersion).

2. Basic Skills of Acupuncture

(1) Needle Insertion

There are basically two methods of inserting the Japanese filiform needle: the direct insertion technique and the insertion tube technique. These techniques will each be explained briefly below.

Direct Insertion Technique
This method of needle insertion is widely used in China, but it is seldom used when inserting the thinner Japanese filiform needles. Japanese needles are sometimes inserted without a tube when needling very superficially and repeatedly. Direct insertion is a useful technique, but it can cause pain during the initial stages of insertion unless a practitioner is quite skilled. To insert a needle directly without an insertion tube, first firmly hold the needle in the right hand with the thumb and

Fig. 30 Direct Insertion Technique

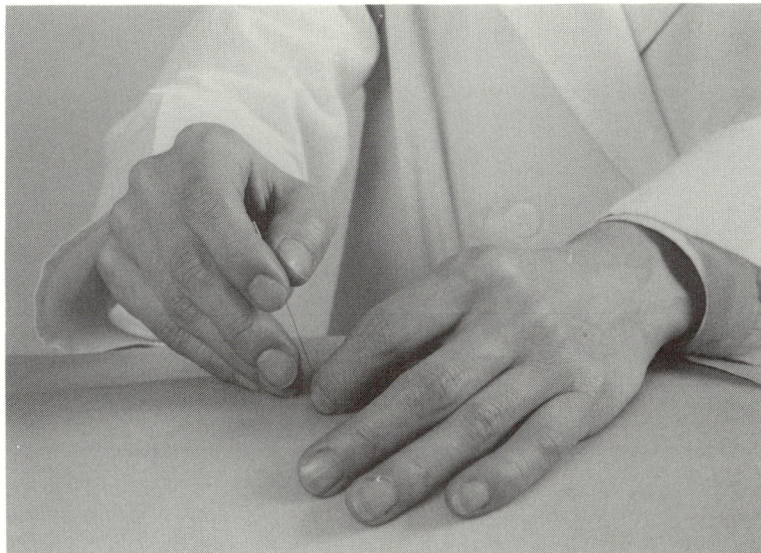

index finger so that both the handle and the needle body are held (Fig. 30). Place the thumb and index finger of the left hand on either side of the point to be inserted and part the skin to create slight tension in the skin between the two fingers. Then gently bring the needle tip up to the skin and swiftly push it through the skin. Continue pushing the needle in slowly to the desired depth and use the left hand to feel for any change in the surrounding tissue. After applying the appropriate needle stimulation, slowly withdraw the needle until the tip is just beneath the skin and then remove it swiftly.

Insertion Tube Technique

The insertion tube was invented to simplify needle insertion and to reduce the pain upon insertion. This method is the most widely used in Japan and it is the easiest way to insert thin Japanese needles. One disadvantage of this method is that the use of insertion tubes complicates sterilization and clean needle practices.

The first step in using an insertion tube is to put the needle into the tube. That is, to load the tube. There are essentially two ways to load an insertion tube. One is the two-handed loading method and the other is the one-handed loading method. In the two-handed loading method the insertion tube is held in the left hand and the needle, in the right, and the needle handle is put into the top end of the tube to load the tube (Fig. 31). This loading method takes more time than the one-handed loading method and it appears less professional. In the one-handed loading method the tube is held with the middle, ring, and little fingers of the dominant hand, and the needle handle is held between the thumb and index fingers (Fig. 32). Then the top end of the tube is moved up toward the end of the needle handle and the needle is dropped into the tube and is stopped by the palm (Fig. 33). After this the tube is turned over with the thumb and the index and middle fingers and the needle is held to keep it from falling out of the tube. The needle is held in the tube by making the handle of the needle stick out about 5 millimeters from the end of the tube and using the index finger to press the handle against the tube as it is turned around. The one-handed loading method is a quick way to

| Fig. 31 | Fig. 32 | Fig. 33 |

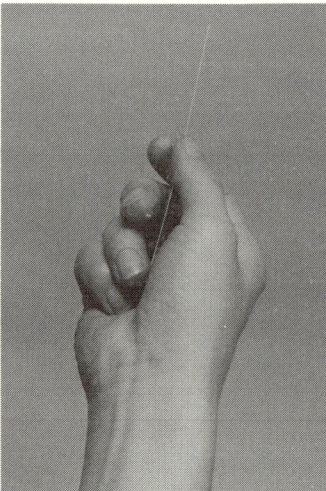 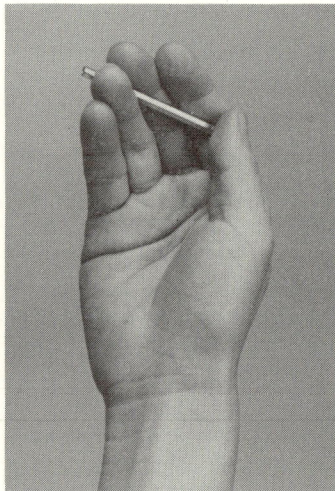 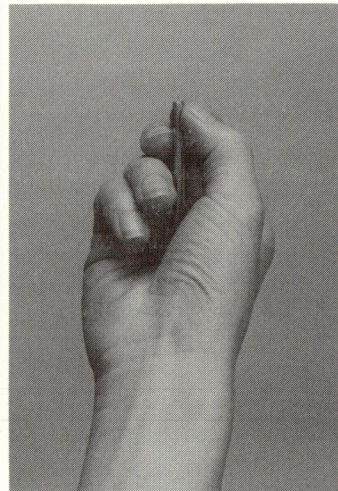

Fig. 34

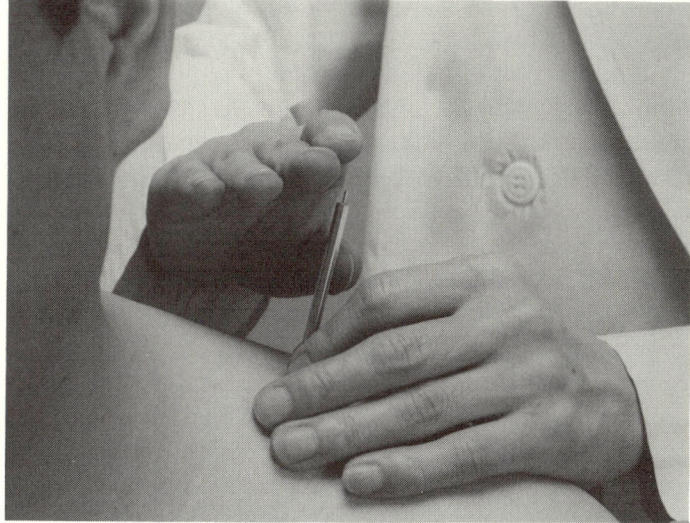

load a tube, and it is the preferred method of professionals. This is because the one-handed method frees the left hand to locate acupuncture points and speeds up the process of needle insertion.

Once the insertion tube is loaded with the right-sized needle, the needle is ready to be inserted. Hold the tips of the left thumb and index finger together and place them over the acupuncture point to be needled. Next put the tube between these fingers. Then lightly tap on the exposed head of the needle a few times using the right index finger (Fig. 34). Tap the head of the needle with a little more force until it becomes flush with the tube. This first stage of insertion is called "tapping in." If there is pain with the first tap, it is best to adjust one's hold on the tube slightly before proceeding. After the skin has been penetrated by tapping in, the thumb and index finger of the left hand are kept in place to hold the needle up as the tube is lifted off the needle with the right hand. The tube is normally held in the ring and little fingers of the right hand while the thumb and index finger take hold of the handle of the needle to continue inserting the needle to the desired depth.

Essential Points for Skillful Needle Insertion

Many fine details of basic needle insertion technique have been defined and emphasized in traditional Japanese acupuncture since the development of the insertion tube. Among the many aspects of basic needling technique, there are some important requirements for point manipulation, the supporting hand, and the needling hand. Only the most essential points which relate to these aspects of basic needle insertion will be presented here. These fundamental principles of needle insertion need to be understood and practiced repeatedly in order to use Japanese acupuncture needles skillfully and effectively.

Point manipulation refers to the stroking and massaging of the acupuncture point before and after the insertion of the needle. Aside from the initial probing to locate the acupuncture point, before the needle is inserted, additional stimulation is provided. Usually the tip of the thumb, index finger, or middle finger of the supporting hand is used to stroke, press, or massage in a circular motion. Such manipulation improves circulation around the point and increases the effect of needle stimulation. Also this manipulation serves to desensitize the skin and reduce the pain during insertion. After the needle is removed the acupuncture point is often massaged or pressed with the supporting hand to "close the point." Massaging a point after needling serves several purposes. It calms down any sensory nerve endings which were excited during the needling, it alleviates any residual needle sensation which may remain, and it facilitates the reabsorption of any bleeding in the tissues caused by the penetration of small blood vessels.

The supporting hand is the hand which supports the skin surrounding the point of insertion. It refers to the left hand for those who are right-handed. Generally, when inserting Japanese needles, the tips of the thumb and index finger of the supporting hand are held together over the point to support the needle body during insertion and withdrawal. There are several ways to hold the needle with the fingers of the supporting hand. The most common way is called the half-moon hold and in this method the thumb and index fingers form a semicircle (Fig. 35).

Fig. 35   Half-moon Hold   **Fig 36   Full-moon Hold**

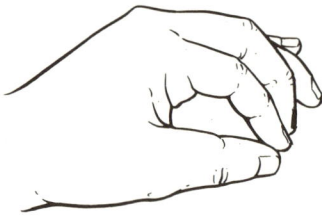

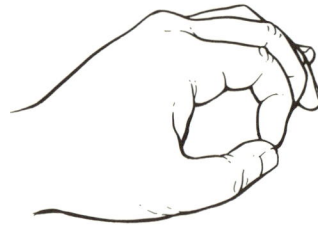

Another common way is called the full-moon hold and in this method the thumb and either the index or middle finger are used to form a circle (Fig. 36). The hold employed largely depends on the part of the body being needled because the supporting hand must conform to the skin surface. The skillful use of the supporting hand is very important for many reasons. It is used to reduce the sensitivity of the skin before insertion, to assist in the process of insertion, to prevent the body part from being moved during needling, and to feel the patient's response to the needle stimulation. Some classical texts even emphasize the skillful use of the supporting hand as being more important than that of the needling hand.

The needling hand is the active hand that inserts and withdraws the needle. The needling hand is the dominant hand, or the right hand for right-handed people. To insert Japanese needles the thumb and index finger of the needling hand need to hold both the handle and body of the needle. Furthermore, the hand and forearm have to be in line with the needle so that the whole arm can be employed in needling. The insertion and manipulation of the needle with the needling hand is the key technique in acupuncture, which can make or break a treatment. For this reason the practitioner must concentrate fully to sense the patient's response. Relaxation and gentleness are the key in providing just the right amount of stimulation. The proper way for the practitioner to concentrate while performing acupuncture is described as follows in the ninth chapter of the *Ling Shu*: "While needling a point, one must remain poised in calmness and quiet to seek the movement of (the patient's) spirit. The doors and windows must be closed to shut out all distractions and one's attention should be totally focused. One should pay no attention to other voices and must concentrate wholly on the needle." This passage teaches that an acupuncturist must avoid all distractions during needling to concentrate fully on the needle so that he can sense and respond appropriately to the changes taking place.

The following basic rules must be observed to render a skillful acupuncture treatment and to achieve the best results:

1. Relax the arms from the shoulders down and allow your strength to issue from your lower abdomen.
2. Rather than thinking of willfully inserting and withdrawing the needle, just let the needling proceed naturally.
3. Set aside the notion of using a physical object, the needle, and penetrate with the feeling that your fingers are actually reaching into the body.
4. Never force the needle in farther when you encounter firm resistance during insertion.
5. If there is pain or resistance when inserting a needle, withdraw it slightly and adjust the angle or withdraw it completely.
6. Avoid forceful or rough handling of the needle during insertion and withdrawal.
7. Do not needle while carrying on a conversation or when there are other distractions.

(2) Needle Manipulation Techniques

A great variety of techniques for manipulating the needle after it is inserted has been developed through the centuries to produce certain effects. Although there are many approaches and variations in needle manipulation techniques, the techniques listed below are the most representative and widely used techniques in Japan today. A practitioner must learn each one of these needle manipulation techniques individually and then master appropriate combinations and variations of these to become capable of rendering the appropriate needle stimulation in each case.

Simple Insertion and Withdrawal
In this most basic needling technique, the needle is inserted to a certain depth without any other manipulation and then withdrawn immediately (Fig. 37). The amount of stimulation is very mild so this technique is often employed for patients who are hypersensitive.

Twisting and Rotating
Twisting the needle is a very common technique employed during insertion and withdrawal of the needle (Fig. 38). Twisting the needle slightly back and forth

Fig. 37   Fig. 38   Fig. 39   Fig. 40

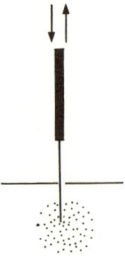   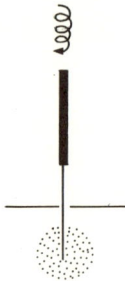   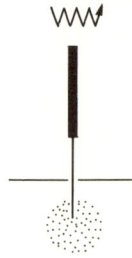   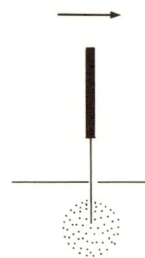

Fig. 41   Fig. 42   Fig. 43

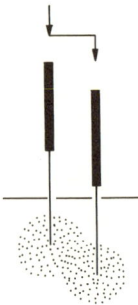   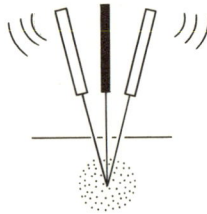   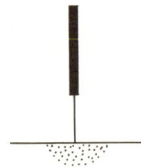

serves to facilitate the vertical movement of the needle. Rotating the needle means to turn the needle around more than 360 degrees. The amount of stimulation in twisting and rotating ranges from mild to fairly strong, depending on the degree of rotation and the depth of the needle.

Lifting and Thrusting

This is a common technique in which the needle, after having been inserted to the appropriate depth, is moved vertically in and out (Fig. 39). This is traditionally referred to as "sparrow pecking" since the movement of the hand resembles a sparrow's head pecking at food. Lifting and thrusting tends to be relatively strong stimulation, but the amount of stimulation depends on the amplitude and speed of the lifting and thrusting movement.

Retaining the Needle

This is a commonly used technique in which the needle is left in place for a certain amount of time after inserting it to a certain depth (Fig. 40). The amount of time for retaining the needle is between five and thirty minutes. Often the skin around the needle will gradually turn red (an area one to three centimeters across). The needling sensation while retaining Japanese needles is usually very mild if felt at all.

Intermittent Insertion

In this needling technique the needle is inserted in stages (Fig. 41). Initially the needle is inserted only a half to a third of the desired depth, after which it is held for a few breaths, and then the next half or third is needled. The amount of stimulation in intermittent needling is mild and this technique is used when extra caution is necessary during needle insertion.

Vibration

This is a technique in which the handle of the needle is flicked or hit after the needle is inserted to the desired depth (Fig. 42). There are a variety of ways in which to produce vibration, from the very subtle vibration of scraping the ridges on the handle to the strong vibration of hitting the handle with the insertion tube. This technique is generally stimulating and is most appropriate for numb and insensitive areas. Traditionally this technique was called the "ki collecting technique" and was used to stimulate areas of hypofunction.

Contact Needling

In contact needling instead of inserting the needle, the tip is gently held against the skin to stimulate a point (Fig. 43). This technique is very useful for applying extremely mild and subtle stimulation. Contact needling is used with brushing and stroking techniques in pediatric acupuncture. For adults this technique is reserved for very sensitive points and patients.

(3) Angle and Depth of Insertion

Regardless of how accurately an acupuncture point is located and how skillfully the needle is manipulated, if the angle, direction, and depth of insertion is wrong, the desired effect cannot be obtained. The rule of thumb for deciding the angle of insertion is vertical insertion for muscular or fleshy parts, oblique insertion for curved parts or places close to bone, and horizontal insertion over bony surfaces (Figs. 44–46).

Fig. 44 Vertical Insertion

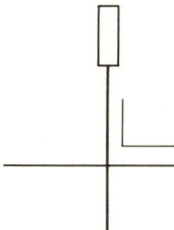

Fig. 45 Oblique Insertion

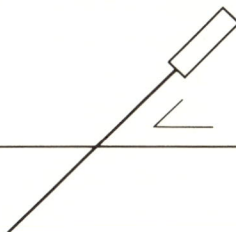

Fig. 46 Horizontal Insertion

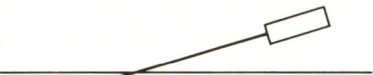

The proper direction of insertion largely depends on the anatomical features underlying the point and tends to follow the lay of the tissue. The depth of insertion generally depends on the part of the body being needled. For example, the proper depth is usually around 25 millimeters for the upper back and 35 millimeters for the lower back. The right depth, however, cannot be stated precisely for every case since this varies according to the patient and the exact depth of the reaction. The needle must reach the tissue that is the site of the cutaneous reaction. Therefore when the reaction is superficial, the point must be needled shallowly; when it is deep, the point must be needled deeply.

Fig. 47   Average Depth of Insertion

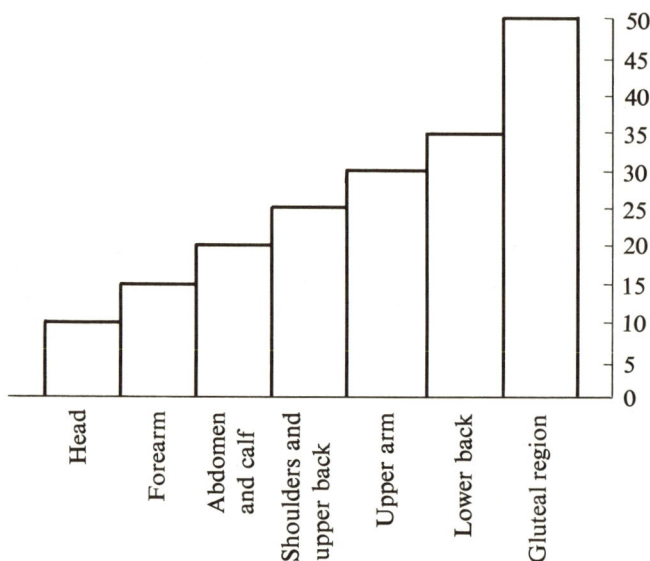

3. The Basic Skills of Moxibustion

(1) Scarring and Non-scarring Moxibustion

In Japan the most commonly applied form of moxibustion both by health professionals as part of acupuncture treatments and by the general public for home remedies is the scarring moxibustion called *tōnetsu-kyū* (penetrating moxibustion). In this form of moxibustion, minuscule cones of high quality moxa are burned consecutively on the skin three or more times depending on what is appropriate for the patient. Even though penetrating moxibustion is a type of scarring moxibustion and it often causes a blister, the skin area burned is usually so small that a scar does not form. Although applied much less often, the other forms of scarring moxibustion practiced in Japan are *shōshaku-kyū* (cautery moxibustion) and *dano-kyū* (suppurative moxibustion). Cautery moxibustion is the burning of moxa directly on the skin for the purpose of burning off unwanted tissue such as warts and corns, and typically many cones of a fairly large size are burned consecutively. Suppurative moxibustion is the burning of one to three large cones (with bases of up to 1 cm in diameter). The purpose is to raise a large blister and cause a localized infection. The subsequent draining of puss removes toxins from the body and the small infection stimulates the immune system.

Fig. 48　Indirect Moxibustion

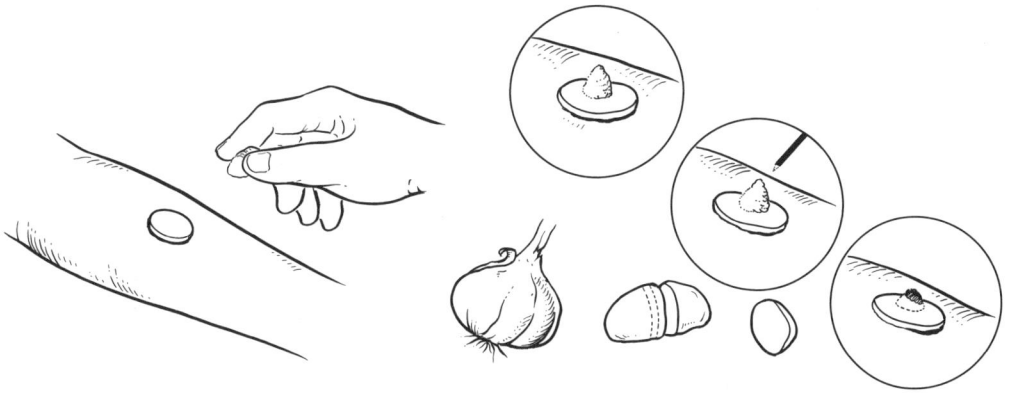

Non-scarring moxibustion is also known as indirect moxibustion and, rather than burning the moxa directly on the skin, something is placed between the skin and moxa to shield the heat (Fig. 48). Some commonly applied heat buffers for moxa in Japan are slices of ginger, garlic, onion, leeks, miso, and pieces of gauze saturated in a salt solution. These substances not only reduce the heat of the moxa to create a milder and more tonifying thermal stimulation but also have some additional effects due to skin osmosis. Another popular form of non-scarring moxibustion is *on-kyū* (warming moxibustion), in which a burning moxa (usually low quality moxa) is held close to the skin to heat certain areas. Moxa sticks are the most widely applied form of warming moxibustion. In recent years many moxa stick holders and other devices have been developed in Japan to simplify the application of warming moxibustion. Another commonly applied form of non-scarring moxibustion, which is actually a type of direct moxibustion, is *chinetsu-kyū* (heat sensing moxibustion). In this method, a very large cone of moxa is burned directly on the skin and removed as soon as the heat is felt. Generally a pair of tweezers or chopsticks are used to remove the burning cone, but some people just quickly remove it with their fingers. This form of moxibustion is applied consecutively on the same point up to five times. This is a very popular method because it is not painful and does not cause a burn.

(2) Application of Penetrating Moxibustion

First the proper moxa material and incense must be obtained. Penetrating moxibustion requires high quality moxa and the incense must be a type which does not break too easily. After selecting the points to be treated by moxibustion, take a small amount of moxa (no larger than the end of the thumb) and roll it between

Fig. 49

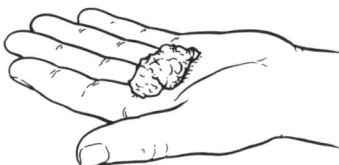

Fig. 50

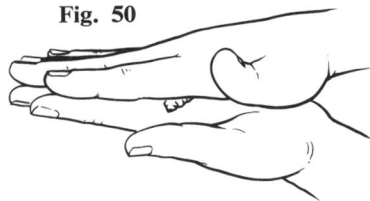

Fig. 51

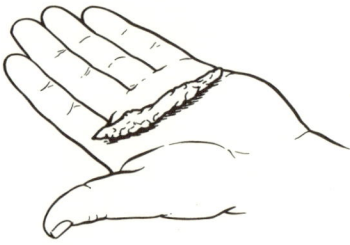

Fig. 52

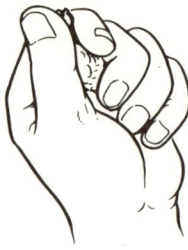

Fig. 53

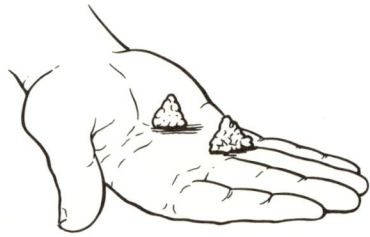

both hands to form a long circular piece (Figs. 49–51). Then lightly role tne ena of this piece of moxa back and forth between the thumb and index finger so that its diameter becomes less than five millimeters. After forming a thin string of moxa, take small pieces off the end to create tiny cones the size of a rice grain (Figs. 52 and 53). The cone must be well formed and of an even consistency. Do not apply cones which are poorly formed because they tend to burn incompletely or cause unnecessary burns.

After forming the cone, place it on the desired point. When the practitioner's hand is moist, the moxa will adhere to the fingers and make it difficult to place the cone on the point. In this case, rubbing some ashes from the incense between the thumb and index finger will make it easier. Also the moxa cone can be made to stand up much easier when the area is moistened with water or alcohol before placing the cone. Any ash on the tip of the incense must be knocked off before using it to ignite the moxa (Fig. 54). Light the moxa cone by bringing the burning tip of the incense just next to the top of the moxa cone (Fig. 55). Rotating the incense stick back and forth with the thumb and index finger while lighting the moxa cone will keep the cone from sticking to the burning tip of the incense stick (Fig. 56). If the moxa cone falls over or lifts off the skin after being lit, remove it immediately and try again with a new cone.

Fig. 54

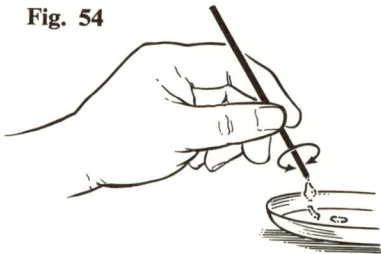

Fig. 56

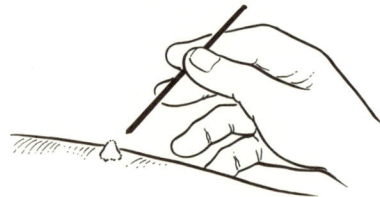

Fig. 55

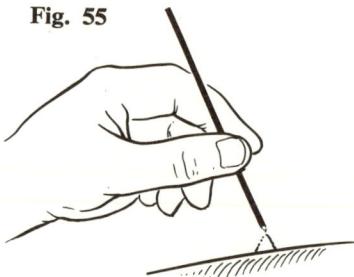

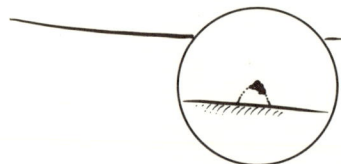

To offset the burning sensation of direct moxibustion, it is useful to press the skin on either side of the moxa cone as it burns. When holding the incense stick in the right hand, the tips of the left index and middle fingers can be used to press the skin on either side of the burning cone. Doing this serves to raise the base of the moxa cone slightly off the skin and moderates the heat stimulation, reduces the sensation of heat, and prevents burns. After the moxa cone is finished burning, either remove the ash and put another cone in its place or put another cone directly on top of the ash. Be careful to place additional moxa cones in the exact same point, or else the burn can become unnecessarily large. After applying the appropriate number of cones on each point, clean the area with cotton swabs soaked in alcohol.

4. Diagnosis for Acupuncture and Moxibustion Treatments

In traditional Chinese medicine there are four methods of examination: looking, listening, questioning, and touching. In the looking examination, the patient's complexion, tongue, body type, and posture, as well as mental disposition are studied. In the listening examination the smell of the patient as well as his voice and respiratory rhythm are noted. In questioning all matters relevant to the patient's condition are asked. In the touching examination the patient's pulse is taken and his body is closely inspected from the surface. All the information obtained from the four examinations is considered as a whole to decide the treatment pattern.

In Japanese acupuncture the information obtained from the touching examination is the primary basis for deciding the treatment strategy. A detailed examination of the patient by touch is what enables Japanese practitioners to determine the appropriate treatment for each patient. Since touching, or the palpatory examination, is the greatest factor in diagnosis in Japanese acupuncture, this technique will be given the primary emphasis in this book. The detailed explanation of the other traditional examinations will be left to other texts of Chinese medicine.

(1) Detecting Reactions in the Skin and Superficial Tissue (Locating Acupuncture Points)

The touching examination most useful in the clinical practice of acupuncture is palpation of the skin surface to detect abnormalities and to determine which meridian and acupuncture points are indicated for treatment. What are the abnormalities, or reactions, that occur in relation to the meridians? To answer this question, the most common types of reactions in the skin and superficial tissue will be described.

Fig. 57   Tender Point

Point painful or tender when pressed

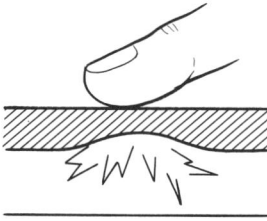

Fig. 58   Induration

Hard or knotted area

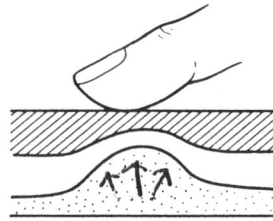

Tender Points (pressure points)

Tender points are places where a subjective sensation of tenderness or pain is felt by the patient when pressed. In many cases the points with underlying hardness, or indurations, are also tender. The amount of pressure required to produce a reaction of tenderness varies, but generally firm pressure with the thumb is sufficient.

Indurations

Indurations are localized areas of tension and hardness palpated in the skin, subcutaneous tissues, and muscles. The size and shape of the induration, or fibro-cytic nodule, in the soft tissue varies greatly. There are rounded indurations from the size of a rice grain to a marble, and also indurations can appear as a tight band of tension.

Fig. 59   Depression

Depressed and hollow areas

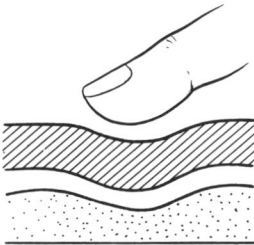

Fig. 60   Superficial Tension

Tense or tight areas at the skin surface

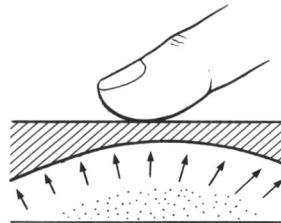

Depressions

Depressions are detected by stroking lightly over the skin surface. They are palpated as areas where the resilience of the skin and subcutaneous tissues is less than surrounding areas. The size of depressions vary from small areas no bigger than the tip of the little finger to areas greater than the ball of the thumb. In some cases depressions appear across a larger area to form a furrow or groove. Depressions are generally regarded as a sign of a deficiency and are a reaction characteristic of chronic cases.

Superficial Tension

Areas of superficial tension are detected by stroking lightly over the skin surface. Superficial tension is palpated as tight areas which offer more resistance to stroking and pressing than other areas. Superficial tension is generally regarded to be a sign of an excess and is a reaction characteristic of acute cases.

Pigmentation (freckles and blemishes)
The points or areas with pigmentation often correspond to the affected meridians. The color varies from black, brown, and gray, to white (lack of pigmentation is also significant). In some cases pigmented points are used directly for treatment.

Paresthesia (hyperesthesia and hypesthesia)
Paresthesia occurs either as hyperesthesia (excessive sensitivity) or as hypesthesia (reduction in sensitivity). Hyperesthetic areas on the skin are painful to the slightest touch, and hyperesthesia can occur across a large area as generalized hypersensitivity or in localized areas as hypersensitive points. Areas with hypesthesia, on the other hand, are insensitive to touch and sometimes there is a sensation of numbness. When the area of hypesthesia on the skin is large, several points with the least sensitivity or greatest numbness must be selected for treatment.

Abnormal Temperature (coolness and hotness)
Areas of abnormal coolness or hotness can sometimes be detected when stroking lightly over the skin surface. Such areas are used for treatment especially when they are also tender or have underlying tension or indurations.

Abnormal Moisture Level (dryness and dampness)
Abnormal moisture can be palpated as dryness or dampness when lightly touching or stroking the skin. The skin tends to feel rough when it is dry, and it tends to feel moist and sticky when it has abnormal moisture. Abnormal moisture levels often appear over a wide area along the affected meridians. In this case a limited number of points lying within this area which are tender or indurated must be selected for treatment.

(2) Standard Procedure for Palpatory Examination

To begin the palpatory examination, have the patient sit down on the end of the treatment table and observe the lateral aspect of the patient's neck from the back. Then start palpating for tension and abnormalities on the lateral aspect of the neck, especially around the sternocleidomastoid muscles on the right and left sides. A substantial number of people show a discrepancy in muscle tone between the sternocleidomastoid muscles on either side. Although this imbalance could be regarded as a habitual condition, it can be observed that many more or less healthy individuals have a slight tendency toward torticollis.

After palpating the lateral aspect of the neck, grasp the top of the patient's shoulders (suprascapular area) from behind on both sides to see if there is a difference in the size and consistency of the muscles. A difference between the muscles on the right and left sides is in many cases just an occupational or habitual condition, but in some cases it can be related to a pathological condition. There is a distinct possibility of scoliosis when the muscles are thick and hard on one side while being thin and soft on the other.

The next step is to palpate the spine from top to bottom. First locate the spinous process of the fourth cervical vertebra and place your hand over the spine so that ball of the middle finger comes directly over this spinous process. Move your hand straight down to palpate the spinous processes of the thoracic and lumbar vertebrae. Note any protrusions or indentations and any irregularities in the spacing between the spinous processes. Repeat the same procedure of sliding the fingers over the spinous processes, but this time keep the fingers pointing down toward the patient's feet. (Instead of dragging the fingers, lightly push them down over the spine.) To do this, you have to change your position to stand next to the patient and face the opposite direction so that your hand can be placed upside down over the patient's spine with the middle finger over the spinous process of the upper thoracic vertebra. Face down slightly to slide the middle finger over the spinous processes down to the fifth lumbar vertebra. This method of palpating the spine makes it easier to detect abnormal alignment of the spine.

After examining the spine, stroke and press the patient's back to examine the condition of the muscles adjacent to the spine as well as the latissimus dorsi muscles. Determine if there are any abnormally tense areas or tender points and mark the location of these reactions. Palpation of the musculature on the back completes the examination in the seated position.

Have the patient assume prone position, lying with his body as straight as possible from head to toe. The patient should face straight down by bringing his arms up by his head and placing his hands under his forehead with the palms facing down. The practitioner starts palpating by stroking down the spine from the upper cervical vertebrae to the sacrum, using three fingers (the index, middle, and ring fingers). The middle finger must be directly over the spinous process as the fingers slide over the spine. Confirm and mark the spinous processes which are out of alignment. Then go down the spine, lightly striking the spinous process of each vertebra with a percussion hammer to see if this causes pain. When a vertebra is out of alignment or it is painful when struck, invariably there is a thin band of tension in the costotransverse ligament on one or both sides of the vertebra.

Next use the index or middle fingers of both hands to palpate the groove on both sides of the spine (the medial margin of the erector spinae muscles) from the upper cervical vertebrae down to the sacrum. Repeat the same procedure and palpate from the neck down to the hips, going over the highest part of the erector spinae and then over the lateral margin of the erector spinae. As the final step of palpating the back, the back is thoroughly inspected by dividing it into three areas. The first area is the interscapular area from the level of the second to the sixth thoracic vertebra, the second area is the lower thoracic area from the level of the seventh to the twelfth thoracic vertebra, and the third area is the lumbar area from the level of the first to the fifth lumbar vertebra. Stroke and press the skin on both sides of the spine at the same time to see if there is any difference. Note any abnormal reactions such as excessive tension, indurations, lack of muscle tone, and depressions. Where there are abnormal reactions, see if the location corresponds to back *shu* points. Also check which spinal dermatome and which sympathetic dermatome the reactive points are associated with. The palpatory examination in the prone position is complete when the upper, middle, and lower portions of the back have been thoroughly inspected.

Have the patient assume the supine position with his body as straight and relaxed as possible. Both arms should be at the patient's side and his mouth should be relaxed and slightly open. The practitioner should stand on the right side of the patient. Begin by palpating the sternocleidomastoid muscle on both sides of the neck once more and confirm any abnormal reactions. Next use the ball of the index or middle finger to feel along the superior border of the clavicle (the supraclavicular fossa). Then palpate along the inferior border of the clavicle from the sternum out to the lateral head of the clavicle. The area above and below the clavicle needs to be inspected closely since reactions often appear in this area as tenderness or induration by the visceromotor reflex or the vascular reflex and also there is a reduction in electrical resistivity due to the viscero-autonomic reflex.

Next palpate down the sternum from the manubrium to the inferior border of the sternal body. Careful attention should be paid here because quite often a reaction can be found in the middle of the sternum. After this palpate the intercostal spaces from the first to the twelfth, working laterally from the sternum. Place the tips of the index, middle, and ring fingers in the same intercostal spaces on both sides and compare the difference. The three fingers are employed side by side to palpate the first five intercostal spaces, but from the sixth intercostal space on down, the three fingers can be placed in three different intercostal spaces to palpate three lines at once. Reactions tend to appear most frequently in the spinal dermatomes from C_3 to C_5 and from T_1 to T_5.

Palpation of the thorax is followed by the examination of the abdomen. In Western medicine the examination of the abdomen is usually done with the patient's knees bent, but in Oriental medicine the patient's knees are kept straight. Bending the knees up is useful for relaxing the abdominal wall, but doing this also makes it harder to locate abnormal reactions on the abdominal wall. Start the examination of the abdomen by checking the amount of tension in the epigastrium. Many patients with chronic problems have great tension and tightness in this area. Next examine the median line from the xiphoid process to the navel. This line corresponds to the linea alba in Western medicine and to the conception vessel in Oriental medicine. Place four fingers side by side and press successively down this line. When there are abnormally soft or hard areas, note which conception vessel points they correspond to. After this, palpate the hypochondriac regions on the right and left sides from the epigastrium out to the tip of the twelfth rib. First palpate the right side and then the left, and after that palpate both sides together to compare each side. Then palpate down the rectus abdominis muscles on both sides from the epigastrium to the level of the navel. Begin by pressing down the medial sides of the muscles with the tips of the three fingers and then check the lateral sides. Next palpate the obliquus abdominis muscles in the flank region in the same manner, comparing the right and left sides. Follow this by palpating the median line (conception vessel) from just below the navel to the pubic symphysis. Then palpate the waistline from both sides of the navel to the flank region. The waistline roughly corresponds to the *dai* vessel (one of the eight extra meridians). Next examine the hypogastric region by palpating the medial and lateral sides of the rectus abdominis muscles as well as the obliquus abdominis muscles in the same way as above. When there is strong tension or tenderness on the left side of the lower abdomen, this is traditionally associated with blood stagnation (a source of gynecological problems). Finish the examination of the abdomen by palpating the inguinal regions on the right and left sides to check for abnormal tension or tenderness.

(3) Deciding the Treatment Based on Palpatory Findings

After completing the palpatory examination detailed above, compare the reactive points on the back with those on the chest and abdomen. Reactive points on the anterior aspect and those on the posterior aspect can be compared directly by having the patient lie on his side. It is useful to mark the most tender or hard points with a soft pencil or a small piece of tape. After finding corresponding reactive points on the upper back and chest and on the lower back and abdomen, determine which type of reflex produced these reactions (e.g., visceromotor, viscerosensory, or visceroautonomic). In some cases reactions appear in relation to the spinal and sympathetic dermatomes as discussed in Chapter 3. In other cases reactions appear in relation to the front *mu* and back *shu* points of the traditional meridian system. At times the reactive points appear in an erratic manner which does not correlate to either system.

If the reactive points on the anterior aspect and those on the posterior aspect largely correspond to either the spinal or sympathetic dermatomes, it can be determined which organ dysfunction is most likely. If the reactive points correspond to the *mu* or *shu* points, the principle of meridians can be applied and points along the related meridians can be palpated on both sides of the body to seek related reactive points. In the author's experience, the viscerocutaneous reactive points much more often correspond to *mu* and *shu* points than they relate to the same dermatomes.

The leg and the arms as well as the neck and head must be inspected closely to locate other reactive points along the meridians showing the greatest reaction. Once all the possible related areas have been examined and distal reactive points have been located, the acupuncture, moxibustion, and massage treatment can be started. Since it is not practical or wise to treat all the reactive points with acupuncture and moxibustion, select ten to fifteen points for treatment which are the most related to the problem or symptoms by traditional and anatomical correlations. The other reactive points can be massaged or treated more generally by the application of heat. The effect of a treatment is usually better when a selective approach is used in treating points. Treating the main reactive points usually has a positive effect on the body as a whole so that the lesser reactive points are normalized without specific treatment. The selection of points for treatment is a subjective process which very much depends on the practitioner's experience and skill in locating the most effective treatment points.

5. Tonification and Dispersion Techniques in Acupuncture and Moxibustion

The *Su Wen*, the oldest classic of acupuncture and moxibustion, states one must "disperse where there is an excess and tonify where there is a deficiency." Tonification and dispersion are fundamental concepts in Oriental medicine and it is essential to have a basic understanding of these to practice acupuncture.

Traditionally tonification means to aid, reinforce, and make complete, while dispersion means to take, reduce, or control. Therefore where there are deficiences in *ki* and *ketsu*, a tonifying treatment is given, and where there are excesses, a dispersing treatment is given. In other words, to tonify means to reinforce a condition of deficient *ki* and *ketsu*, to invigorate a person whose vitality has declined, and to aid the natural powers of the body for maintaining a homeostatic balance. To disperse means to reduce *ki* in cases where there is an excess of *ki* (hyperfunction) and to control the pathological overactivity of certain physiological mechanisms.

Nevertheless, accurate diagnosis of deficiencies and excesses and the appropriate use of tonification and dispersion techniques are no simple matter. This problem is stated as follows in the classics of acupuncture and moxibustion: "Deciding the deficiency and excess is a tenuous affair because one moment it seems clear and then it becomes very elusive." "Deficiencies arise from an inner need to be deficient and excesses arise from an inner need to be excessive. These follow a natural law, but when the mediocre physician unwisely attempts to interfere in this process, these qualities become very hard to discriminate."

What tonification and dispersion mean in practical terms is the positive and negative influence brought to bear on the body in order to rectify the imbalance in the physiological equilibrium and to help the body maintain a functional balance. Tonification and dispersion are opposite effects sought in employing various needling techniques, and it is a general concept related to providing the appropriate amount of stimulation in acupuncture treatments. Tonification and dispersion are, like deficiencies and excesses, a concept of antagonistic effects and they do not indicate specific levels or quantities. Therefore, it is not accurate to define a particular method or amount of stimulation as being tonification or dispersion. A given amount of stimulation can act either as tonification or dispersion depending on the situation and the sensitivity of the patient.

Since tonification and dispersion are relative concepts, some types of therapy can be defined as being more tonifying and others, more dispersing. Between acupuncture and moxibustion, acupuncture is considered to be relatively dispersing, moxibustion, relatively tonifying. Of course there are more tonifying methods and more dispersing methods within each of these therapeutic modalities. Simple insertion with a filiform needle is considered tonifying in relation to micropuncture with a three edged needle which is a dispersive technique. Warming moxibustion using a moxa stick is considered tonifying in relation to direct suppurative moxibustion which is very dispersive. The best known traditional rules concerning tonification and dispersion techniques in acupuncture and moxibustion are listed below for reference.

Tonification and Dispersion by Yin and Yang
Illnesses arising from internal causes (e.g., emotions, fatigue, and poor diet) manifest more in the yin meridians and tonification techniques are used to treat them. Illnesses coming from external causes (e.g., injury or exposure to elements) affect the yang meridians and dispersion techniques are used to treat them. As a general principle, when there is both a deficiency (yin) and an excess (yang), the yin is treated first and the yang is treated later. In other words, tonification always comes before dispersion.

Tonification and dispersion by acupuncture and moxibustion
TONIFICATION—A chronic disease leads to depletion (deficiency) so moxibustion is the preferred method of treatment.
DISPERSION—In acute diseases the pathogenic influence causes an excess so acupuncture is the preferred method of treatment.

Tonification and dispersion by type of needle used
TONIFICATION—thin needle and shallow insertion
DISPERSION—thick needle and deep insertion

Tonification and dispersion by direction of needling
TONIFICATION—needle pointed with the flow of the meridian
DISPERSION—needle pointed against the flow of the meridian

Tonification and dispersion by needling with breathing
TONIFICATION—Insert while the patient exhales and withdraw while the patient inhales.
DISPERSION—Insert while the patient inhales and withdraw while the patient exhales.

Tonification and dispersion by heat and cold
TONIFICATION—Warm needles are used for cold conditions and the needles are retained.
DISPERSION—Needles are used at room temperature for heat conditions and quick insertion and withdrawal is applied.

Tonification and dispersion by manipulation of the point
TONIFICATION—Before insertion stroke the point to be needled, and then flick it with a nail. After withdrawing the needle quickly cover the point with a finger and massage it.
DISPERSION—Do not manipulate the acupuncture point before insertion. Instead of covering the point after withdrawing the needle, place two fingers on either side and spread the skin.

Tonification and dispersion by speed of needling

TONIFICATION—Insert the needle slowly and painlessly in stages and withdraw it quickly and smoothly.

DISPETSION—Insert the needle quickly to the desired depth and withdraw it slowly in stages.

Tonification and dispersion in moxibustion

TONIFICATION—Form the moxa cone loosely, place it lightly on the skin, let it burn naturally, and burn successive cones on the ashes of previous cones.

DISPERSION—Form the moxa cone tightly, press it firmly onto the skin, fan it as it burns, and remove the ash before burning another cone.

6. Special Needling Methods

(1) Moxa Needling

Moxa needling is a method of burning a ball of moxa on the handle of a needle after inserting a needle. In this method, either the ball of moxa is packed tightly onto the handle of the needle or it is placed in a special holder which fits over the handle. Moxa needling is used for its warming and tonifying effect on acupuncture points. Moxa needling has the combined effect of acupuncture (especially that of retaining the needle) and that of indirect moxibustion. The heat of the burning moxa is conducted through the needle and is also radiated to the surrounding skin surface.

In moxa needling, thicker stainless steel needles (4 or 5 gauge) and poor quality moxa for warming moxibustion are used. The poor quality moxa burns longer and hotter than good quality moxa, so it is actually better suited for moxa needling. To perform moxa needling, first needles are inserted in selected points and are retained after obtaining a fair amount of needle sensation. Next compact balls of moxa are formed by compressing and rolling moxa in the palms of the hands.

Fig. 61   **Fig. 62**

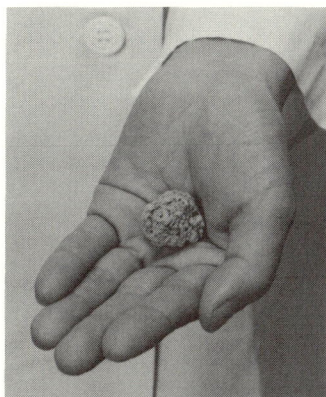
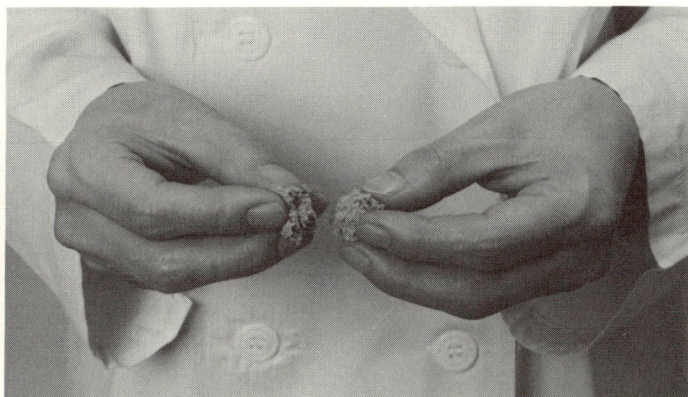

Fig. 63   Fig. 64

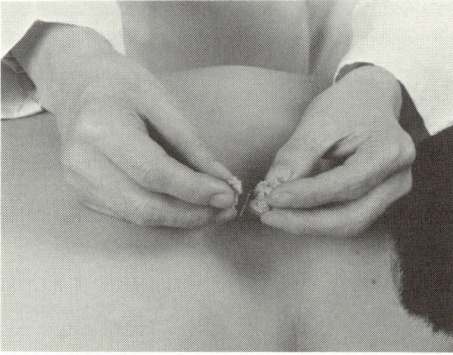
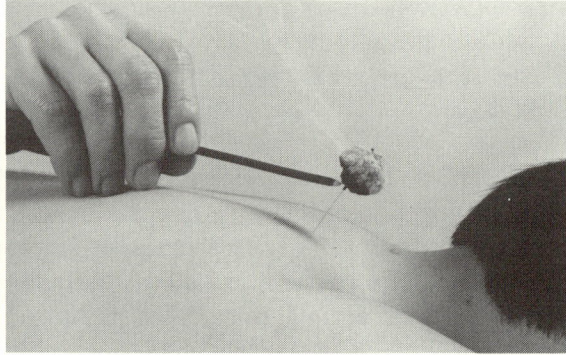

Then the balls of moxa are split in half and the two halves are pressed back together over the handle of the needles to form a ball once more (Figs. 61–63). Various holders have been invented to simplify the process of fixing the moxa on the handle of the needle. The ball of moxa is ignited after it is firmly in place on the needles (Fig. 64). After the moxa finishes burning, always allow a little extra time before removing the ashes from the handle of the needle. Up to three balls of moxa can be burned consecutively on one retained needle.

There are several points of caution in applying moxa needling. If the moxa is to be placed on the needle without a holder, special care must be taken so that the moxa is firmly in place. The size of the ball of moxa and the distance from the skin surface determines the amount of heat, so these factors must be taken into consideration. As a rule, the ball of moxa must be at least an inch away from the skin. When thin needles are used, for moxa needling, they tend to bend under the weight of the moxa, so be sure to use needles of sufficient thickness. Even when a holder is used, the practitioner must pay attention while the moxa is burning to make sure that the heat does not become too intense and also that hot ashes do not accidentally fall onto the skin. Special care must be taken when removing the ashes, because hot ashes can fall off and burn the patient.

Moxa needling is applied for many conditions, especially for cold conditions. The most common applications are for shoulder tension, frozen shoulders, low back pain, neuralgia, diarrhea, gastrointestinal disorders, menstrual irregularity, and chilling of the extremities.

(2) Scatter Needling

Scatter needling is a technique of random needling over a broad area without particular relation to meridians or acupuncture points. It is generally applied on parts of the interscapular area or lumbar area in relation to superficial tension, indurations, and tender points. In scatter needling thin needles are inserted superficially and quickly withdrawn on many points in and around the reactive area. The depth of insertion is usually little more than that of a tapping insertion with a tube (4 mm), and never exceeds one centimeter. The key to scatter needling is quick and rhythmical insertion and withdrawal of the needle. The scatter needling technique stimulates the sensory nerve endings close to the skin surface and increase local circulation and facilitates the reabsorption of exudate substances. This method is commonly applied around the affected area in cases of osteo-arthritis of the knee, eczema, and muscular tension in the neck and shoulders.

(3) Intradermal Needling

The use of minuscule intradermal needles is very widespread among Japanese acupuncturists, and a large variety of intradermal needles are used. The simplest ones to use are the ring-type intradermal needles, which are shaped like tiny tacks. Otherwise, many varieties of pin-type intradermal needles are commonly used (Fig. 65). The inserted portion of the ring-shaped intradermal needles extends two to five millimeters vertically into the skin. The pin-type intradermal needles are inserted horizontally so that they remain within the epidermis. Intradermal needles are usually imbedded for a minimum of two days for the prolonged effect of the minute stimulation of the retained intradermal needles.

Fig. 65   Varieties of Intradermal Needles

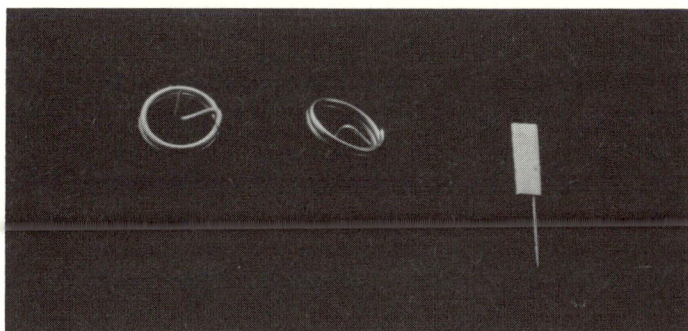

Fig. 66   Imbedded Intradermal Needles

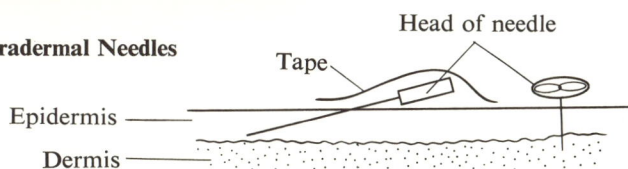

To insert a pin-type intradermal needle, first place a small piece of bandage tape just next to the point the needle is to be imbedded. Then hold the head of the needle with a pair of tweezers and use the fingers of the free hand to draw apart the skin over the point of insertion (Fig. 67). Insert the intradermal needle horizontally so that the head comes right over the piece of tape. Then place another larger piece of tape over the imbedded needle and the exposed head (Fig. 68). To avoid movement and irritation after they are imbedded, pin-type intradermal needles should always be inserted at right angles to the direction of skin stretch (parallel to the direction of skin folds). To remove pin-type intradermal needles, peel the tape off toward the head of the needle when the needle is imbedded in an area of great movement, such as near the elbow. Peel the tape off toward the tip of the needle when the needle is imbedded in an area of little movement.

Fig. 67   **Fig. 68**

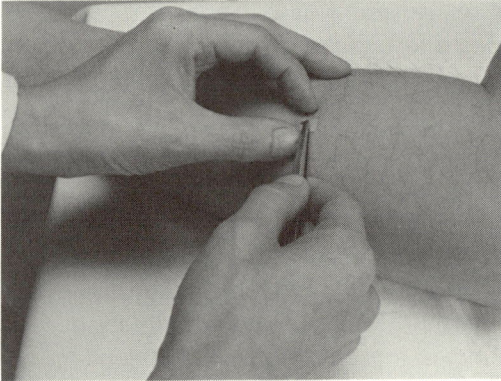
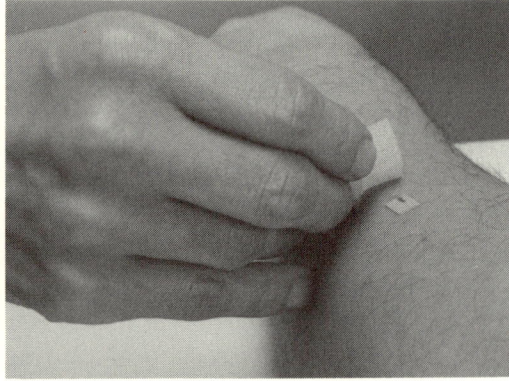

The insertion of a ring-type intradermal needle is much simpler. Ring-type intradermal needles are also called press needles because all you have to do is find the point and put the needle in like a tack. Tweezers may be used to hold the ring portion of the needle for insertion, but larger-sized ring needles can be held in the fingers. After the needle has been inserted and pressed in as far as it will go, a small piece of adhesive tape is placed over the ring portion to hold the needle in place. A faster method of applying the ring-type intradermal needle is to cut square pieces of tape and place one needle upside down on each piece. This way the needles can be inserted and fixed in place with one quick press.

After placing intradermal needles, have the patient move those parts to see if any needle causes pain or discomfort. If there is any problem with any intradermal needle, remove the needle and reinsert it so that it cannot be felt. Advise the patient to remove intradermal needles which cause undue irritation or pain later on.

(4) Pediatric Acupuncture

Pediatric acupuncture is performed on one-month old infants to five-year olds that have a hypersensitive or irritable disposition. In pediatric acupuncture, special needles are used to stimulate the skin surface with pressure and friction (Fig. 69). Treatments generally last from three to five minutes and the needling is considered sufficient when the stimulated area becomes damp or reddened.

The two main techniques employed for pediatric acupuncture are contact needling and friction. To perform contact needling, hold a needle close to its tip between the thumb and index finger. The tip of the needle should protrude between the thumb and index finger so that pushing the tip of these fingers against the skin brings the tip of the needle in contact with the skin to provide a very slight prick. Contact and release from one point to the next in a rhythmical fashion to stimulate a certain area or meridian. The plum blossom needle, cluster needle, and roller needle enable the practitioner to provide contact needling over a wide area quickly. Special pediatric needles are used to provide friction, and the amount of stimulation differs greatly by the size and shape of the needle. The pediatric needle

Fig. 69 Varieties of
Periatric
Needles

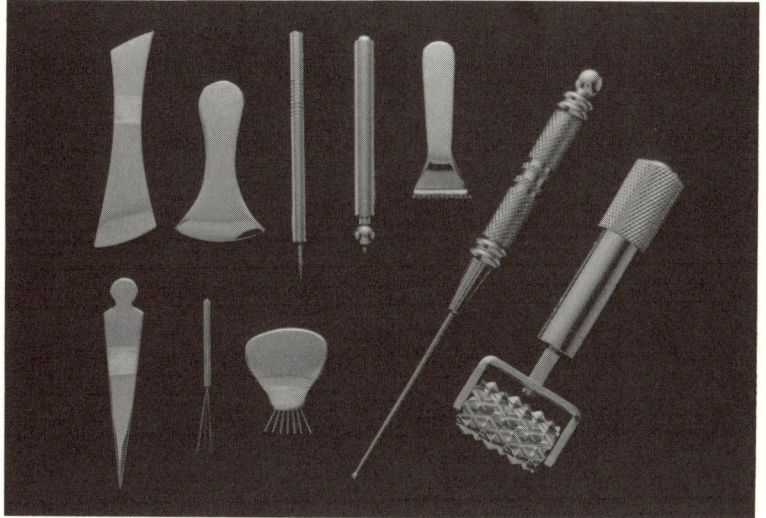

is brushed or scraped over the skin to stimulate superficial circulation. Care is
required in applying friction so as to keep from injuring the delicate skin of
infants and children.

Generally contact needling is performed first and this is followed by some
friction. It is good to end the treatment on a certain part by stroking over the
treated area with the hands. This serves to normalize the sensitivity of the skin and
soothe the child. Infants and children are very sensitive, so a little stimulation
goes a long way. Special care must be taken to keep from giving excessive stimulation. It is best to keep the first treatment very gentle and short and to gradually
increase the amount of stimulation as a child becomes accustomed to acupuncture.
Pediatric acupuncture is known to be effective for a variety of childhood conditions
including irritability, abdominal pain, bronchial asthma, tonsillitis, nocturnal
enuresis, and asthenic constitutions.

Fig. 70   Areas of Stimulation in Pediatric Acupunture

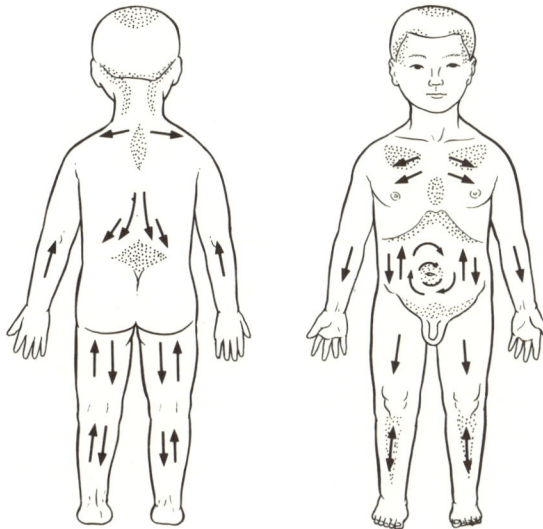

(5) Micropuncture

Micropuncture has a long history as one of the oldest forms of acupuncture. Although micropuncture may be considered to be a form of venesection (blood letting), the methods used in Oriental medicine involve only a small amount of bleeding, so it is appropriately termed micropuncture. Generally a three-edged needle (Fig. 67) is used in micropuncture to make a small cut over reactive skin areas such as tender or indurated points, localized inflammation, end points of the fingers and toes, and dilated capillary endings. A few drops to a thimblefull of blood is drawn out either by squeezing the area or using a suction cup. Since large needles are used to make a cut, micropuncture acts as fairly strong stimulation, so usually it is performed on only a few points near the end of an acupuncture treatment. Micropuncture is a very efficacious method for pain and other excessive symptoms. Also sometimes it is used as an emergency resuscitation method.

Fig. 71   Three-edged Needle

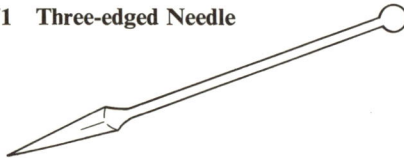

To perform micropuncture on dilated capillaries (telangiectasis), a few points over the more prominent vessels are selected. Telangiectases are also known as vascular spiders and they appear in many forms, but they differ from varicose veins in that they are fine dark blue or purple lines appearing through otherwise normal skin. The needle must penetrate through a fatty layer beneath the skin to reach the capillary, but it never has to go deeper than a centimeter. After breaking the skin with a quick prick, if necessary, press and squeeze the area around the cut to facilitate bleeding. A suction cup (introduced in the next section) can be placed over the cut to induce hyperemia and draw out more venous blood. Allow the bleeding to stop by itself, but if bleeding continues over ten minutes, press a cotton swab soaked in alcohol over the cut to stop the bleeding. Micropuncture on dilated capillaries is effective for older overweight and hypertensive women with chronic headaches, shoulder tension, or low back pain. In this case dilated capillaries in the back of the knees and the sides of the legs are treated. Bleeding dilated capillaries is also effective for young women with menstrual irregularity and chilling in their lower extremities. In this case capillaries appearing below the inner malleolus are treated.

The procedure for performing micropuncture on reactive points is similar to that for dilated capillaries, but since there is very little tissue under some reactive points, the depth of penetration is an important consideration. Pinching up the skin and then piercing it prevents injury to cutaneous nerves and superficial blood vessels. Micropuncture is applied on GB-21 to relieve strong shoulder tension. BL-10 is likewise used for occipital headaches and hypertension. Otherwise BL-40 is used in cases of sciatica and GV-20 is used for vertex headaches.

Performing micropuncture on end points of the hands and feet is different than that for other areas because the points used are distal acupuncture points. These traditional "well" points at the bases of the finger and toenails are extremely sensitive. The needle does not have to penetrate more than one millimeter at these points to cause bleeding. It is better to pierce the skin very shallowly and then squeeze or "milk" the finger to obtain blood, instead of piercing deeply to cause spontaneous bleeding. The amount of blood drawn is much less than for other points. Allow no more bleeding than can be absorbed by a few cotton swabs. Micropuncture at end points is most commonly applied at LU-1, HT-9, and SI-1. LU-1 is used for stifling sensations in the epigastrium and sore throats. HT-9 is used for angina pectoris, hypertension, and shock. SI-1 is used for cerebral hyperemia (hotness of the head) and for reducing fevers.

Micropuncture is contraindicated for bleeding disorders such as hemophilia as well as for deficient conditions such as anemia, hypotension, and general weakness. Also, due to the more invasive nature of the technique, micropuncture must not be performed on patients who have been exposed to viral hepatitis or AIDS. It goes without mention that the equipment, the practitioner's hands, and the part to be treated must be thoroughly sterilized before and after performing micropuncture.

(6) Cupping

Cupping is a method used as an adjunct to acupuncture in which a glass ball is used to form a "vacuum" over a small area of the skin to create negative pressure. The negative pressure causes the skin under the cup to bulge upward and blood is drawn to the area and eventually a dark red spot forms. The "vacuum" is created in the glass cup by burning some paper or flammable object in the cup and quickly placing it on the skin, or otherwise by using a pump to suction the air out after placing the cup on the skin. In China, simple glass cups are used for cupping, but

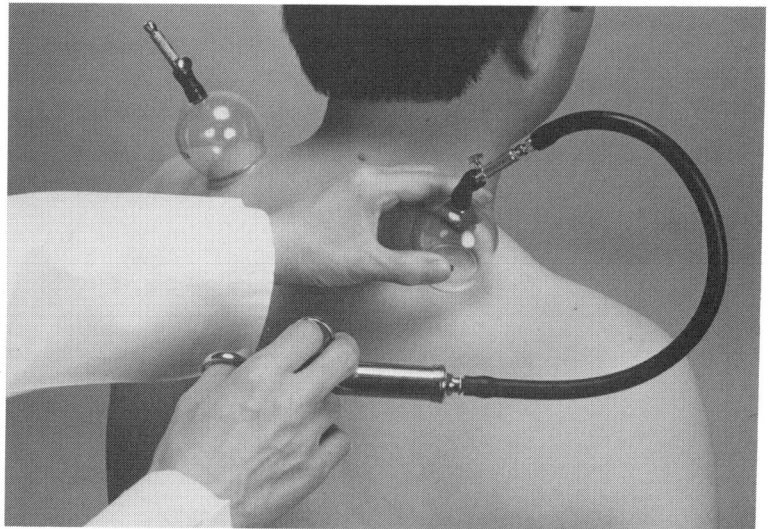

Fig. 72 Cupping by
Use of
Manual Pump

in Japan glass cups with a nipple on the end are in common use. Instead of using a flame to form a "vacuum," with these glass bulbs, a manual pump or an electric compressor is used to suction air out through the nipple. The nipple has a valve in it which prevents air from entering the glass bulb once it is placed on the skin. To use these glass bulbs, first a hose from the pump is connected to the nipple and then the bulb is firmly placed on the skin. Suction is applied manually or electrically until the desired negative pressure is achieved, and then the hose is removed. After leaving glass bulbs on for about ten minutes, they are removed by pressing in the skin next to the rim to allow air into the bulbs.

There are two basic approaches in cupping. One is to provide only the negative pressure of cupping on specific skin areas to cause localized hyperemia. The other is to use the negative pressure of cupping to facilitate the flow of blood in micropuncture. Cupping by itself serves to dispel stagnation of *ki* and blood and is applicable for a wide variety of problems ranging from atherosclerosis to gastro-intestinal disorders. Cupping by itself is primarily applied on *shu* points and other reactive points on the back. The number of cups applied at one time should be six or less. Generally the cups are left on for ten to fifteen minutes. Since cupping leaves red marks on the skin which remain for up to a week, the patient should be made aware of this in advance. Cupping with micropuncture is more dispersing than cupping alone, and all the cautions in the previous section on micropuncture apply. Usually, only a few points are treated with micropuncture and cupping. All cupping is contraindicated during menstruation and pregnancy as well as for tumors and injuries.

(7) Carotid Sinus Stimulation

Direct stimulation of the carotid sinus, located close to the division of the common carotid artery into its external and internal branches, is a technique developed by a prominent modern Japanese acupuncturist Bunshi Shirota. The acupuncture point used to reach the carotid sinus is ST-9, which lies directly over the common carotid artery. The carotid sinus is the dilated portion of the internal carotid artery which has special parasympathetic nerve endings. The carotid sinus has pressor-receptors which control blood pressure by reducing the heart rate as the blood pressure in the carotid artery rises. Stimulating the carotid sinus is thought

Fig. 73 Anatomical Location of Carotid Sinus

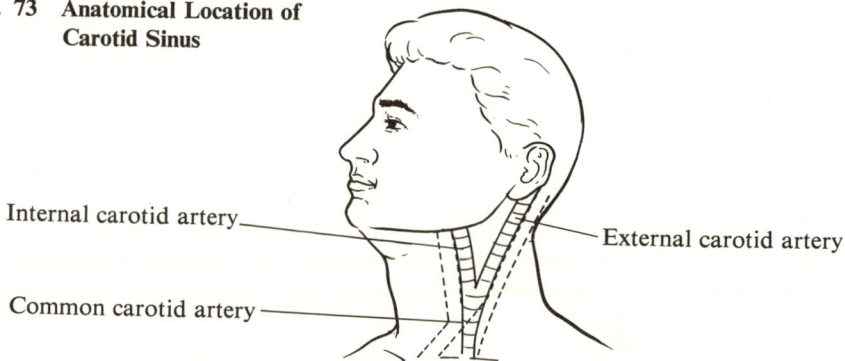

Internal carotid artery

External carotid artery

Common carotid artery

to have a therapeutic effect by regulating the autonomic nervous system through the autonomic fibers of the ninth cranial nerve (glossopharyngeal nerve).

Carotid sinus stimulation has a direct effect of lowering the blood pressure, and it is a useful technique for cases of essential hypertension. The effect, however, is not sustained and the technique is not very useful for advanced cases of athero-sclerosis or renal hypertension. Be that as it may, carotid sinus stimulation is useful for a wide variety of disorders and pain syndromes including tachycardia, asthma, arthritis, gastrospasms, and acute tonsillitis.

Carotid sinus stimulation is best done with a thin silver or stainless steel needle (2 or 3 gauge). The patient must be in the supine position without a pillow and his head should be tilted back so his chin points up. ST-9 is two to three centimeters lateral to the laryngeal prominence on the anterior border of the sternocleido-mastoid muscle where the pulsation of the carotid artery can be felt the strongest. Slowly insert the needle vertically toward the artery until the arterial wall is reached (at a depth of 1 to 2 cm). Letting go of the needle, the handle should move back and forth with the pulsation of the artery. Retain the needle for no more than a minute. Withdraw the needle gently and briefly massage the point with one finger.

(8) Stellate Ganglion Stimulation

Stimulation of the stellate ganglion, located in the anterior cervical region, is a widely used needling technique with a variety of applications. In this method, the stellate ganglion, also known as the cervicothoracic ganglion, on the cervical sympathetic nerve trunk is stimulated with a needle to affect the function of the autonomic nervous system. The stellate ganglion is composed on the inferior cervical ganglion and the first thoracic ganglion, which are usually fused. The postganglionic fibers of the stellate ganglion are distributed to the head, neck, heart, and upper limbs. Stellate ganglion stimulation is used in cases of tinnitus, vertigo, headaches (both vascular and tension headaches), cervicobrachialgia, and circulatory problems in the upper limbs (e.g., Raynaud's disease).

Fig. 74   Anatomical Location of the Stellate Ganglion

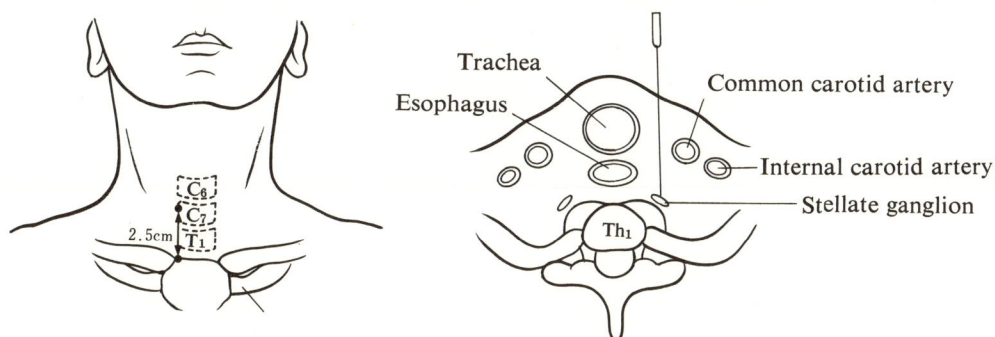

Stellate ganglion stimulation is performed with a longer than average stainless steel needle (6 cm) of standard thickness (4 gauge). The patient must be in the supine position, and it is helpful to place a small pillow under the patient's neck to extend the neck. The point of insertion is 2.5 centimeters above the sternoclavicular joint, just medial to the sternocleidomastoid muscle. The needle must be inserted toward the transverse process of the seventh cervical vertebra. The anterior tubercle of this transverse process can be palpated by pressing deeply over the above point. When forming the supporting hand to receive the guide tube to begin the insertion, use the thumb and index finger to push the sternocleidomastoid muscle and the carotid artery to the side, out of the way. Slowly insert the needle vertically and be careful to avoid the trachea. After coming up against the transverse process of the seventh cervical vertebra at a depth of about five centimeters, withdraw the needle about a centimeter and apply gentle lifting and thrusting. The patient should feel a dull or heavy sensation deep down, which sometimes reaches the interscapular region. Each side is stimulated about five minutes, but the symptomatic side is usually stimulated longer. Often there is immediate relief from symptoms after stellate ganglion stimulation.

The needle should be withdrawn and reinserted in the following cases: when a strong pulsation is felt at the tip of the needle, when the needle moves every time the patient swallows, and when a sharp pain radiates to the patient's chest, head, or arms. The patient should be able to speak all during the procedure, so it is best to stimulate the point gently while confirming the effect with the patient from time to time.

(9) Auricular Acupuncture

Auricular acupuncture is a traditional method of treatment, but it was not widely used until the introduction of the fetal model for auricular points by a French physician Dr. Paul Nogier. Dr. Nogier illustrated the resemblance of the distribution of auricular points to the anatomical parts of the fetus in the normal inverted position (Fig. 75). Auricular acupuncture is based on the concept that the condition of the whole body is reflected in the ears. Thus all the internal organs as well as parts of the body are correlated to points on the surface of the auricle. Just as on the body surface, the surface of the auricle has reactive points reflecting

Fig. 75 Correlation of Fetus to Auricle

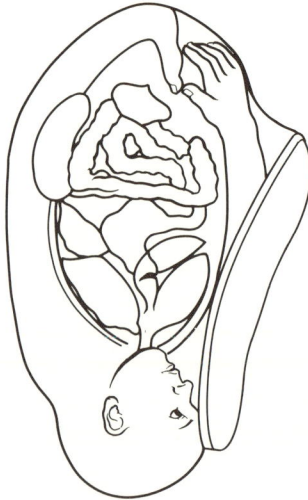

disorders of the body, and the same reactive points can be used for treatment. Some practitioners probe for points of low electrical resistance using special point location devices.

The outer ear is known to be densely supplied with nerve endings from the somatic nervous system as well as the autonomic nervous system. Auricular acupuncture is considered to have a reflexive effect on various organs by regulating the function of the autonomic nervous system and by stabilizing the homeostatic function of the body. Auricular acupuncture is widely used for the treatment of pain syndromes and organic diseases as well as for weight control and withdrawal symptoms from smoking and drugs.

The first step in performing auricular acupuncture is to locate reactive points on the auricle. This can be done in a number of ways, but the simplest way is to visually inspect the ear for abnormally dilated capillaries and small eruptions as well as areas of different pigmentation such as erythema, freckles, and dark spots. Another simple method to detect reactive points is to press points of the ear with a small blunt object such as the end of a hair pin to locate tender points. Another popular method for finding auricular points is to use an electrical point locator which detects points with low resistivity. Regardless of which method is used, the practitioner should narrow down the area of search, because probing the entire surface of both ears can be very time-consuming. The reactive points tend to appear most clearly in the ear on the side of the body with the symptoms. Probe the ear on the other side only if significant reactive points cannot be located on the auricle of the affected side. Reactive points tend to appear in certain parts of the ear in relation to the disease condition of the patient, so search a particular part of the ear according to the problem.

The following are the general reactive areas associated with problems in various parts of the body:

1. Auricular lobule—face and sense organs
2. Antitragus—head and brain
3. Anterior portion of helix—external genitalia
4. Helix crus—diaphragm
5. Antihelix—spine
6. Superior antihelix crus—lower limbs
7. Inferior antihelix crus—hips and pelvis
8. Triangular fossa—uterus
9. Medial aspect of tragus—throat and nasal passages
10. Lateral aspect of tragus—external nose
11. Scapha—upper limb
13. Cymba conchae—visceral organs
14. Cavum conchae—heart and respiratory organs
15. Intertragic notch—endocrine system

Many different types of stimulation are applied on auricular points for treatment including intradermal needles, filiform needles, and metal grains. The most widespread method used in Japan is to implant intradermal needles in auricular

Fig. 76 Surface Anatomy of the Auricle

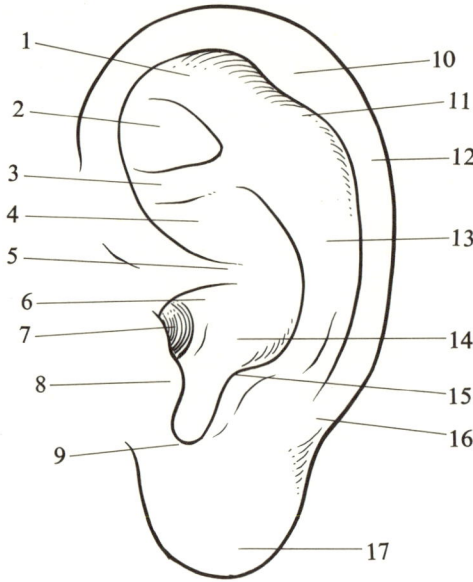

1. Superior antihelix
2. Triangular fossa
3. Inferior antihelix crus
4. Cymba chonchae
5. Helix crus
6. Supertragic notch
7. External auditory meatus
8. Tragus
9. Intertragic notch
10. Auricular tubercle
11. Scapha
12. Helix
13. Antihelix
14. Cavum conchae
15. Antitragus
16. Helix cauda
17. Auricular lobule

Fig. 77 Auricular Acupuncture Points

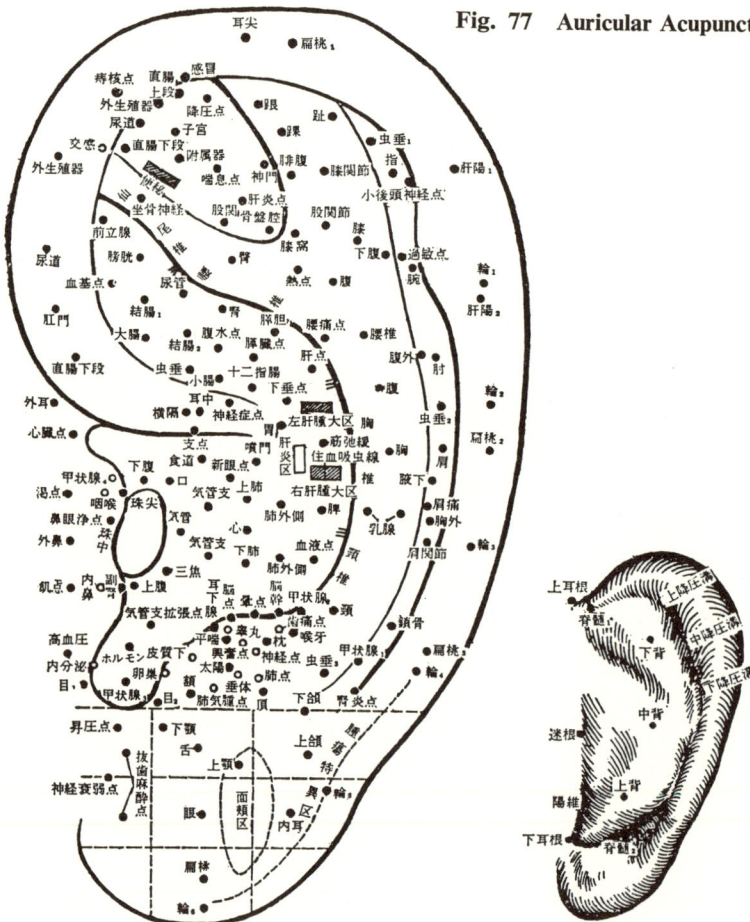

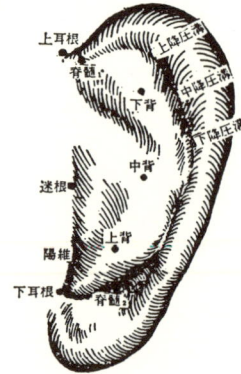

points along with other acupuncture points. Ring-type intradermal needles are most popular for this purpose. Another common approach is to place short filiform needles (1.5 cm) for up to twenty minutes and also to applying electrical stimulation with or without needles. Some practitioners tape tiny metal balls on auricular points and have their patient's press on these from time to time. Regardless of the form of stimulation, five to six auricular points are usually sufficient for one treatment.

(10) Electroacupuncture

In electroacupuncture needles are used as electrodes to apply electrical stimulation to specific areas. Electroacupuncture came into practice in Japan in the 1950s with the development of the Ryōdō-Raku acupuncture system, which is still the most popular electroacupuncture method in Japan. In this system of acupuncture resistivity measurements are taken at all the source points as a way of diagnosing the condition of the twelve major meridians. The main treatment modality used in Ryōdō-Raku is electrical stimulation through needles inserted in acupuncture points. The most widespread mode of electrical stimulation used in acupuncture clinics in Japan is low frequency alternating currents. In recent years the use of electrode pads instead of needles for applying electrical stimulation, a method known as TENS (Transcutanéous Electrical Nerve Stimulation), is also increasing in popularity.

Electroacupuncture is applied in acupuncture clinics in Japan for a variety of purposes including pain control, improving muscle tone, and general regulation of physiological functions. The pain killing effect of acupuncture is enhanced by electrical stimulation, and vasodilation and improved circulation is obtained by the rhythmical muscle contractions induced by electroacupuncture. Also the effect of acupuncture in regulating the autonomic nervous system is increased by electro-acupuncture. Regardless of the aim, applying electrical stimulation in addition to the simple mechanical stimulation of needle insertion produces a stronger and more lasting effect.

There are such a wide variety of electroacupuncture devices on the market today that it is difficult to recommend one specific type or to elaborate on the various features. Only the basic principles applicable to all devices for low frequency electrical stimulation will be presented here in order to discuss the clinical applications of electroacupuncture. For specific instruction on the use of a certain device, study the owners manual carefully. Most devices have a minimum of two output jacks. In direct current devices the positive lead is inserted into one jack and the negative lead is inserted into the other jack. The negative lead is also called the stimulation electrode and the positive lead, the indifferent electrode. In some direct current devices the polarity of the two leads can be switched back and forth. In alternating current devices, both leads are similar in terms of polarity. There are some devices which provide both direct and alternating currents. Although there are many different applications of various currents depending on the capabilities of the device, when a direct current electroacupuncture device with fixed polarity is used, the negative lead must be connected to the point which is

Fig. 78 Electroacu-
            puncture

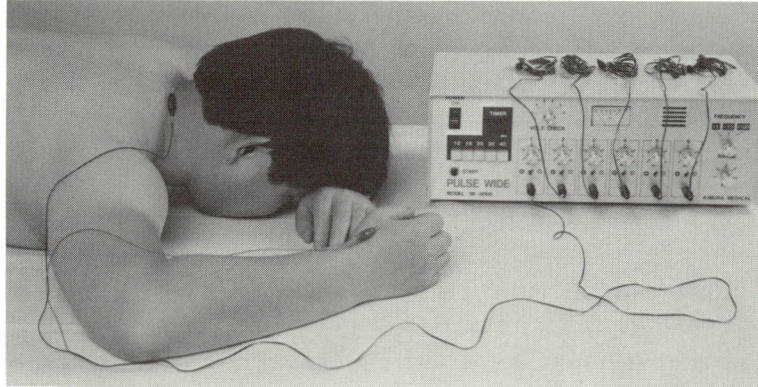

most in need of stimulation and the positive lead should be connected to another point to complete the circuit. Regardless of the polarity or type of current applied, the two leads must never be placed in such a way that the electrical current crosses the heart, brain, spinal cord, uterus or testicles. Also, if the patient is wearing a pace maker or has arrhythmia, electroacupuncture is contraindicated.

In order to perform electroacupuncture, first needles must be inserted in the points to be stimulated. The needles used for electroacupuncture must be relatively thick stainless steel needles (5 gauge or thicker). It is advisable to keep needles used for electroacupuncture separate and to carefully inspect them after each use since they are more prone to damage. Turn the electroacupuncture device on after inserting the needles, making sure that the intensity level is at zero, or the lowest possible setting. Then clip or attach the leads to the needles at the handles. Adjust the frequency setting (generally between one and three Hertz). Begin turning the intensity level up gradually until the highest level is reached in which there is twitching of the muscles but no pain. Set a timer for the appropriate amount of time for stimulation (generally between fifteen and thirty minutes).

It is important when doing electroacupuncture that the individual differences in sensitivity to electrical stimulation be taken into account. The general principles for determining the appropriate amount of stimulation outlined in the beginning of the next chapter are applicable. Also, as a rule, the level and duration of stimulation should be reduced for patients who have little or no experience with electroacupuncture. Another important consideration when providing electroacupuncture is to have the patients assume a position which is as comfortable as possible since they must remain in the same position for up to half an hour.

A moderate amount of localized muscle contractions (twitching) produced by electroacupuncture is very useful for improving circulation and reducing discomfort in tense and indurated muscle tissue. Electroacupuncture is also very useful for controlling pain for conditions like neuralgia. The effects and aims of electroacupuncture can be viewed from three angles from the standpoint of clinical application. The first is the effect of electroacupuncture in causing localized muscle contractions, which is used to stimulate muscle tissue. The second is the effect of electroacupuncture on nerves and pain reception, which is used to control pain. And the third is the general effect of electroacupuncture in physiological regulation, which is used to improve the functional condition of the body. These three approaches will each be explained below in greater detail with some practical examples. Although specific clinical applications of electroacupuncture are presented below, be sure to refer to Part II for a more thorough discussion of treatment for specific conditions.

Electroacupuncture Directed at Muscle Tissue
The aim of this approach is to facilitate circulation and to promote relaxation of muscle tissue by causing rhythmical contractions. The points of stimulation are in major muscles at specific motor points (which generally correspond to acupuncture points). In the figures and discussion below, point A represents the main point of stimulation (negative lead attached) and point B is a secondary point for completing the circuit (positive lead attached). The exact location of these points should be determined by localized reactions of tenderness or muscular tension. This approach to electroacupuncture is effective for musculoskeletal conditions including neck and shoulder stiffness, cervicobrachialgia caused by tension in soft tissues, and low back pain due to muscle strain.

(A)   Stimulation of upper fibers of the trapezius muscle
Insert needles vertically up to two centimeters in points A and B and then connect the leads to the needles. Slowly raise the intensity of stimulation to cause mild contractions of the upper fibers of the trapezius. This procedure is effective for pain or tension in the occipital region, stiffness in the neck and shoulders, and eye-strain.

Fig. 79   Upper Portion of Trapezius

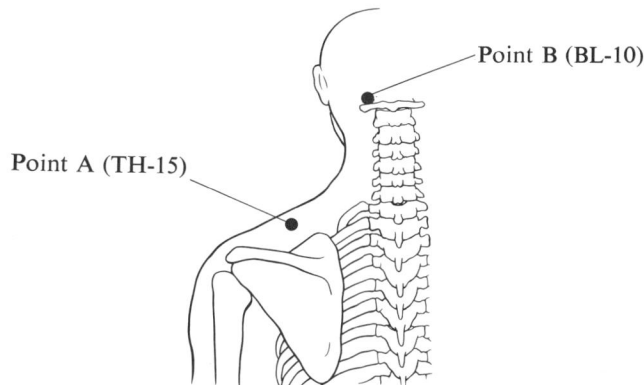

Point B (BL-10)

Point A (TH-15)

(B)   Stimulation of levator scapulae muscle
Insert a needle vertically up to two centimeters in point A (medial to the sterno-cleidomastoid muscle and lateral to the splenius capitis muscle). Insert a needle vertically up to two centimeters in point B (in the tensest point of the trapezius muscle). The muscle contractions caused by the electrical stimulation should make the scapula move up slightly each time. This procedure is effective for tension or stiffness in the neck and shoulders.

Fig. 80 Upper Portion of Levator Scapulae

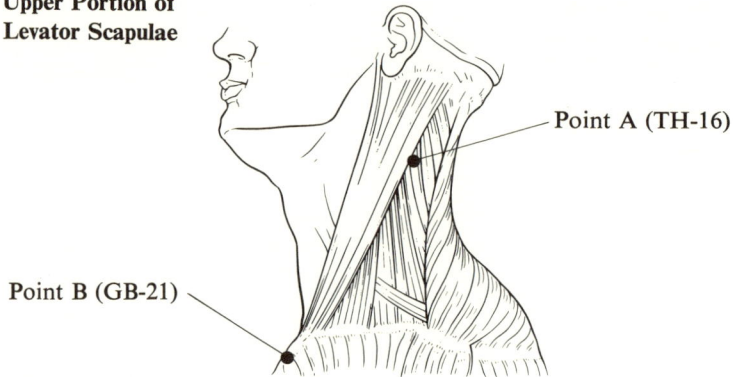

Point A (TH-16)

Point B (GB-21)

(C) Stimulation of rhomboideus muscles
Aim the needles laterally and insert obliquely in points A and B up to two centimeters. Deep insertion at these points can cause pneumothorax so caution must be exercised. The muscle contractions should cause slight adduction of the scapula each time. This procedure is effective for pain and stiffness in the interscapular region.

Fig. 81 Minor and Major Rhomboideus Muscles

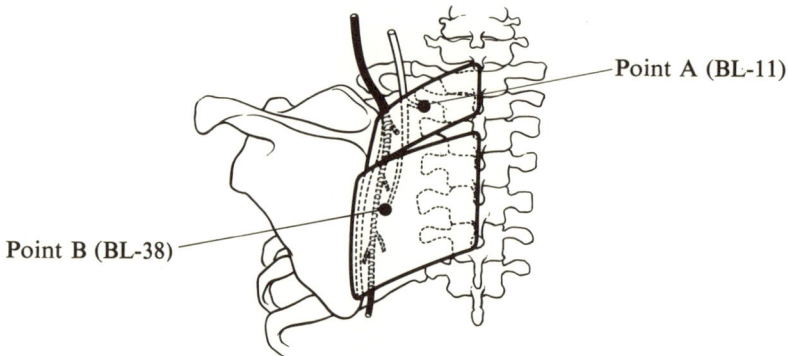

Point A (BL-11)

Point B (BL-38)

(D) Stimulation of erector spinae muscles
Insert the needles vertically three to four centimeters in points A and B. Raise the

Fig. 82 Erector Spinae Muscles in the Lumbar Region

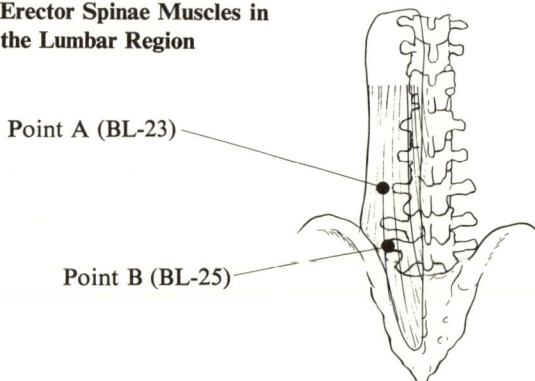

Point A (BL-23)

Point B (BL-25)

intensity of stimulation gradually to cause mild contractions in the erector spinae muscles. This procedure is effective for pain and tension in the lumbar and sacral region.

(E)   Stimulation of quadratus lumborum muscle
Insert the needles vertically at the lateral margin of the erector spinae muscles to a depth of about four centimeters. The muscle contractions should cause slight elevation of the iliac. This procedure is effective for pain and tension in the lumbar area.

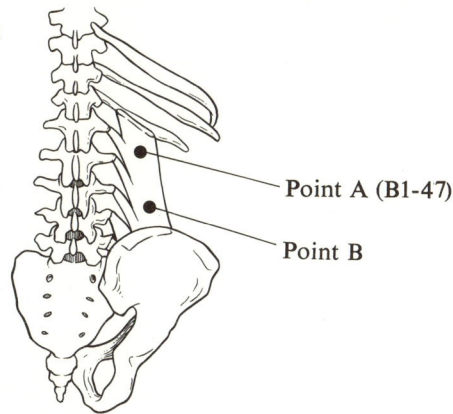

Fig. 83   Quadratus Lumborum Muscle

Point A (B1-47)

Point B

Electroacupuncture Directed at Peripheral Nerves
The aim of this approach is to reduce the excitation or sensitivity of specific peripheral nerves. In the case of paralysis or numbness in the extremities, however, the aim is to increase the excitability of the affected nerves. The electrical stimulation is applied between the root of a spinal nerve and a peripheral point on the same nerve. The needle must be inserted carefully just adjacent to the nerve to be treated. The exact depth varies according to the individual, but a strong needle sensation must be obtained before beginning stimulation. This approach to electroacupuncture is effective for pain syndromes of the peripheral nerves (neuralgia) and for certain types of peripheral nerve paralysis. It is most often employed for trigeminal neuralgia, neurogenic cervicobrachialgia, sciatica, and facial paralysis.

(A)   Stimulation of the radial nerve
Point A is located three centimeters lateral to the median line between the fifth and sixth cervical vertebrae. Insert the needle three to five centimeters in this point until a deep sensation is obtained. Use vertical insertion for both point A and point B. Raise the intensity of stimulation gradually to a point where the pain decreases or otherwise to the highest tolerable level. Check the intensity after five minutes to make sure that the stimulation is at the optimum level and is not causing undue discomfort.

(B)   Stimulation of the median nerve
Point A is located three centimeters lateral to the median line between the sixth

Fig. 84   The Radial Nerve

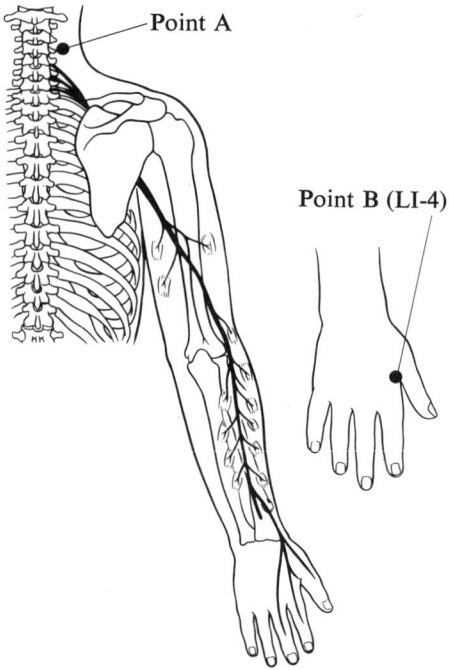

Point A

Point B (LI-4)

Fig. 85   The Median Nerve

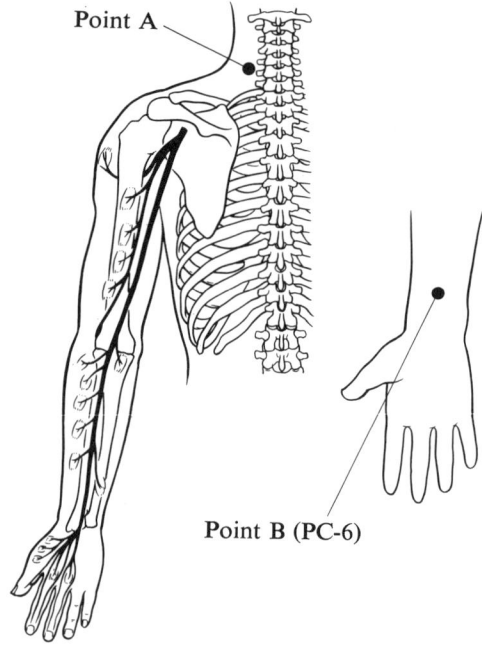

Point A

Point B (PC-6)

Fig. 86   The Ulnar Nerve

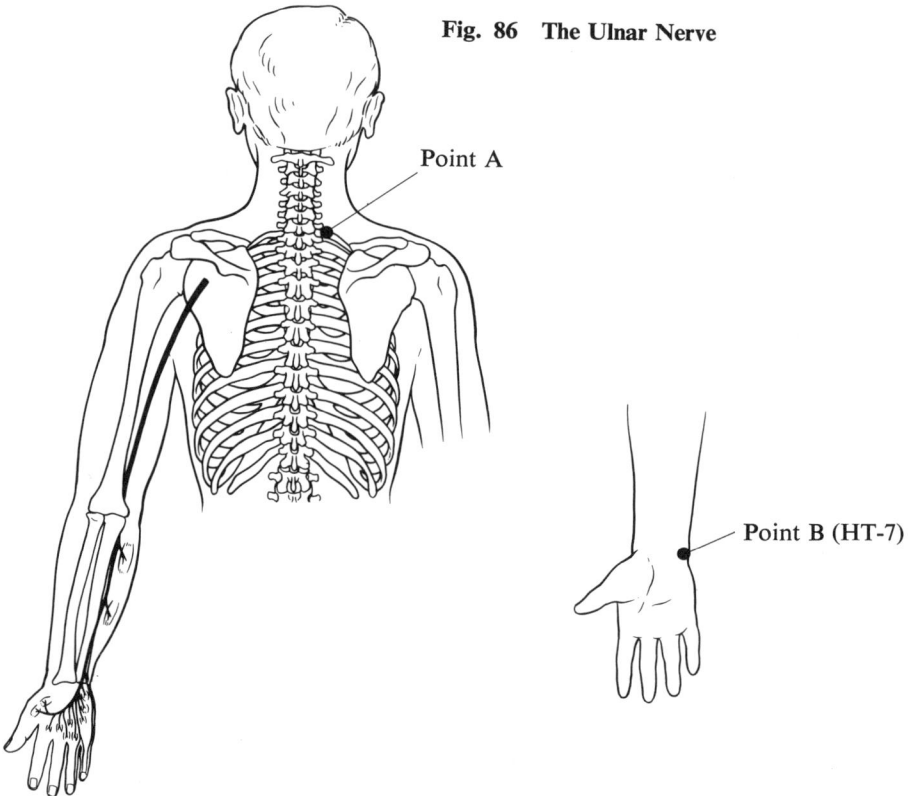

Point A

Point B (HT-7)

and seventh cervical vertebrae. Insert the needle three to five centimeters in this point until a deep sensation is obtained. Use vertical insertion for both point A and point B. Raise the intensity of stimulation to a point where the pain decreases or otherwise to the highest tolerable level. Check the intensity after five minutes and make adjustments if necessary.

(C) Stimulation of the ulnar nerve

Point A is located three centimeters lateral to the median line between the seventh cervical and first thoracic vertebrae. Insert the needle three to five centimeters in this point until a deep sensation is obtained. Use vertical insertion for both point A and point B. Raise the intensity of stimulation to an appropriate level and check after five minutes to see if any adjustments are necessary.

(D) Stimulation of upper lumbar plexus

The stimulation of the upper lumbar plexus can be done with the patient in the prone or side-lying position. In this procedure the femoral and lateral femoral cutaneous nerves are stimulated. Point A is located about five centimeters lateral to the inferior border of the spinous process of the second lumbar vertebra (BL-23). Insert the needle vertically five to seven centimeters to obtain a needle sensation. Point B is located about halfway between the superior border of the greater trochanter and the inferior border of the lateral epicondyle of the femur (GB-31). Insert the needle three to five centimeters to obtain a needle sensation. Raise the intensity of stimulation gradually to a point where the pain sensation is decreased. This procedure is effective for pain and neurological symptoms in the upper lumbar region as well as along the path of the femoral nerves.

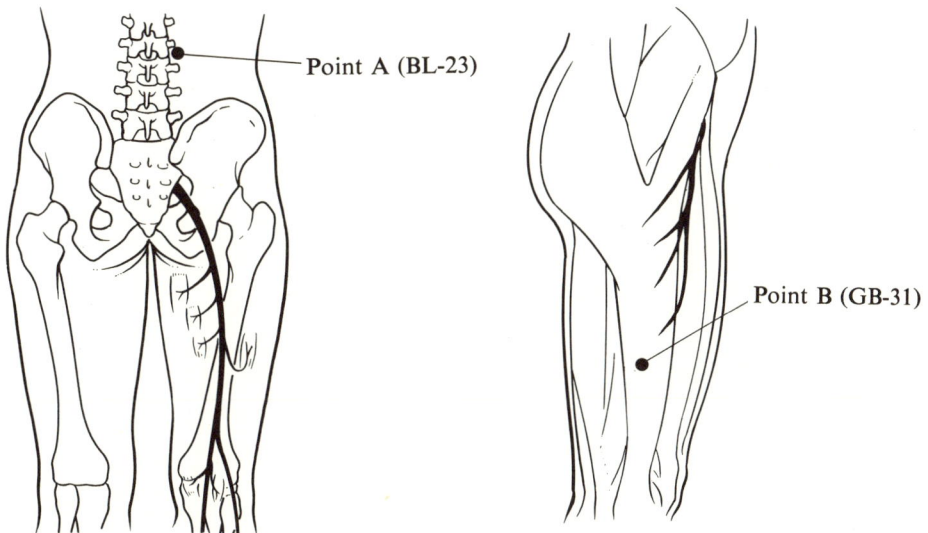

Fig. 87   The Lumbar Plexus and Femoral Nerves

Point A (BL-23)

Point B (GB-31)

(E) Stimulation of the lower lumbar plexus

The stimulation of the lower lumbar plexus is done with the patient in the prone position. In this procedure the lumbosacral trunk and sciatic nerve are stimulated.

Point A is located about five centimeters lateral to the inferior border of the spinous process of the fourth lumbar vertebra. Insert the needle vertically five to seven centimeters to obtain a needle sensation. Point B is located in the center of the posterior aspect of the thigh about fifteen centimeters (six cun) below the gluteal crease. Insert the needle vertically three to five centimeters to obtain a needle sensation. This procedure is effective for pain and neurological symptoms in the lower lumbar region and down the back of the thigh.

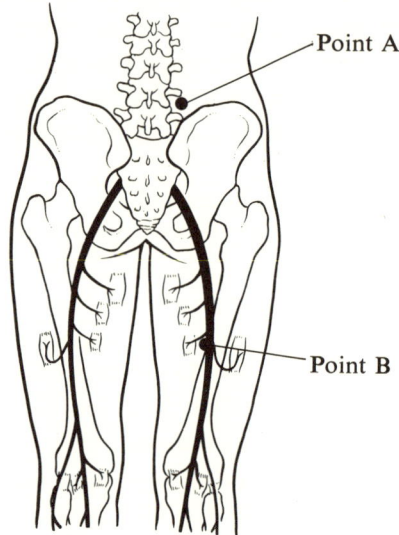

Fig. 88   The Lumbar Plexus and
             Sciatic Nerve

Point A

Point B

(F)   *Stimulation of the sciatic nerve*

The stimulation of the sciatic nerve is done with the patient in the side-lying position. Point A is located about three centimeters (one cun) medial and inferior to a point halfway between the greater trochanter and the posterior superior iliac spine. Insert the needle vertically seven to eight centimeters in this point and obtain

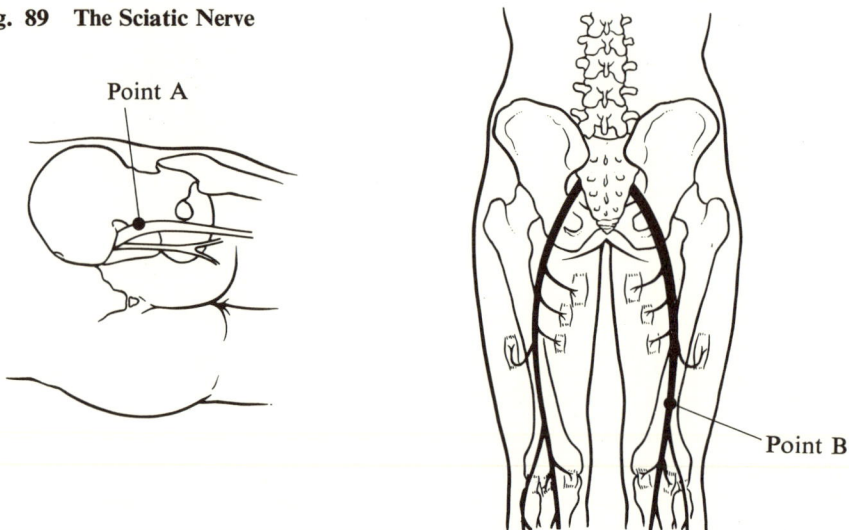

Fig. 89   The Sciatic Nerve

Point A

Point B

a strong sensation which radiates down the back of the thigh. Point B is located in the center of the posterior aspect of the thigh, about halfway between the gluteal crease (BL-36) and the popliteal fossa (BL-40). Insert the needle vertically three to five centimeters in this point and also obtain a strong sensation. Raise the intensity level gradually to a point where the pain decreases or otherwise to the highest tolerable level.

(G)   Stimulation of the trigeminal nerve
The stimulation of the trigeminal nerve is done by utilizing one of the three points accessing the affected branch of the trigeminal nerve. Point A, located at the lower border of the zygomatic arch, is used in every case. This point is ST-7, which is in the depression occupied by the condyloid process of the mandible when the mouth is opened wide. Insert the needle vertically two to three centimeters. There are three possible points for point B depending on which branch of the trigeminal nerve is affected. When the pain is in the area between the eye and forehead, use the point above the top margin of the orbit (a tender point over the supraorbital foramen). When the area between the eyes and upper lip is painful,

Fig. 90   The Trigeminal Nerve

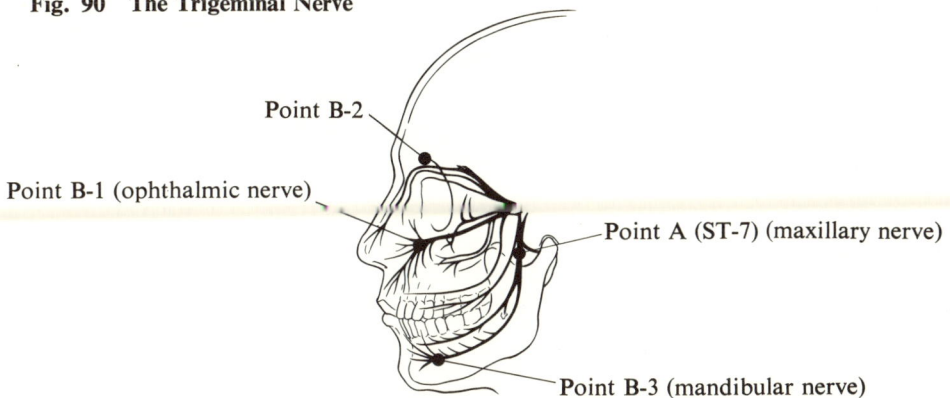

Point B-2

Point B-1 (ophthalmic nerve)

Point A (ST-7) (maxillary nerve)

Point B-3 (mandibular nerve)

use the point in the depression below the lower margin of the orbit (ST-2: over the infraorbital foramen). When the area over the lower jaw and just in front of the ear is painful, use the point just lateral to the midline on the lower jaw (a tender point over the mental foramen). The needle in point B must be inserted obliquely one to two centimeters. Raise the intensity of stimulation gradually to a level where the pain sensation is decreased.

(H)   Stimulation of the facial nerve
The stimulation of the facial nerve is done by using any one of a number of points to penetrate the facial muscles with motor impairment. Point A is located in the depression under the ear lobe (TH-17: over the trunk of the facial nerve). Insert the needle vertically two to three centimeters. Locate point B over the most impaired muscle and insert the needle horizontally up to five centimeters to penetrate as much of the muscle as possible with the needle. The treatment is even more effective if two or more muscles can be threaded by one needle. Raise the intensity

Fig. 91 The Facial Nerve

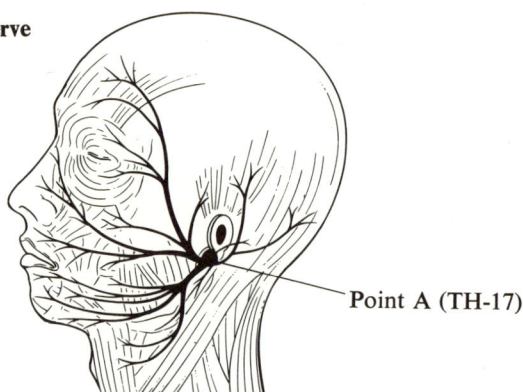

Point A (TH-17)

of stimulation to a tolerable level which causes mild rhythmic contractions in the facial muscles.

Electroacupuncture for General Physiological Regulation

The aim of this approach is to enhance the functional capacity of the body by applying mild electrical stimulation between major acupuncture points. This approach is usually used in cases of general weakness or deficiency involving autonomic dysfunction such as general malaise, climacteric disorders, and neurasthenia. Unlike the other approaches, the level of stimulation must remain well below the threshold of discomfort, and localized muscle contraction should not be induced.

(A)   Stimulation of LI-4 and LU-6

This procedure is applied to relieve multiple symptoms in the cervical and cranial area. It is also very effective for the treatment of chronic cases of tonsillitis, pharyngitis, and laryngitis.

(B)   Stimulation of LI-4 and PC-6

This procedure is applied for symptoms in the facial area as well as the thoracic region. It is very effective for the treatment of nasal congestion and chronic rhinitis or sinusitis.

(C)   Stimulation of ST-36 and SP-6

This procedure is useful for alleviating various symptoms in the lumbosacral region as well as the lower limbs. It is most often used for idiopathic gynecological symptoms and circulatory problems in the lower extremities. It can be effective for any condition involving autonomic dysfunctions with symptoms in the abdomen, pelvis, or the lower limbs.

Chapter 5
Guidelines for the Clinical Application of Acupuncture and Moxibustion

1. Guidelines for the Application of Acupuncture

(1) Amount of Stimulation and Sensitivity of the Patient

The amount of stimulation is a very important consideration in the clinical application of acupuncture just as the dosage of medication is a very important consideration in the practice of medicine. The two fundamental rules concerning the amount of stimulation in traditional acupuncture is to apply tonifying stimulation for deficient conditions and to apply dispersing stimulation for excess conditions. Therefore when physiological functions are hypoactive, mild acupuncture stimulation is applied for an invigorating or exciting effect, and conversely when physiological functions are hyperactive, strong stimulation is applied for a sedative or inhibiting effect. In order to give acupuncture treatments for an invigorating (tonifying) effect, or otherwise for a sedating (dispersing) effect, a practitioner must provide just the right dosage of needle stimulation. This dosage is a function of the amount of stimulation at each point, the number of points needled, and the total duration of the acupuncture treatment. A variety of factors must be taken into consideration to provide the optimal stimulation including the length and thickness of the needle, the depth of insertion, the duration (i.e., quick insertion and withdrawal, or retaining the needle), and the selection of needling techniques (e.g., contact needling, simple insertion, pressing the point after withdrawal, etc.). Generally the decision regarding the optimal amount of stimulation in each case is based on the practitioner's experience and sensitivity to the reactions of the patient. The following are the basic factors involved in acupuncture stimulation which determine the amount of stimulation:

Length and thickness of needle
The longer and thicker the needle is, the more tissue it displaces when it is inserted and the greater an effect it has on the nervous system. In other words, long and thick needles act as stronger stimulation than short and thin needles.

Speed of insertion and needle manipulation
The faster the needle is moved during insertion and withdrawal, the greater the friction is between the needle and the surrounding tissues. This means that quick

insertion and withdrawal and rapid needle manipulation act as stronger stimulation compared with slow and gentle needling.

Choice and application of needling techniques
The needling techniques involving greater movement provide more stimulation than those techniques involving very slight movement. The degree of stimulation can vary even with the same technique. For example, in lifting and thrusting the amplitude and speed of needle movement can be varied to provide very mild or very strong stimulation.

Duration of needle stimulation
The stimulation is greater when the needle is left in place for a certain length of time, rather than when quickly inserted and withdrawn immediately.

Continuity of needle stimulation
When a specific amount and quality of stimulation is applied over a period of time, the physiological effect is greatest in the beginning and the effect diminishes with time as the body becomes accustomed to the stimulation. When, on the other hand, a weak stimulation and strong stimulation is applied alternately, the body does not become as accustomed to this form of stimulation as readily as it does to continuous forms of stimulation. In other words, intermittent and periodic variation of stimulation produces a greater effect than continuous stimulation.

Location of needling
The body is more sensitive in the anterior aspect of the torso, the flexor muscles of the four limbs, and the peripheral areas (fingers and toes). The body is less sensitive in the posterior aspect of the torso and the extensor muscles of the four limbs.

Type of tissue
There is a considerable difference in the sensitivity of various types of tissues in the body to acupuncture stimulation. Tissue of the nervous system is most sensitive and muscle tissue is the next most sensitive.

Sensitivity
The effect of the same acupuncture stimulation varies considerably according to the sensitivity (receptivity, excitability) of the patient. Therefore, in the clinical application of acupuncture, special attention must be paid to the following factors which determine the sensitivity of a patient:

Age and sex
In general men are more tolerant of strong stimulation than woman. Young children are more sensitive to stimulation than adults. Infants in particular are very sensitive and have strong reflexes so that sometimes even mild needle stimulation can cause muscle spasms.

Constitution and temperament
Those with a nervous temperament are more sensitive to thin acupuncture stimulation than those who have a relaxed disposition. Thin people tend to be more sensitive to acupuncture stimulation compared with those who are overweight.

Type of disease
What is a moderate level of stimulation for a healthy person is strong stimulation for patients with neuralgia or hyperesthesia and is weak stimulation for patients with hypesthesia or partial paralysis.

Experience with acupuncture
Patients who receive acupuncture treatments on a regular basis are able to tolerate stronger stimulation simply because of habituation. Those patients who are new to acupuncture or have little experience with it tend to be more nervous about it and sometimes even mild stimulation is felt to be very strong. As a general rule, new patients should be given weak stimulation for the first few treatments and then the amount of stimulation can be gradually increased in subsequent treatments so that they have a chance to get used to stronger needle stimulation.

Appropriate Amount of Stimulation
Acupuncture stimulation generally follows the same principle as other types of physical stimulation, in which mild stimulation excites the function of the nervous system and continuous or strong stimulation inhibits the function of the nervous system. Nevertheless, there are times when this simple principle does not apply in clinical situations. For example, when trying to relieve pain of a nervous origin such as neuralgia or hyperesthesia, good results are often obtained by applying a very mild and soft stimulation for a long time, which tends to produce a pleasant sensation. Furthermore, sometimes in cases of neuralgia or convulsions only one treatment, in which just one part of the body is needled, proves effective. Also in the case of paralysis, when the function of the nervous system has declined, the application of mild and soft stimulation for extended periods is often beneficial. In this manner the clinical application of acupuncture requires an understanding of what degree of stimulation is appropriate for each patient, and since the appropriate amount of stimulation can only be grasped through practical experience, the acupuncturist must constantly strive to improve his skill and practical knowledge.

(2) The Therapeutic Effects of Acupuncture

The therapeutic effects of acupuncture refer to the various effects of acupuncture which serve to correct the functional abnormalities in the tissues and organ systems of the body. The following effects of acupuncture can be listed as being the main therapeutic principles for treating various conditions, and to satisfy specific objectives in treatment:

Regulating effect

Applying an appropriate amount of acupuncture stimulation to the tissues and organ systems serves to regulate various physiological functions of the body. There are two different effects contained in the regulating effect of acupuncture. One is the sedating (inhibiting) effect by which hyperfunctions such as pain and muscle spasm are controlled and returned to a normal state. The other is the invigorating (exciting) effect by which the weakening or loss of nerve functions such as numbness and paralysis is reversed and the function of nerves is restored.

Induction effect

The direct acupuncture stimulation of the affected area and otherwise the stimulation of a distal area affects the vascular network to cause hyperemia in the stimulated area. This effect is used to regulate blood flow to the affected area. There are two different ways to apply the induction effect of acupuncture. One way is to induce blood flow to the affected area. In this approach the affected area is needled directly to increase circulation in the affected area. This approach is useful for localized anemia, muscle atrophy, and paralysis. The other way is to induce blood flow to a distal area. In this approach a part far removed from the affected area is needled when there is localized hyperemia or inflammation to reduce the circulation in the affected area. This approach is utilized in cases of cerebral hyperemia by needling the back of the neck, the shoulders, and upper back. It is also applied for catarrhal inflammation of the digestive organs by needling the sacroiliac region and the legs.

Anti-inflammatory effect

Very slight needling (especially the use of intradermal needles) causes reflexive vasoconstriction in the stimulated area and this reduces the blood flow in the area and facilitates the absorption of pathological secretions. Also, since slight needling serves to attract white blood cells to the stimulated area and causes an increase in the number of blood cells in the surrounding tissues, it is very useful in treating simple inflammation.

Hematinic effect

Acupuncture treatments directly and indirectly affect the function of the autonomic nervous system and generally creates a condition of parasympathetic tonus. This condition heightens the activity in reticuloendothelial tissue, which brings an increase in red blood cells, white blood cells, and platelets. Also this condition stimulates the production of antibodies and facilitates recovery from various illness.

(3) Indications for Acupuncture

The range of diseases that are treatable with acupuncture is very wide. In ancient China acupuncture was apparently used for almost every kind of disease. The main feature of acupuncture therapy is that it acts to correct dysfunctions of the nervous system, especially that involving the autonomic nervous system. Also the effect of acupuncture can be directed at specific areas of the body and there are no undesirable side effects. Even when treatments are not effective, the negative effects are negligible.

The best known effects of acupuncture therapy are the analgesic effect and the physiological regulating effect. The analgesic effect is greater where the pain is due to functional causes. When there is extreme pathology at the origin of the pain, acupuncture is often ineffective in relieving the pain. Acupuncture is also very effective in relieving physical discomfort which borders on pain (e.g., feeling of pressure, tension, stiffness, muscle fatigue). The physiological regulating effect of acupuncture occurs most notably in relation to the functioning of the autonomic nervous system. Regular acupuncture treatments have been proven as being helpful for reaching optimum body weight, sleeping better, improving appetite, controlling allergic reactions, increasing circulation, calming down, and enjoying a greater sense of well-being. The modulating effect on the nervous system is responsible for bringing relief from the various symptoms of the general adaptation syndrome (the so-called semi-sick condition).

Based on the above two therapeutic effects of acupuncture, the diseases which can be most effectively treated with acupuncture are those of a functional nature. The following are the commonly encountered conditions and symptoms, which are not only safe for acupuncture but respond well to acupuncture.

Disorders of the nervous system
Various types of neuralgia of the peripheral nerves, spasms, paralysis, neurasthenia, hysteria, migraine, tetany, writer's cramp

Disorders of the circulatory system
Cardiac neurasthenia (e.g., nervous palpitation, nervous cardialgia), essential hypertension, various symptoms of arteriosclerosis (e.g., headache, dizziness, tinnitus, neck and shoulder tension, constipation, insomnia, lassitude)

Disorders of the musculoskeletal system
Acute and chronic arthritis, acute and chronic muscular rheumatism, lumbago, interscapular pain, contusions, sprains (useful primarily for the analgesic effect)

Disorders of the digestive system
Parotiditis, esophageal spasm and paralysis, acute and chronic gastritis, gastro-atony, gastric neurosis (gastrospasm, nervous indigestion), acute enterocolitis, intestinal atony, hepatic congestion, constipation, diarrhea, hemorrhoids

Disorders of the respiratory system
Chronic bronchitis, bronchial asthma

Disorders of the urogenital organs
Edema due to chronic nephritis, cystitis, cystospasm, urethral inflammation, testitis

Pediatric disorders
Pediatric dyspepsia, night terror, convulsive fits, nocturnal enuresis

Gynecological disorders
Uterospasms, menstrual irregularities, menstrual pains

Although acupuncture is effective for the conditions listed above, acupuncture and moxibustion are generally used to treat traditional syndromes or symptom complexes, so it must be kept in mind that acupuncture therapy, rather than being effective against specific disease entities, is effective in alleviating or relieving a variety of symptoms which appear as a result of disease.

(4) Contraindications for Acupuncture

Conditions Not Suited for Acupuncture
The conditions not suited for acupuncture refer to those conditions which do not respond well to acupuncture or those cases which may be aggravated by acupuncture stimulation despite the positive effects of acupuncture. The main conditions in this category are skin diseases, febrile diseases, parasites, denaturation or hypertrophy, necrosis, neoplasms, syphilis, and leprosy.

Conditions Contraindicated for Acupuncture
The conditions contraindicated for acupuncture are those conditions in which acupuncture can actually cause harm. The main conditions in this category include the legally designated communicable diseases, tetanus, erysipelas, hemophilia, scurvy, and purpura. Otherwise there are the following conditions and temporary situations for which acupuncture must be avoided:

1. Extreme emaciation
2. Very unstable stage of diseases
3. High fevers
4. Very high blood pressure
5. Extremes of emotion such as during great anger or grief
6. Immediately after a massive hemorrhage
7. Violent mental illnesses
8. During strong palpitations or dizziness
9. Right after a meal or on a very empty stomach
10. After drinking alcohol

Parts of Body Contraindicated for Acupuncture

There are certain parts of the body in which needles must not be inserted under ordinary circumstances. The areas not to be penetrated in acupuncture are the fontanelle, medulla, eyeballs, ear drums, pharynx, trachea, lungs, heart, pleura, peritoneum, testicles, major blood vessels, and the uterus during pregnancy.

(5) Sanitation and Sterilization for Acupuncture

Every acupuncturist must take appropriate steps to insure against possible infection by preventing contamination of the needles and equipment before treatment and by safely disposing used needles and materials. For general sanitation the practitioner's gown should be clean at all times and any linen used by the patients must be washed after each use. Also all working surfaces and tables on which acupuncture equipment is kept must be cleaned regularly with a disinfectant. A variety of cleaning agents can be used to disinfect equipment, but usually a 0.1 percent solution of corrosive sublimate is used to sterilize glass and steel and 3 percent solution of lysol is used to clean plastic and other materials. To maintain asepsis in the process of needling, the practitioner's hands must be washed thoroughly with soap and water before and after each treatment. All the needles and equipment coming in contact with needles (needle trays, needle tubes, etc.) must be sterilized by a reliable means before use. The area to be needled must first be disinfected with sterile cotton saturated with a 70 percent solution of ethyl alcohol. The practitioner's hands and fingers must also be disinfected just prior to needle insertion with cotton saturated with alcohol. Once the needles are removed, they should immediately be placed in a special container for used needles. In order to prevent accidental infection, needles to be disposed must be placed in a closed container for disposal clearly marked with a warning that contaminated needles are enclosed. If the needles are to be reused, they should be soaked in a disinfecting detergent solution prior to being sterilized.

The recent spread of AIDS has greatly increased public concern regarding the cleanliness and safety of health care professions including acupuncture. AIDS and Hepatitis B pose a serious threat to the health and safety of practitioners as well as patients, and the highest standards of hygiene and sterilization must be used to prevent infection through acupuncture. The following sterilization procedures are considered effective in preventing infection from viruses of AIDS and Hepatitis B as well as other microbes:

> Steam heat sterilization of 250°F at 15 pounds pressure
>   for thirty minutes
> Dry heat sterilization of 338°F for two hours
> Ethylene oxide sterilization

(6) Body Positioning for Acupuncture

During the treatment the patient must be positioned in such a way that the tension or relaxation of the part being needled can be adjusted according to need. When the lateral aspect of the limbs, the upper back, the lumbar region, or the buttocks are to be needled on one side, the patient should assume the side-lying position with the area to be needled facing up. In this case the arms should be slightly bent and placed in front. Also the patient's knees should be comfortably bent. The natural flexion of the limbs in this way allows the muscle tension to be increased or decreased as needed. The practitioner can stand on either side of the patient, but it is usually more convenient to stand in back of the patient.

When the anterior aspect of the neck, the anterior thoracic region, or the medial aspect of the legs are to be needled, the patient should assume the supine position. When needling the anterior aspect of the neck, the skin tends to move around so a small pillow can be placed under the neck and occipital area to extend the neck backward and stretch out the skin on the anterior aspect of the neck. When the scalp, occipital area, or scapular region are to be needled, the patient should assume the seated position and place both hands on their lap in a relaxed manner. The practitioner generally stands behind the patient, but it is also possible to needle while sitting in a chair.

(7) How to Avoid Problems in Acupuncture

Problems which occasionally arise from inserting an acupuncture needle, such as subcutaneous bleeding and the needle becoming stuck, are preventable with the proper precautions. Before an acupuncture needle is used on a patient, it must be inspected closely for imperfections. If the tip of the needle is blunted or damaged or if the body of the needle is bent or marred in any way, the needle must be discarded since its use could cause unnecessary pain and there is greater possibility of it becoming stuck or breaking. Sometimes even inserting a good acupuncture needle can prove quite difficult because the underlying tissues are tightly contracted. If this ever happens, do not force the needle in. Forcing the needle often causes pain and there is greater risk of needle breakage. In such a case it is best to thoroughly massage the tense area with the fingertips to relax it before needle insertion. Also, rather than inserting the needle directly into the tense point, insert it just next to the tense point. Needling adjacent points should relax the tense point enough so that a needle can be inserted in the focal point of tension.

Sometimes a needle will become stuck after insertion and the needle will not come out because of a localized muscle spasm around the needle. If this happens, do not pull the needle out by force. Pulling the needle forcefully is painful to the patient and is damaging to the surrounding tissues, and in rare instances it can cause the needle to break. When a needle becomes stuck and cannot be withdrawn easily, try inserting the needle a little deeper (where this can be done safely). Briefly twist and rotate the needle at the deeper level and then try to withdraw it again. If the needle is still stuck, tap the skin around the inserted needle with a fingertip or a guide tube to relax the tissue and then try to withdraw it once more. If the needle will not budge after tapping the surrounding skin, insert a few needles just adjacent to the stuck needle and apply some lifting and thrusting on them. This procedure should enable the stuck needle to be removed easily.

Occasionally, after a needle is removed there is some bleeding, subcutaneous hemorrhaging, or formation of a small node at the point needled. If there is any bleeding, the point should be immediately wiped with a cotton swab soaked in alcohol and the point should be pressed firmly and massaged with a fingertip in a circular motion for about a minute. Massaging the point of insertion in advance is useful for preventing the above mentioned problems, and massaging the point after needling serves to stop bleeding and node formation.

(8) How to Deal with Needle Breakage

In rare instances an acupuncture needle will break because the patient makes a sudden movement during needling or because a damaged needle is used. If it should ever happen that a needle breaks during insertion, press on either side of the point with the thumb and index finger of the pressing hand so as to spread the skin and expose the end of the broken needle. Do not say anything if the patient is unaware of the situation, because this could upset the patient and further complicate matters. After locating the exposed end of the needle, remove it with a pair of tweezers.

If the needle breaks below the skin and the end cannot be brought to the surface by pressing around it, simply press the point of insertion gently and leave it. Leaving a broken needle in the body usually does not have any adverse effects especially if the needle that broke was thin and short. A dull needle sensation may remain for a few days afterward, but other than this nothing should happen. When the broken needle is a number two or three gauge needle and it is not much more than one cun in length, it remains in the superficial muscles without harm. Over time the needle curls into a tiny ball by the repeated contraction and expansion of the muscles. New connective tissue forms around the curled-up needle so that it becomes a harmless small mass imbedded between the layers of muscle.

The situation is more serious if a needle breaks close to a vital organ or a major blood vessel, or if a deeply inserted long and thick needle breaks. If this happens, a physician must be consulted to surgically remove the needle. The surgical removal of the needle can be expedited by inserting another needle adjacent to the site of the broken needle and taking radiographs to precisely locate the buried needle in reference to the adjacent needle.

2. Guidelines for the Application of Moxibustion

(1) Amount of Stimulation in Moxibustion

Just as in acupuncture, attention must be paid to provide the optimal amount of stimulation in the application of moxibustion. The amount of heat stimulation in moxibustion can be regulated by controlling the size of the moxa cone, the number of cones applied, and the compactness of the moxa material. The appropriate amount of stimulation for each patient is decided based on the age, sex, constitution, weight, and other factors relating to sensitivity as well as the aim of the treatment. Generally a limited number of cones of a smaller size is applied on older and weaker patients as well as on those patients who tend to be nervous or hypersensitive. A greater number of cones of a larger size are applied on those patients who are better able to tolerate heat stimulation. The factors which deter-

mine a patient's sensitivity to moxibustion are basically the same as those listed
for acupuncture stimulation.

The general standard for the number of cones to be applied is three to ten cones
for children around the age of ten and seven to twenty cones for adults. The standard size of moxa cones for direct moxibustion (tōnetsu-kyū) is the size of a grain of
rice. Sometimes larger moxa cones are applied, but they are rarely made larger
than a soybean. Moxa cones of a larger size are applied only for suppurative moxibustion. In most situations which require more stimulation, it is better to keep
the size of the cones small and increase the number of cones for mild but sustained
heat stimulation.

Normally moxibustion treatments are applied once a day and a course of treatments lasts from three to seven days. Usually the moxibustion treatment is discontinued for the same number of days before resuming with another course of
treatment. There are some chronic conditions in which daily moxibustion treatments without intervals are beneficial. However, when the patient does not respond
well to continuous moxibustion treatments or shows undesirable reactions, the
treatments must be discontinued. Be that as it may, daily moxibustion is practiced
widely in Japan because it is very useful for treating chronic conditions and
improving health. The best approach in daily moxibustion treatments is to teach
patients or their family members to apply moxa on a few points everyday so that
the effects are mild but consistent and sustained. It is interesting to note that the
Chinese character for moxibustion is composed of two parts. The top portion
means a long time and the bottom means fire. This implies that the moxibustion
must be continued for a long time to be effective.

(2) The Therapeutic Effects of Moxibustion

The therapeutic effects of moxbustion, in the same manner as in acupuncture, serve
to adjust any functional abnormalities in the organs and tissues of the body to
restore a normal physiological equilibrium. The following therapeutic effects of
moxibustion can be listed according to various aims of treatment:

Regulating Effect
The regulating effect of moxibustion is obtained by applying the appropriate
amount of heat stimulation on the body to arouse and promote those functions
that are weakened or lacking and to sedate and reduce those functions that
are abnormally heightened. The size of the moxa cones and the number of cones
are determined according to whether the functons of the organs and tissues are to
be aroused or sedated. Abnormal function of the sensory nerves such as hyperesthesia and paresthesia can often be cured by this effect of moxibustion. The
regulating effect is also beneficial for conditions like polio in which there is an
abnormal increase or decrease in peristalsis.

Induction Effect
The primary (initial) effect of moxibustion is to cause vasoconstriction, and the
secondary (delayed) effect is to cause vasodilation. This effect can be utilized to
draw blood from one part to another part. For example, in cases of congestive

headaches or cerebral hemorrhage, moxibustion is applied to the extremities to cause vasodilation in the peripheral areas and thus reduce the circulation to the head. Also, when there is localized hyperemia (inflammation) deep inside the body, moxibustion is applied to the surrounding skin surface to cause vasodilation in the superficial capillary networks to draw blood to the skin (away from the inflammation).

Reflexive Effect

The heat stimulation of moxibustion has a reflexive effect which can arouse or sedate the functioning of organs and tissues, and this effect also enhances endocrine function. Applying moxibustion on the back, for example, serves to alleviate various nervous disorders of the visceral organs. The reflexive effect is commonly utilized by stimulating corresponding organ points on the back to cure functional disorders.

Cardiovascular Effect

Moxibustion has been shown to increase blood cell count, especially red blood cells. An increase in red blood cells causes a marked increase in plasma hemoglobin. In addition moxibustion reduces blood clotting time and increases the contractile strength of the cardiovascular system. For these reasons, moxibustion is said to have a hematinic (blood building) effect, a blood coagulation enhancing effect, and a cardiotonic effect.

Immunological Effect

Aside from the positive effect of moxibustion on the cardiovascular system, it produces immunogens which stimulate and strengthen the immunological response. This increases the body's resistance to disease and is instrumental in preventing illness. This effect of moxibustion accounts for the widespread application of moxibustion from ancient times for the purpose of preventing illness.

(3) The Indications and Contraindications for Moxibustion

The indications for moxibustion treatment are essentially the same as those for acupuncture treatment, but moxibustion is known to be particularly effective for chronic conditions. The contraindications for moxibustion treatment are also very similar to those for acupuncture treatment. Since those conditions treatable with moxibustion and those not to be treated with moxibustion are more or less the same as those conditions already listed as indications and contraindications for acupuncture, refer back to the previous section for specific indications and contra-indications.

(4) Precautions in Applying Moxibustion

Before giving moxibustion treatments, the practitioner must judge whether moxibustion is indicated or not based on the patient's complaints and the examination. When moxibustion is indicated, the patient's sex, age, constitution, and physical problem must be taken into consideration to decide the number of points and the size and number of cones to be applied. Before applying any moxa, all the areas to be treated must first be disinfected with alcohol.

When administering a moxibustion treatment, whether seated or standing, the practitioner should maintain a good posture. Idle conversation must be avoided to enable the treatment to proceed in a quiet and serious manner. During the moxibustion treatment the patient should assume a comfortable and relaxed position. The points should be marked in advance so the moxa cones can be placed accurately. During the burning of the first few moxa cones, it is helpful to press the skin on both sides of the cone so that the pain is reduced.

A moxibustion treatment consists of making small burns on the skin so there is not the same need for thorough sterilization as in acupuncture, but since communicable diseases can be transmitted, the practitioner's hands and any equipment should be kept clean and sterile. Also, for good measure, the point on which moxa is applied should be disinfected with alcohol before and after applying the moxa.

(5) How to Prevent Infection after Moxibustion

Sometimes it happens that the area treated with moxibustion becomes infected. This usually happens because the blister raised by the moxibustion is scratched and bacteria enter from the break in the skin. Infections are more likely when the burn left by moxibustion is large. Large burns cause localized skin inflammation and blisters (lymph secretions under a thin layer of skin) which can be quite irritating. Scratching this blister damages the skin, which acts as a barrier to microorganisms, and this can lead to an infection. When the burn left by moxibustion is small, however, infections are rare because the blister is very small, there is very little irritation, and it heals rapidly.

Therefore, in order to prevent infection in the area treated by moxibustion, the burn must be kept as small as possible. So it follows that the size of the moxa cones applied should be very small except in special cases. Further, when applying moxa repeatedly on the same point, special attention must be paid to place the cones on the exact same point. Since blisters form more often when the combustion temperature of the burning moxa is low, the same point should be treated repeatedly with moxa cones which burn quickly and efficiently. It is also important to warn the patient against scratching the points treated with moxibustion. If a blister is broken accidentally, the area should be disinfected with alcohol or mercurochrome.

(6) How to Deal with Infections

If the area treated with moxibustion should become infected and there is marked redness and swelling in the surrounding area, a zink borate paste (5 percent boric acid, 5 percent zink oxide, 90 percent unguentum simplex) can be applied to disinfect the area. The application of penicillin paste or mercurochrome is also quite effective for disinfecting and reducing the inflammation. Sometimes when the burned area is very small and the redness and swelling is very slight, applying several more cones of moxa on the infected point will speed up the healing process.

Part II

Clinical Application

1. Occipital Neuralgia (Pain and Tension in Occipital Region)

Description

Occipital neuralgia is characterized by paroxysmal pain occurring in the occipital region, which radiates from the nuchal region up to the vertex. The pain is usually aggravated by brushing the hair or turning the head. The majority of simple headaches are caused by circulatory disorders in the cerebrum, but pain from occipital neuralgia is felt in the scalp since this condition is a functional disorder of the nerves innervating the scalp. For this reason, just touching the hair on the scalp can cause a prickling pain. The pain is usually localized in the back of the head and neck. Another feature of occipital neuralgia is that there is tenderness along the course of the occipital nerves.

The cause of occipital neuralgia, just as in other forms of neuralgia, varies widely from common colds, infectious diseases, strain and tension in the occipital region, to spinal disorders (e.g., caries and tumors). Because the cause of occipital neuralgia could be serious, x-rays of the cervical vertebrae must be obtained to rule out spinal disorders. Occipital neuralgia is usually seen in those who tend to have a nervous disposition, and the pain is often aggravated by mental stress.

Acupuncture points

Behind ear—GB-11, GB-12
Occipital region—GV-15, GV-16, GV-17, BL-9, BL-10
Lateral neck—GB-20, SI-17
Upper back—BL-11, BL-12
Shoulders—GB-21, SI-13
Hands—LI-4
Legs—GB-34

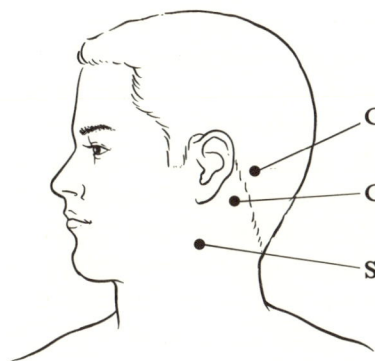

GV-17 (Nōko)
BL-9 (Gyokuchin)
GV-16 (Fūfu)
GB-20 (Fūchi)
GV-15 (Amon)
BL-10 (Tenchū)
GB-21 (Kensei)
BL-11 (Daijo)
BL-12 (Fūmon)

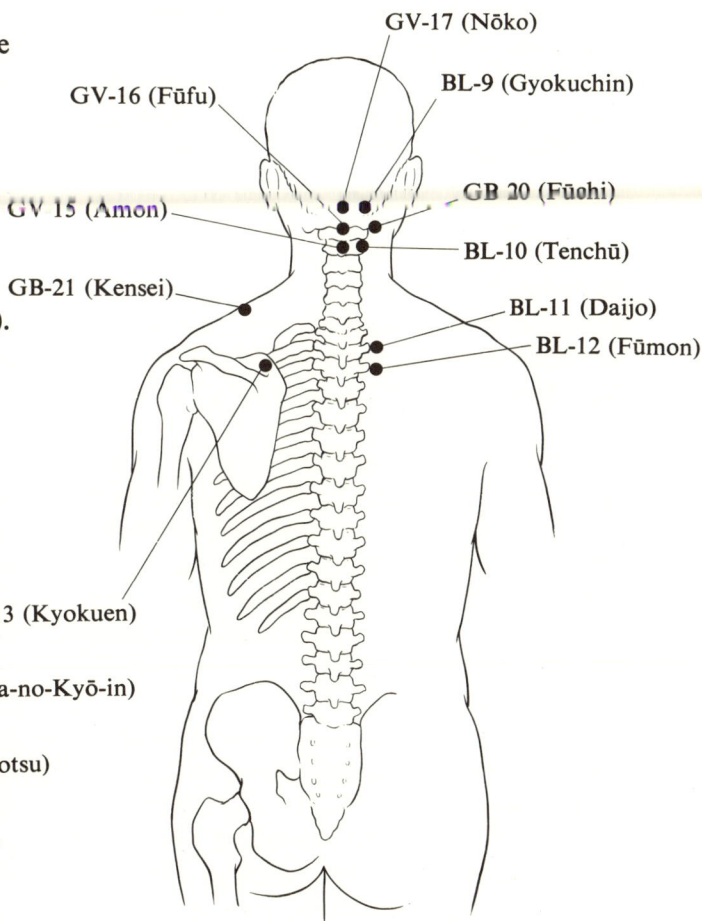

SI-13 (Kyokuen)
GB-11 (Atama-no-Kyō-in)
GB-12 (Kankotsu)
SI-17 (Tenyō)

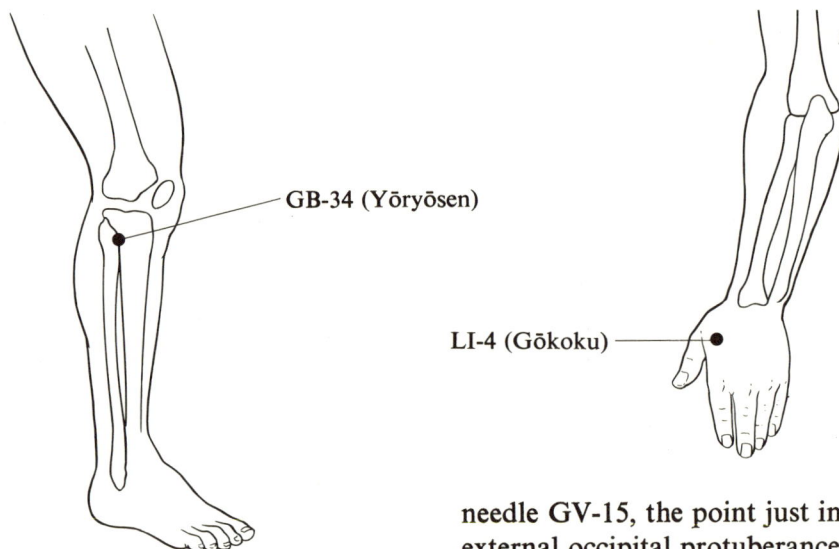

GB-34 (Yōryōsen)

LI-4 (Gōkoku)

Treatment

The occipital nerve consists of the greater and lesser occipital nerves. The greater occipital nerve (under BL-10) innervates the scalp on the medial portion of the occiput. It surfaces around the inferior border of the occiput, passes about 2.5 centimeters lateral to the external occipital protuberance, and goes up to the vertex. The lessor occipital nerve (under GB-20) travels a similar course about 2.5 centimeters lateral to the greater occipital nerve and innervates the scalp on the lateral aspect of the occiput, which is known as the retroauricular region.

In acute cases of occipital neuralgia, when the pain is so intense that combing the hair is unbearable, begin the treatment by applying a warm compress on the occipital region. Have the patient assume the prone position for the acupuncture treatment and insert needles in BL-11, BL-12, GB-21, and SI-13 to a depth of about two centimeters until a slight needle sensation is obtained and then retain the needles. Next insert needles vertically into BL-10 and GB-20 in the occipital region (to a depth of 1 to 1.5 cm) and apply some lifting and thrusting on the needles after obtaining a slight needle sensation and then retain the needles. Next

needle GV-15, the point just inferior to the external occipital protuberance. This point is traditionally forbidden to acupuncture so do not insert the needle very deep. Needle this point for the purpose of reducing tension in the occipital region, but do not go deeper than five millimeters.

In cases of lesser occipital neuralgia, with the pain in the lateral aspect of the occiput behind the ears, needle GB-11 and GB-12 on the posterior margin of the mastoid process. In cases of greater occipital neuralgia, with the pain extending from the posterior aspect of the neck up to the vertex, needle GV-17, GV-16, and BL-9 horizontally with the tip of the needle aimed up toward the vertex and retain the needles. Insert the needles in BL-9 so that the needle passes between the skull and scalp. These needles should be retained five to ten minutes.

If the method of retaining needles described above does not bring relief, another effective approach that can be used in the follow-up treatment is to select a few points with the greatest tenderness and to apply low frequency electrical stimulation through needles inserted in these tender points. In treating occipital neuralgia, it is also useful to needle LI-4 on the back of the hand and GB-34 on the side of the leg as distal points of stimulation.

2. Trigeminal Neuralgia

Description

Trigeminal neuralgia is characterized by paroxysmal attacks of intense pain along the course of the trigeminal nerve on the face. Trigeminal neuralgia is most common among middle-aged women. Sometimes trigeminal neuralgia occurs spontaneously for no apparent cause (idiopathic trigeminal neuralgia), and on other occasions it occurs as a symptom of other pathology (e.g., brain tumors, aneurysms, sinusitis, and infectious diseases). Idiopathic cases of trigeminal neuralgia usually involve just one branch of the trigeminal nerve and only rarely is the whole nerve affected. Also idiopathic cases are most common among older individuals, there is no motor impairment, and only one side is affected. Symptomatic cases of trigeminal neuralgia, on the other hand, quite often affect all branches of the trigeminal nerve, and occurs equally often in all age groups. In symptomatic cases, aside from pain, there is sensory impairment on facial skin, loss of the corneal reflex and the mandibular reflex, and spasm or atrophy in the temporal and masseter muscles. Idiopathic cases tend to occur sporadically, but in symptomatic cases the pain persists and

intensifies with paroxysmal attacks. In both types of trigeminal neuralgia, however, there are paroxysmal attacks of pain and there is marked tenderness at the point where the affected branch of the trigeminal nerve emerges from the cranial fossa to the skin.

There are characteristic tender points for each type of trigeminal neuralgia according to the branch affected. Tenderness is present at the supraorbital foramen if the first branch is affected (ophthalmic neuralgia). Tenderness is present at the infraorbital foramen and zygomaticofacial foramen with second branch involvement (maxillary neuralgia) and likewise at the mental foramen with third branch involvement (mandibular neuralgia). Attacks of pain in trigeminal neuralgia are often induced by exposure to cold, talking, chewing, and vibration. The mucous membranes of the facial region become inflamed during attacks

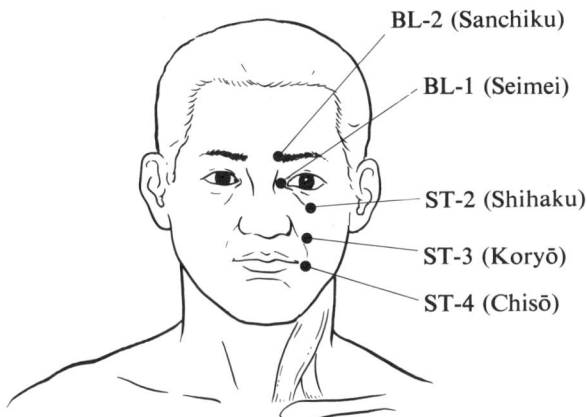

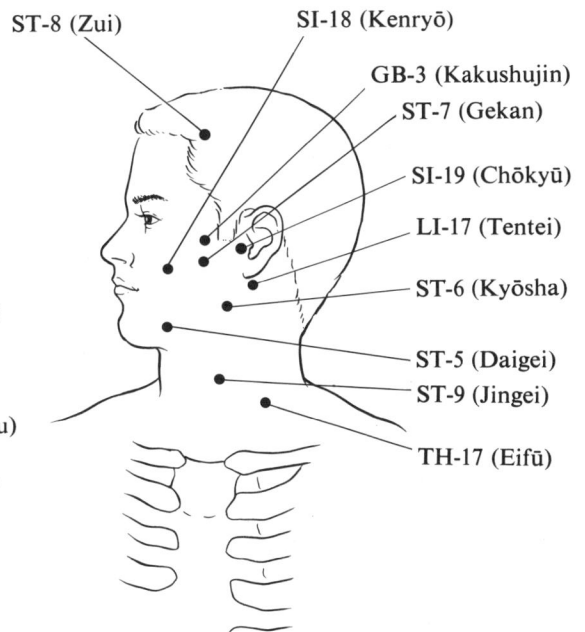

BL-2 (Sanchiku)
BL-1 (Seimei)
ST-2 (Shihaku)
ST-3 (Koryō)
ST-4 (Chisō)

ST-8 (Zui)
SI-18 (Kenryō)
GB-3 (Kakushujin)
ST-7 (Gekan)
SI-19 (Chōkyū)
LI-17 (Tentei)
ST-6 (Kyōsha)
ST-5 (Daigei)
ST-9 (Jingei)
TH-17 (Eifū)

of trigeminal neuralgia and there is an increase in excretions such as sweat, tears, and saliva along with a substantial increase in nasal discharge.

Acupuncture points
Face—BL-1, BL-2, ST-2, ST-3, ST-4, ST-5, ST-6, ST-7, ST-8, SI-18, SI-19, GB-3, GV-24
Ear—TH-17
Anterior neck—ST-9, LI-17
Posterior neck—GB-20, BL-10
Shoulders—GB-21, SI-13
Hands—LI-4
Legs—GB-40

Treatment
It is important to distinguish idiopathic

trigeminal neuralgia from symptomatic manifestations of other pathology. Idiopathic trigeminal neuralgia has the following characteristics:

(1) It occurs sporadically by fatigue or exposure to cold.
(2) There is tenderness at specific sites such as the supraorbital foramen,

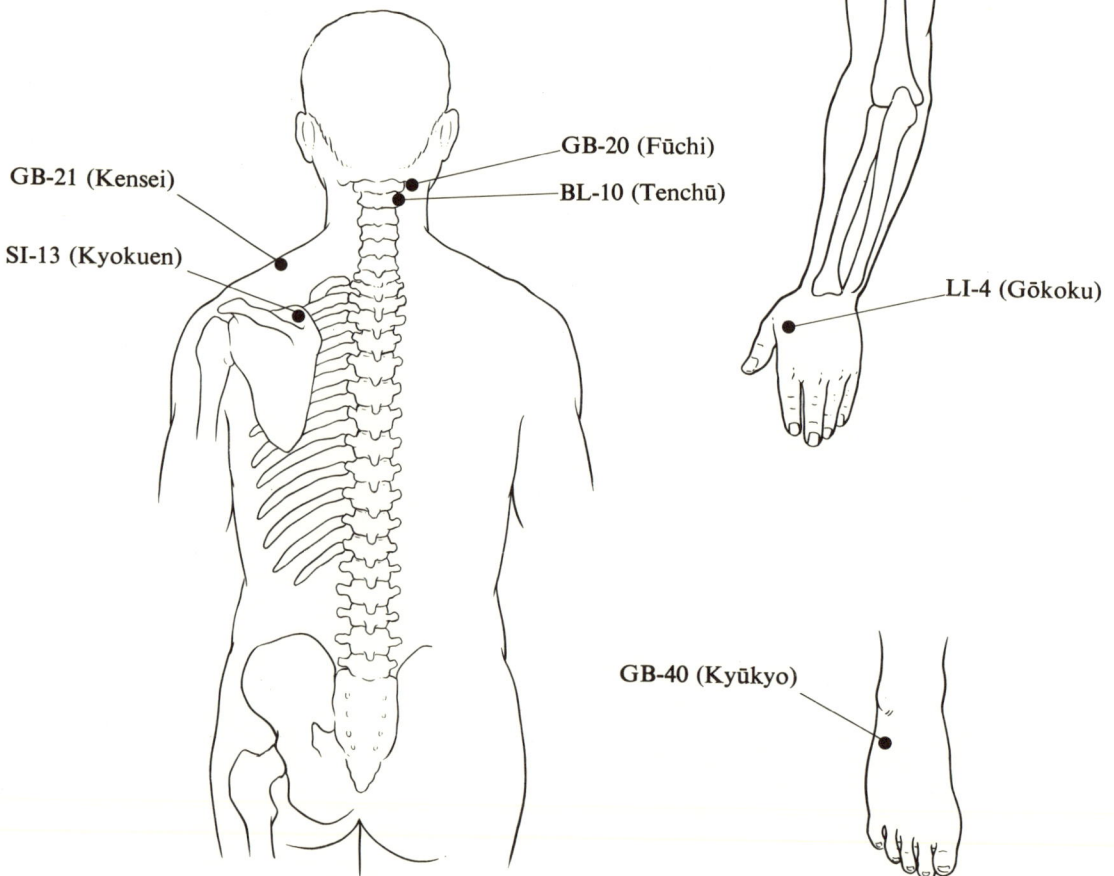

GB-21 (Kensei)

SI-13 (Kyokuen)

GB-20 (Fūchi)

BL-10 (Tenchū)

LI-4 (Gōkoku)

GB-40 (Kyūkyo)

infraorbital foramen, and mental foramen.

(3) The pain occurs on one side only.
(4) There is no paralysis of facial muscles.

In ophthalmic neuralgia the pain occurs in the frontal region, upper eyelids, and bridge of the nose. In this case needle BL-1 (shallow vertical insertion with a slight medial slant), BL-2 (horizontal insertion with needle directed laterally under the eyebrow), and GV-24 (horizontal insertion with needle pointing downward). In maxillary neuralgia the pain occurs in the lower eyelids, cheeks, upper lip, and teeth. In this case needle ST-2 (oblique insertion pointing upward at a 45 degree angle so as to reach the infraorbital foramen), ST-3 (horizontal insertion pointing downward), ST-4 (horizontal insertion pointing downward or toward the ears; be careful not to penetrate into the oral cavity), and SI-18 (oblique insertion pointing downward). In mandibular neuralgia the pain occurs in the temporal region in front of the ear and in the lower lip and teeth. In this case needle ST-8 (horizontal insertion pointing toward vertex), SI-19, GB-2, and ST-7 (vertical insertion with slight upward angle), and ST-5 (oblique insertion aimed posteriorly).

No matter which branch of the trigeminal nerve is affected, it is useful to needle TH-17, which is in the depression behind the earlobe (oblique insertion pointing upward). Needling TH-17 is especially important in cases of trigeminal neuralgia because this point is located directly over the ganglion of the trigeminal nerve. After finding out which branch is affected and inserting needles in the appropriate points, apply gentle lifting and thrusting and twisting on the needles and then retain them for ten to fifteen minutes. Good results can also be obtained by applying low frequency electrical stimulation to the needles. The electrical stimulation should cause a mild sensation and slight twitching around the needle (apply frequency of one Hz for about twenty minutes).

Aside from the points mentioned above, ST-9 and LI-17 on the neck should be needled gently for the purpose of improving circulation in the head and facial region as well as for relaxing the sternocleidomastoid muscle. Also BL-10 and GB-20 on the back of the neck and GB-21 and SI-13 on the shoulders should be needled lightly to relieve the muscular tension in the shoulders resulting from facial pain. It is important to always needle distal points such as LI-4 along with other local points. Often patients with trigeminal neuralgia experience chilling in their feet. Neuralgic pain in the face tends to decrease once circulation is improved and the feet warm up. Another way to enhance the effect of the acupuncture treatment is to use moxibustion. The gallbladder meridian covers the entire temporal region, so applying moxibustion to GB-40 (source point of the gallbladder meridian) usually increases the effect. For this point, consecutively apply ten to thirty moxa cones the size of a rice grain.

Applying warm compresses on the occipital region and giving light finger pressure also helps to relieve the facial pain. Generally the pain is largely alleviated after one treatment, but the pain tends to return in several days. Therefore repeat the treatments at appropriate intervals to control the pain, and continue giving treatments until the pain is completely gone.

3. Trauma to Cervical Vertebrae (Whiplash Injury)

Description

The most common cause of trauma to the cervical vertebrae is traffic accidents. Whiplash, in particular, is a common injury which occurs during rear end collisions. In whiplash the neck undergoes hyperextension and hyperflexion which traumatizes the cervical vertebrae. In most cases the symptoms characteristic of whiplash do not appear immediately after the injury. In 70 to 80 percent of the cases the symptoms of whiplash start to appear from several hours to twenty-four hours after the accident, and in 10 to 15 percent of the cases the symptoms begin between twenty-four and forty-eight hours later. Occasionally there are cases where the symptoms do not appear for up to a few weeks. A chronic case of whiplash presents symptoms very similar to herniation of intervertebral disks in the cervical vertebrae. The typical symptoms of whiplash are as follows:

(1) Pain in the neck and occipital region which is strongest when extending the neck
(2) Muscular tension and stiffness in neck and shoulders
(3) Pain, numbness, and paresthesia extending down the arm
(4) Pain in the upper back
(5) Neuralgia of greater occipital nerve
(6) Autonomic dysfunction including headache, nausea, dizziness, ocular pain, lacrimation, tinnitus, and disturbance in visual accommodation

Acupuncture points

Posterior neck—BL-10, GB-20, GB-12, points adjacent to spaces between spinous process of the cervical vertebrae
Lateral neck—SI-17, LI-17
Shoulders—SI-11, SI-13, GB-21, LI-16, TH-15

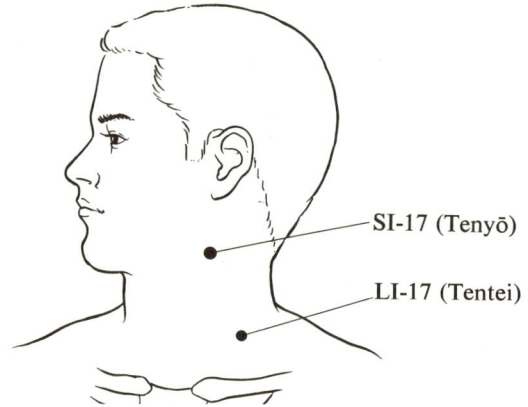

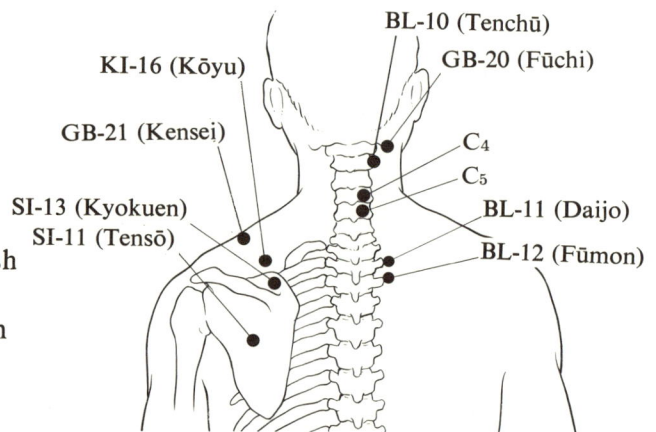

SI-17 (Tenyō)
LI-17 (Tentei)

BL-10 (Tenchū)
GB-20 (Fūchi)
KI-16 (Kōyu)
GB-21 (Kensei)
SI-13 (Kyokuen)
SI-11 (Tensō)
C₄
C₅
BL-11 (Daijo)
BL-12 (Fūmon)

Upper back—BL-11, BL-12
Arms—LI-7, LI-10, LI-11, TH-5, SI-6, LU-5, HT-3, PC-4, PC-6
Wrists—SI-5, TH-4, LI-5, PC-7, HT-7
Hands—LI-4

Treatment

The most important thing in the acute phase of whiplash is to immobilize and rest the cervical area for about one week. The symptoms vary according to the site and extent of damage to the tissues, and therefore points to alleviate these symptoms must be selected for treatment. For symptoms of soft tissue damage, such as headaches, difficulty in turning the head, and pain and stiffness in the shoulders, start the treatment by

LI-11 (Kyokuchi)

LI-10 (Te-no-Sanri)

LI-7 (Onryū)

TH-4 (Yōchi)

LI-5 (Yōkei)

LI-4 (Gōkoku)

TH-5 (Gaikan)

SI-6 (Yōrō)

SI-5 (Yōkoku)

LI-16 (Koketsu)

LU-5 (Shakutaku)

PC-4 (Gekimon)

PC-6 (Naikan)

PC-7 (Dairyō)

HT-3 (Shōkai)

HT-7 (Shinmon)

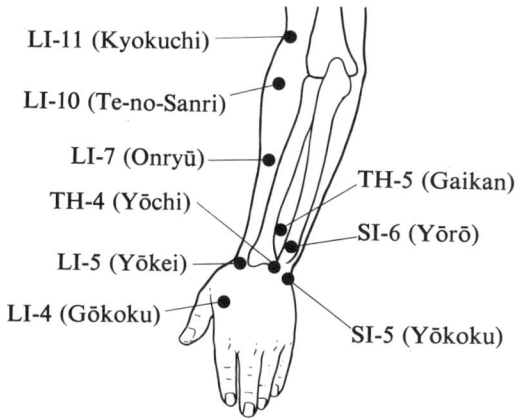

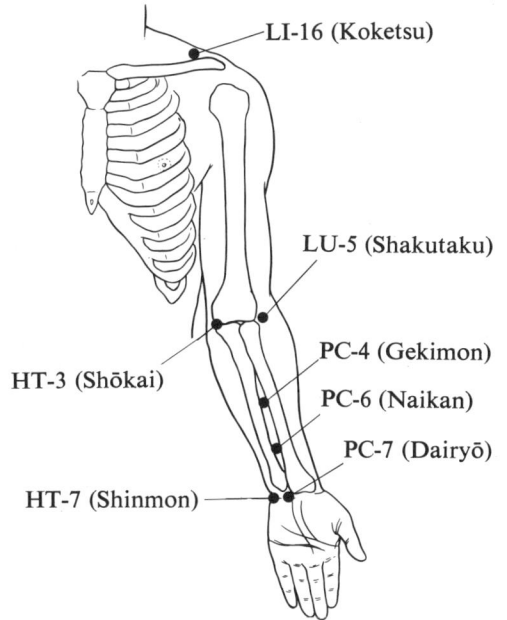

applying a warm compress to the back of the neck. Follow this by needling BL-10 and GB-20 in the occipital region, SI-11, SI-13, GB-21, LI-16, and BL-11 on the shoulders and back.

When there is numbness or loss of sensation in the hand, this is a sign of impingement of the spinal cord at the level of the cervical vertebrae, and this symptom is usually difficult to cure. When there is numbness in the thumb and index finger, the radial nerve is affected. In this case needle LI-11, LI-10, LI-7, LI-5, LI-4, and points just next to the space between the spinous processes of the fifth and sixth cervical vertebrae. When the numbness is in the middle finger, the medial nerve is affected, so needle LU-5, PC-4, PC-6, TH-5, PC-7, and points just next to the space between the spinous processes of the sixth and seventh cervical vertebrae. When the numbness is in the ring finger and little finger, the ulnar nerve is affected, so needle HT-3, HT-7, SI-5, SI-6, and points just next to the space between the spinous processes of the seventh cervical and first thoracic vertebrae. The purpose of needling the above points is to reduce the excitation of the affected nerve. Therefore, after inserting the needles apply rather vigorous lifting and thrusting and rotation on the needles. Then retain these needles for ten to fifteen minutes. Another effective method is to apply a low frequency

electrical current of one Hz through a few of these needles for about twenty minutes.

When there is tinnitus or dizziness, most likely there is some impediment in the vertebral artery passing through the cervical vertebrae. Before treating such a case, obtain x-rays of the head and neck to make sure that the structural damage is minimal. After confirming that these symptoms are due to minor disturbances in circulation, needle points on the back of the neck such as BL-10, GB-20, GB-12, and points just to either side of the space between the cervical vertebrae and retain the needles for five minutes. When there is nausea or palpitations, there is some disturbance in the sympathetic nerves or vagus nerve which lie next to the cervical vertebrae. In this case gently needle SI-17 and LI-17 on the side of the neck. The above needle stimulation is aimed at improving the disturbance in circulation caused by the damage to soft tissue surrounding the cervical vertebrae. Therefore it is important to apply gentle stimulation and continue the treatment over a long period of time. Applying moxibustion on points on the wrist such as TH-4 and LI-4 is also effective in cases of whiplash.

4. Scapulohumeral Periarthritis (Frozen Shoulder)

Description

Scapulohumeral periarthritis is a condition associated with aging. It results from degenerative changes in the ligaments, tendons, and muscles surrounding the scapulohumeral joint which causes the shoulder joint to become slightly inflamed. Scapulohumeral periarthritis is sometimes seen in younger individuals in association with a shoulder injury. It is most frequently seen in individuals between the ages of forty and sixty, and the main symptoms are restrictions in the movement of the shoulder joint and motor pain. In terms of occupational predisposition scapulohumeral periarthritis tends to occur among those whose work involves light physical work rather than those who engage in heavy physical labor. Although in some cases this condition is brought on by a minor injury or strain on the shoulder, there are many cases where there is no identifiable cause.

The characteristic of scapulohumeral periarthritis is that abduction and internal rotation causes pain while adduction and lateral rotation is not difficult. For this reason it becomes difficult to get one's hand around to the back or to comb one's hair. In the acute phase the pain often radiates down the arm to the forearm, and the pain

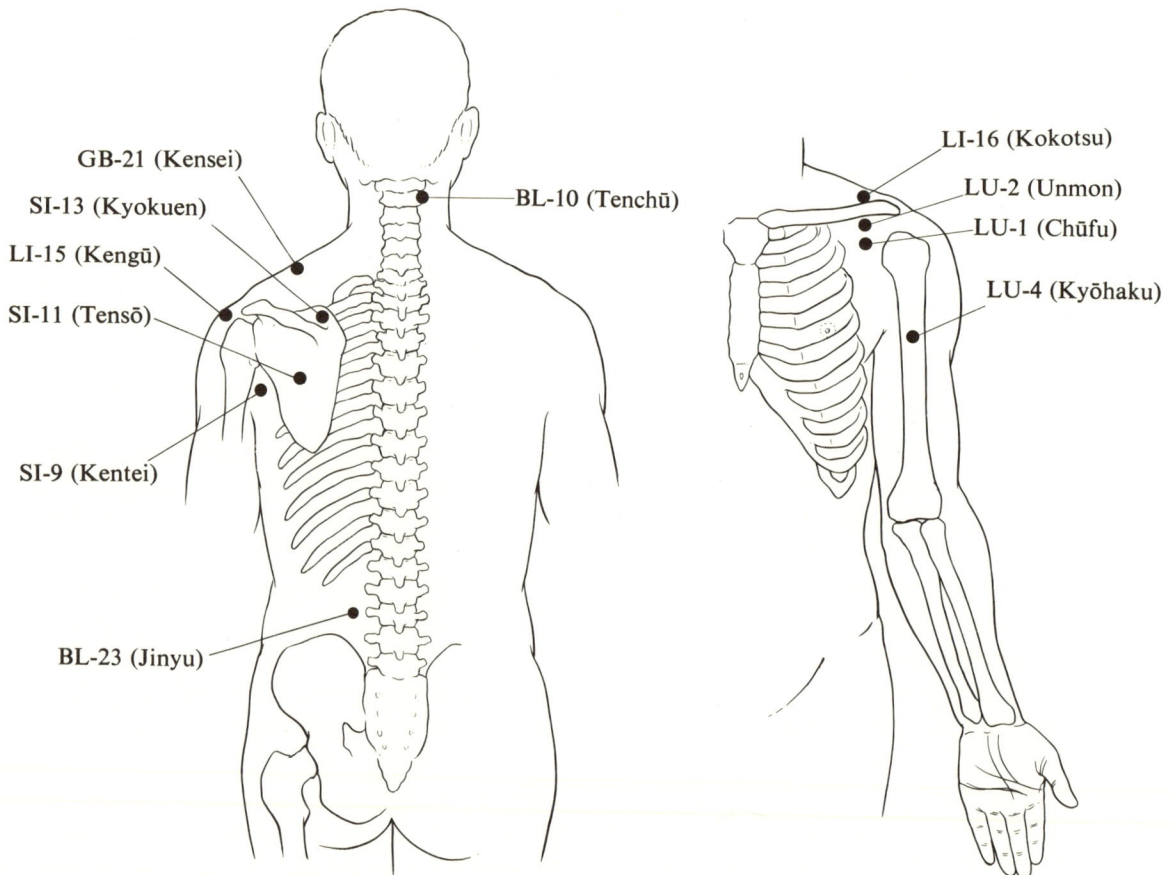

GB-21 (Kensei)
SI-13 (Kyokuen)
LI-15 (Kengū)
SI-11 (Tensō)
SI-9 (Kentei)
BL-10 (Tenchū)
BL-23 (Jinyu)

LI-16 (Kokotsu)
LU-2 (Unmon)
LU-1 (Chūfu)
LU-4 (Kyōhaku)

Shoulders—GB-21, LI-16, LI-15, SI-13, SI-11, SI-9
Arms—LU-4, TH-12, LI-14, LI-11, LI-10

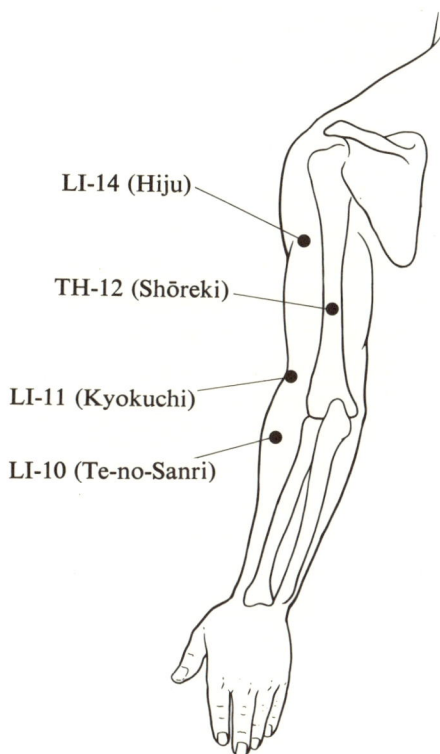

Treatment
The main symptoms of scapulohumeral periarthritis are shoulder pain and restricted shoulder movement. Acupuncture is effective in relieving the pain, but it cannot increase the range of motion. Therefore the key to treatment is to reduce the pain and then have the patient perform therapeutic exercises to restore the range of motion in the shoulder joint. The shoulder should not be treated in the acute phase when there are obvious signs of inflammation such as swelling and abnormal warmth. In the chronic phase it is best to begin the treatment by applying warm compresses or ultrasonic stimulation to warm the affected area and relax the soft tissues. It is good to follow the thermal stimulation with a massage of the muscles around the shoulder (e.g., latissimus dorsi, deltoid, teres major and minor, supraspinatus, infraspinatus, pectoralis major, trapezius, subscapularis, and triceps brachii muscles).

Before performing acupuncture carefully examine which movements of the shoulder joint are restricted (problems in abduction, internal rotation, and extension are most common). The origins and insertions of the muscles involved in the restrictions must be given special attention in needling. On the back of the neck needle BL-10 (origin of the superior fibers of the trapezius muscle; vertical insertion in a slightly upward direction) and on the shoulder, SI-13 (origin of levator scapulae muscle: oblique insertion in an upward direction) and GB-21 (vertical insertion). On the scapula needle SI-11 (vertical insertion) and also SI-9 (vertical insertion pointing slightly upward). Around the shoulder joint, needle the point between the head of the humerus and the coracoid process together with LI-15, which is just

LI-14 (Hiju)

TH-12 (Shōreki)

LI-11 (Kyokuchi)

LI-10 (Te-no-Sanri)

is strongest in the domain of the lateral cutaneous nerve of the arm. The motor pain and radiated pain can be quite intense in the acute phase and sometimes it disrupts sleep. The shoulder joint is moved less and less because of this pain and this eventually causes myogenic contractures to form. This brings a marked reduction in mobility and it becomes difficult to abduct and internally rotate the arm. X-rays of the shoulder often yield findings such as atrophy in ligaments and the origins of tendons, calcium deposits, and bursitis. But such findings are not rare among older individuals, and these findings cannot be regarded as being distinct features of scapulohumeral periarthritis.

Acupuncture points
Posterior neck—BL-10
Lumbar region—BL-23
Upper chest—LU-2, LU-1

lateral to the acromion (vertical insertion going between the bones by reach the joint capsule). Also needle LI-16 (insertion of supraspinatus muscle: oblique insertion going underneath the acromion), LU-2 (oblique insertion toward the acromion to penetrate the coracobrachialis muscle), LU-1 (obliquely toward the acromion), LI-14 (oblique insertion aimed upward), LU-4 (oblique insertion aimed upward), LI-11 (vertical insertion), and LI-10 (vertical insertion). The point at the lowest origin of the latissimus dorsi muscle, BL-23, is also an effective point (vertical insertion).

Once the needle is inserted in the above points lifting and thrusting and rotation should be applied to provide strong stimulation. Needle stimulation alone is usually sufficient, but another method for stronger stimulation is to have the patient move his arm with needles inserted. To do this insert the needles shallowly with the patient in the seated position and have him perform internal and external rotation movements of his arm with his elbow held against his torso and his arm bent. This movement should be repeated slowly back and forth about ten times. Since moving a part with needles inserted acts as very strong stimulation, it is advisable to massage the area thoroughly afterward. After the pain has been reduced or relieved by acupuncture treatments, the patient must begin therapeutic exercises to increase the range of motion. Therefore teach the patient some therapeutic exercises that can be performed at home (e.g., moving the arm through the full range of motion while holding some heavy object such as an iron).

5. Brachialgia (Tennis Elbow and Brachial Neuralgia)

Description

Tennis elbow is the most common type of elbow injury which can be effectively treated with acupuncture. Tennis elbow is known technically as lateral humeral epicondylitis and it occurs most among athletes and those whose occupations involve repeated extension of the elbow and pronation of the forearm. In epicondylitis a localized pain occurs at either the lateral or medial epicondyle of the humerus, but the restriction in movement is usually not substantial. The pain is felt when the elbow is extended and the forearm is rotated, and it results from tenosynovitis or inflammation in the periosteum at the place where the flexor muscles of the forearm attach to the humerus. Although there is tenderness in the affected lateral or medial epicondyle, there is no tenderness when pressing into the joint cavity.

Brachial neuralgia occurs with exposure to cold or as a result of overwork and fatigue. Often it is felt as a dull pain radiating down the arm, but occasionally there are paroxysmal attacks of intense pain. With brachial neuralgia there is marked tenderness all along the course of the affected nerve (radial, median, or ulnar nerve). The pain is produced by the irritation of a nerve and this can be caused by many things. The treatment for brachial neuralgia described below is for conditions associated with the cervicobrachial syndrome in which there is impingement of the nerve due to subluxations in the cervical vertebrae or by bone spurs (osteophytes).

GB-20 (Fūchi)

SI-13 (Kyokuen)

GB-21 (Kensei)

SI-11 (Tensō)

BL-10 (Tenchū)

BL-11 (Daijo)

BL-12 (Fūmon)

LI-15 (Kengū)

TH-14 (Kenryō)

LI-14 (Hiju)

LI-11 (Kyokuchi)

LI-10 (Te-no-Sanri)

LI-7 (Onryū)

TH-5 (Gaikan)

TH-4 (Yōchi)

LI-5 (Yōkei)

LI-4 (Gōkoku)

LI-16 (Kokotsu)

LU-5 (Shakutaku)

PC-4 (Gekimon)

HT-3 (Shōkai)

PC-6 (Naikan)

PC-3 (Kyokutaku)

HT-7 (Shinmon)

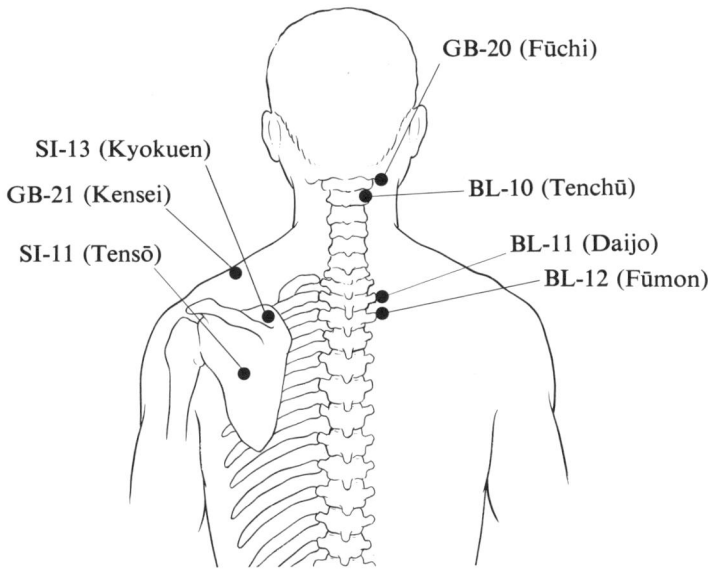

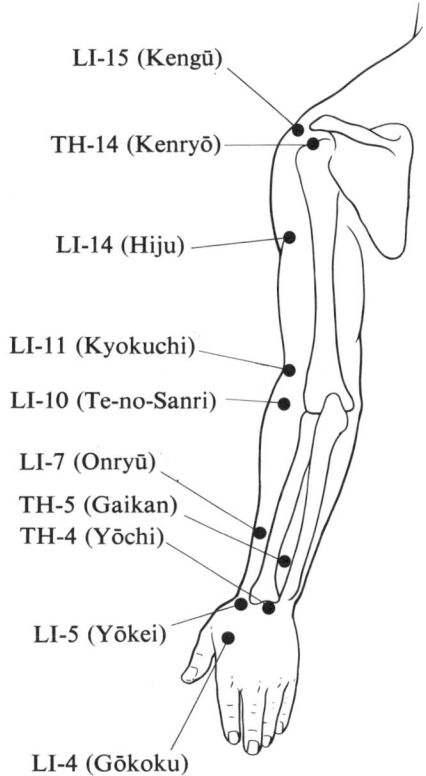

Acupuncture points

Posterior neck—GB-20, BL-10, points
adjacent to spaces between spinous
process of the cervical vertebrae

Upper back—BL-11, BL-12

Shoulders—GB-21, LI-15, LI 16, SI-11,
SI-13, TH-14

Upper arms—LI-14

Elbows—LI-11, HT-3, PC-3, LU-5

Forearms—LI-10, LI-7, PC-4, PC-6

Wrists—TH-4, TH-5, LI-5, HT-7

Hands—LI-4

Treatment

The treatment of tennis elbow will be explained first. Tennis elbow is most often
caused by baseball players or tennis players
straining their arms by extending and rotating their arms suddenly and forcefully. In
the acute phase it is better to rest the arm
until the inflammation subsides. After several
days supinating the forearm from a pronated
position will cause a strong pain. In this
case warm up the elbow with a warm compress and begin the acupuncture treatment
after the painful muscle (pronator teres

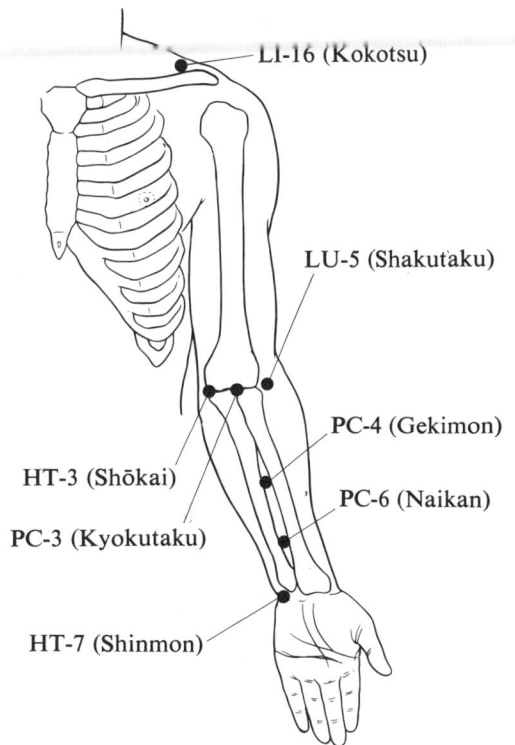

muscle) has been thoroughly relaxed. Insert needles in PC-3, PC-4, PC-6, LI-11, LI-10, LI-7, and LI-5 to a depth where a moderate needle sensation is felt, and then apply gentle lifting and thrusting and retain the needles about fifteen minutes.

The treatment of brachialgia associated with the cervicobrachial syndrome will be explained next. When the neuralgic pain is in the lateral side of the arm, the posterior aspect of the forearm, and the back of the hand, the radial nerve is involved. When the pain is in the palmar aspect of the forearm and the palm, the median nerve is involved. When the pain is on the medial side of the palmar aspect of the forearm, the ulnar nerve is involved. Before acupuncture, apply warm compresses on the neck to reduce the tension in the area where the brachial nerve leaves the cervical spine. To treat neuralgia of the radial nerve, insert needles vertically to a depth of about five centimeters into the points just next to the spaces between the spinous processes of the fourth, fifth, and sixth cervical vertebrae. Also needle LI-14, LI-11, LI-10, LI-7, LI-5, and TH-5 and retain the needles about fifteen minutes. For neuralgia of the median nerve, insert needles into the points adjacent to the above mentioned spinous processes, and needle PC-3, PC-4, and PC-6 and retain the needles. For neuralgia of the ulnar nerve, insert needles deeply into the points just next to the spaces between the spinous processes of the sixth and seventh cervical vertebrae and the first thoracic vertebra. Also insert and retain needles in HT-3 and HT-7. Massage the neck, shoulder, and arm well after removing the needles.

Low frequency electroacupuncture is also effective for treating the cervicobrachial syndrome. Apply low frequency electrical stimulation by connecting two thick needles inserted in the affected side. For neuralgia of the radial nerve, connect a needle inserted just next to the space between the spinous process of the fifth and sixth cervical vertebrae and another needle in LI-4. For neuralgia of the median nerve connect a needle inserted next to the space between the spinous process of the sixth and seventh cervical vertebrae and another needle in PC-6. For neuralgia of the ulnar nerve connect a needle inserted next to the spaces between the spinous processes of the sixth cervical vertebra and the first thoracic vertebra and another needle in HT-7. The pain and numbness extending down the arm should subside or disappear after applying a current of one Hz frequency for twenty minutes. Lightly massage the affected area after removing the needles.

6. Intercostal Neuralgia

Description

It is rare for the posterior roots of the thoracic nerves to become neuralgic, in almost all cases of intercostal neuralgia the anterior roots (the intercostal nerves) are affected. Most frequently the fifth to the ninth intercostal nerves are involved. Some cases of intercostal neuralgia are symptomatic (secondary to other pathology such as neuropathy due to tuberculosis or syph-

ilis, pressure from an aortic aneurysm, and bone cancer), while other cases of intercostal neuralgia are idiopathic (without an identifiable cause). Cases of idiopathic intercostal neuralgia are indicated for acupuncture.

The intercostal nerves follow the ribs from the vertebrae to the sides and reach the sternum in the center of the chest. The main symptom of intercostal neuralgia is paroxysmal pain which either wraps halfway around or completely around the thoracic region along the affected nerves. The pain is usually distributed in a band over the domain of several nerves on one side only and it tends to be on the left side. Normally the pain is greatest while inhaling and somewhat relieved while exhaling. The pain is quite intense and deep breathing, coughing, and talking usually aggravates it.

Acupuncture points

(1) Tender points just lateral to the spine
(2) Tender points just lateral to the sternum
(3) Tender points just below the axilla

Anterior thorax—ST-12, ST-18, LU-1, KI-23, CV-17

Abdomen—KI-21, KI-20, KI-19, KI-17, KI-16, CV-5

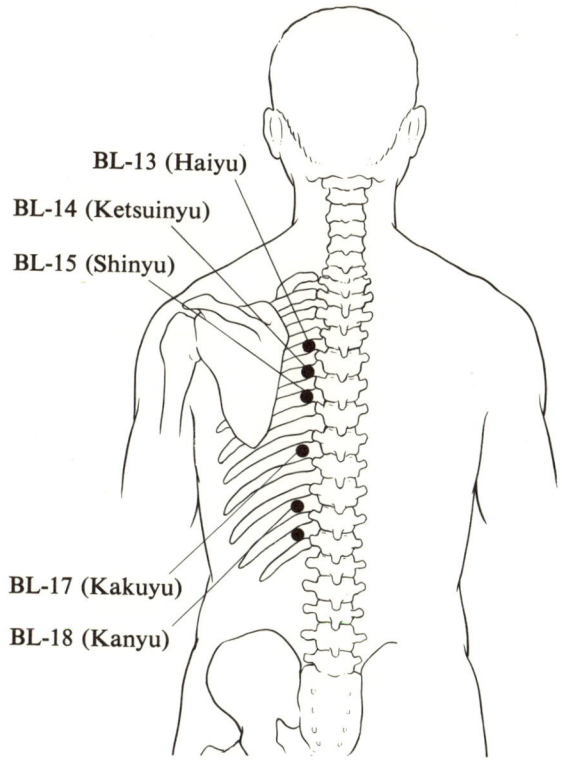

BL-13 (Haiyu)
BL-14 (Ketsuinyu)
BL-15 (Shinyu)
BL-17 (Kakuyu)
BL-18 (Kanyu)

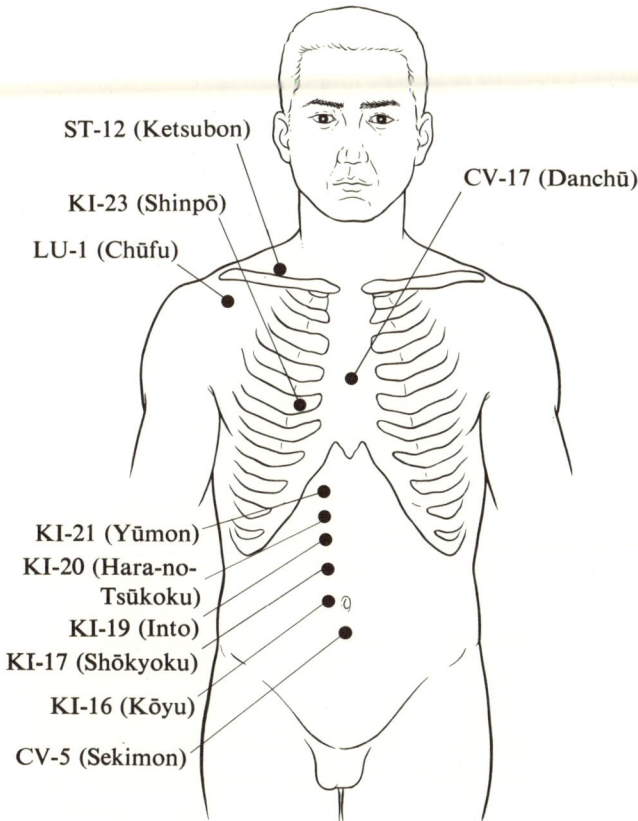

ST-12 (Ketsubon)
KI-23 (Shinpō)
LU-1 (Chūfu)
CV-17 (Danchū)
KI-21 (Yūmon)
KI-20 (Hara-no-Tsūkoku)
KI-19 (Into)
KI-17 (Shōkyoku)
KI-16 (Kōyu)
CV-5 (Sekimon)

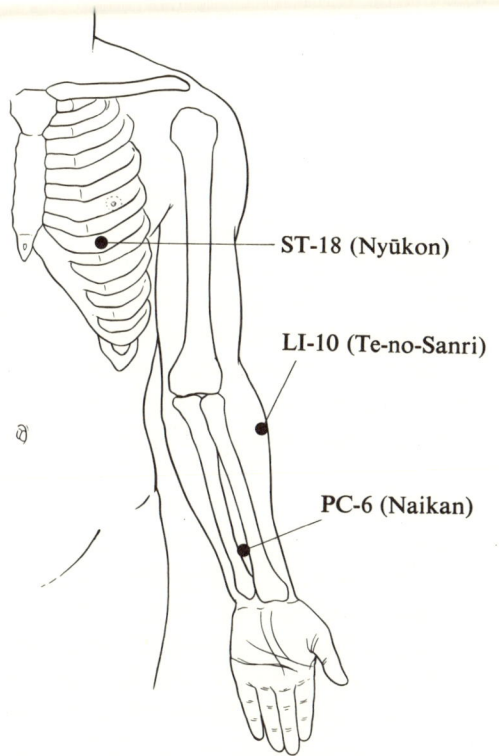

ST-18 (Nyūkon)
LI-10 (Te-no-Sanri)
PC-6 (Naikan)

Back—BL-13, BL-14, BL-15, BL-17, BL-18
Arms—LI-10, PC-6

Treatment
In intercostal neuralgia usually there are three areas with marked tenderness. The areas of tenderness are adjacent to the spine, adjacent to the sternum, and below the axilla. Tender points in these areas are extremely sensitive and even slight pressure can be unbearably painful. All these tender points serve as treatment points.

Have the patient assume the side-lying position with the affected side up and locate the tender points. When needling tender points right next to the spine, insert the needles vertically and relatively deeply (about 4 cm). When there is tenderness down the axillary line, insert the needles horizontally in an anterior direction, following the bottom of the rib in the direction of radiated pain, and retain the needles about ten minutes. When needling tender points along the lateral margin of the sternum, insert the needles vertically and shallowly (5 mm to 1 cm) and retain the needles. In addition to needling the tender points, needle BL-13, BL-15, BL-17, and BL-18. Also, for the purpose of relieving muscular tension in the chest area, needle ST-12, LU-1, KI-23, and CV-17. When there is abdominal pain needle the reactive points between KI-21 and KI-16. To complete the treatment, needle the distal points LI-10 and PC-6.

The effect of the treatment can be increased by applying a warm compress on the painful area before starting the acupuncture. Generally intercostal neuralgia is relatively easy to cure up to six months after the initial occurrence, but once it becomes chronic, intercostal neuralgia becomes difficult to cure and the treatment period becomes greatly prolonged.

7. Osteoarthritis of the Lumbar Vertebrae

Description
Lumbago is more common as people become older since the lumbar vertebrae bear the greatest load of all the vertebrae and also because they move more than the other vertebrae. In osteoarthritis abnormal bone growth on the vertebrae tends to occur more on the lumbar vertebrae, and this is a major cause of lumbago. Loss of elasticity in the intervertebral disks and the formation of bone spurs (osteophytes) can lead to circulatory problems such as the occlusion of arteries in the vertebral body and localized ischemia, as well as impingement of the nerve root. Bone spurs form most often on the fourth lumbar vertebrae, and after this the fifth, third, second, and first are the most likely sites for bone spur formation. Usually bone spurs form on either the in-ferior or superior border of the vertebral body.

Lumbago can occur for many different reasons, and often pain and neuralgic symptoms are caused by the compression of nerve roots with herniated disks, deformed intervertebral foramen, abnormal bone growth on the vertebral arch, or formation of posterior osteophytes. Lumbago can also occur as so-called "postural back pain" from fatigue in the paravertebral muscles associated with deformation of the vertebrae.

Acupuncture Points
Back—BL-18, BL-22, BL-23, BL-25, BL-26, BL-27, BL-52
Buttocks—BL-32, BL-53, BL-36, GB-30
Abdomen—CV-12, KI-16, ST-25, ST-27

BL-18 (Kanyu)

BL-22 (Sanshōyu)

BL-23 (Jinyu)

BL-25 (Daichōyu)

BL-26 (Kangenyu)

BL-27 (Shōchōyu)

GB-30 (Kanchō)

BL-53 (Hōkō)

BL-32 (Jiryō)

BL-36 (Shōfu)

CV-12 (Chūkan)

KI-16 (Kōyu)

ST-25 (Tensū)

ST-27 (Daiko)

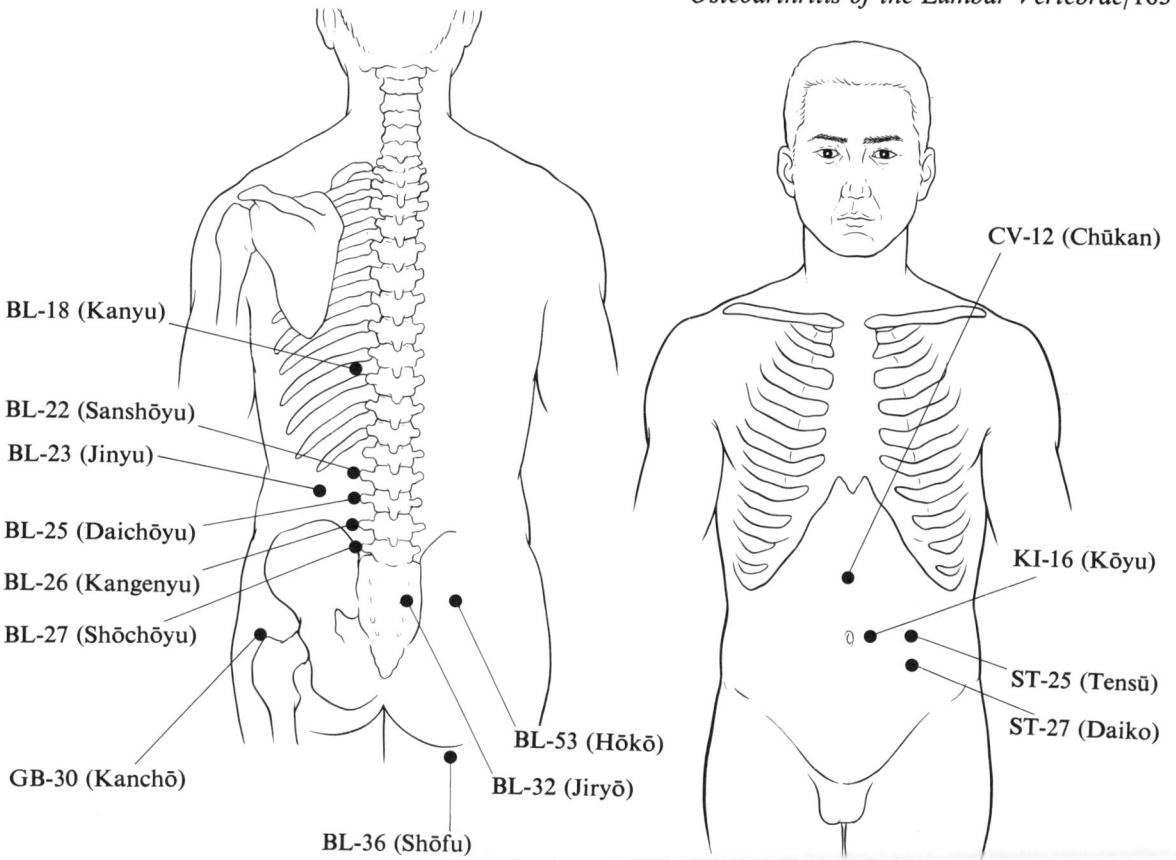

Legs—BL-37, BL-57, KI-1, KI-3, ST-36, SP-6, SP-9

Treatment

The primary cause of pain in osteoarthritis is the formation of bone spurs around the opening for the spinal nerves (the inter-vertebral foramen) which produces an abnormal tension in the surrounding ligaments and muscles. Bone spurs and deformation of the vertebrae cannot be corrected by acupuncture, but treatments can be provided for the purpose of relieving the abnormal tension in the surrounding soft tissues, improving circulation in the area and reducing the excitation of the affected nerves.

Before doing acupuncture it is useful to obtain x-rays of the lumbar region to determine whether there are any bone spurs or

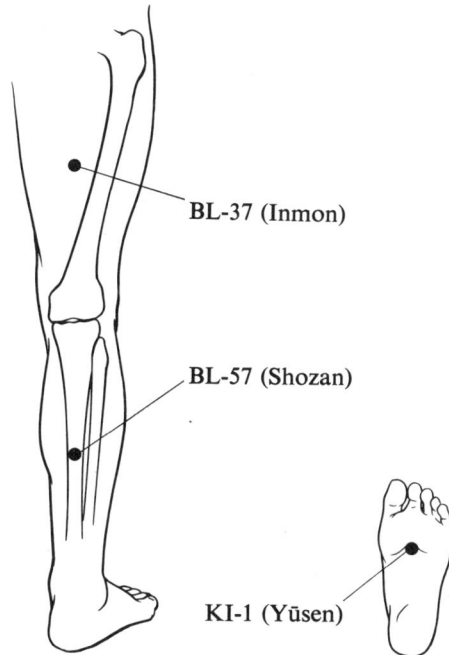

BL-37 (Inmon)

BL-57 (Shozan)

KI-1 (Yūsen)

ST-36 (Ashi-no-Sanri)

SP-9 (Inryōsen)

SP-6 (Saninkō)

KI-3 (Taikei)

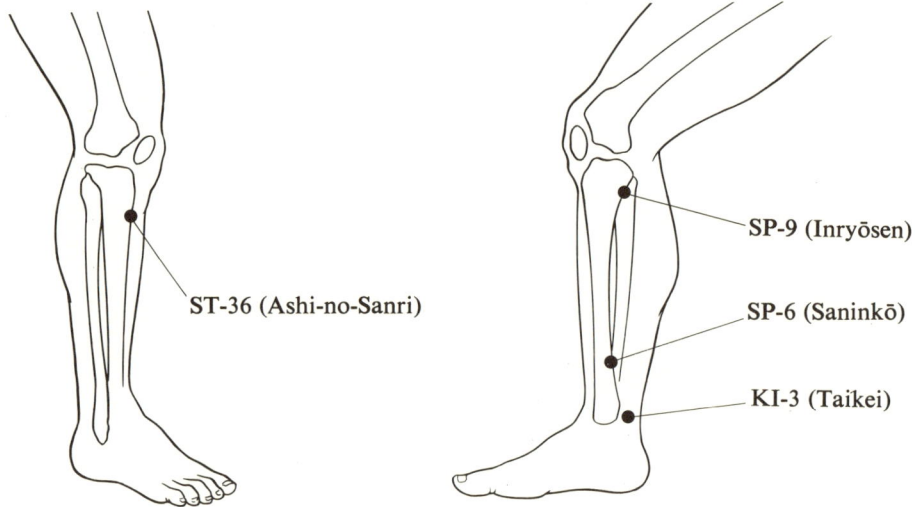

deformities. In addition, manual tests (e.g., Lasègue's test, muscle tests, cutaneous sensitivity test) should be performed to pinpoint the problem area. The first thing to do is to reduce the tension in the muscles of the lumbar region by applying a warm compress. After this begin by needling both sides of the abnormal vertebra (either the back *shu* points or directly adjacent to the vertebra). Aim the needles slightly medially and insert them deeply (about 6 cm) and lift and thrust to provide relatively strong stimulation and then retain the needles.

Deformities in the lower lumbar vertebrae often compress the sciatic nerve, and this produces pain and numbness along the course of the sciatic nerve, and sometimes there is chilling in the legs. If this condition goes untreated for a long time the muscles in the leg will begin to weaken and paresthesia can result. Also the back pain may become worse as time goes on. Even when there are such symptoms as chilling and numbness in the leg, first insert needles as explained above, aiming for the nerve root, and then needle BL-36 (deep vertical insertion), BL-37 (relatively deep vertical insertion), BL-57 (over the tibial nerve: shallow vertical insertion), KI-1 (rapid and shallow simple insertion), and ST-36 (directly over

the common peroneal nerve: vertical insertion). When needling the above acupuncture points, the most tender points must be palpated and needled. Vigorous lifting thrusting should be applied on all points except KI-1 to obtain a strong needle sensation and then the needles should be retained for about fifteen minutes.

Another very effective method for treating osteoarthritis of the lumbar vertebrae is to apply low frequency electrical stimulation through needles inserted next to the affected nerve root and the most tender points along the sciatic nerve. In this case apply a frequency of one Hz for about twenty minutes. As a means of improving circulation in the legs and warming them up, insert needles in ST-36, SP-9, SP-6, KI-3, and KI-1 and provide light stimulation. Whenever there is back pain, the abdominal muscles react and become tense, so also needle the points KI-16, ST-25, ST-27, and GV-20 to prevent additional symptoms. Osteoarthritis of the lumbar vertebrae is a difficult condition to cure completely, but acupuncture can be performed as soon as symptoms appear. Timely treatments will reduce the pain of lumbago and increase circulation in the lower extremities to warm the feet up and prevent other symptoms.

8. Herniated Disk in Lumbar Vertebrae (Slipped Disk)

Description

Herniated disks refer to the extrusion of the nucleus pulposus, which is the core material of intervertebral disks. Herniated disks usually occur with trauma or degeneration of the intervertebral joint and the weakening of the annulus fibrosus, the outer layer of the intervertebral disk. The disk tends to herniate posterolaterally to either side of the posterior longitudinal ligament, and this compresses the spinal cord or the root of the spinal nerve. Herniated disks occur most frequently in the intervertebral joint of the fourth and fifth lumbar vertebrae. Herniated disks in the lower lumbar vertebrae can produce neurologic symptoms such as sciatica, a decline in the patellar tendon reflex, and hypesthesia of corresponding dermatomes in the lower leg and foot.

One of the major causes of herniated disks in middle-aged individuals is lifting heavy objects with bad posturing. Intervertebral disks often begin to show signs of degeneration at the age of thirty, and by the age of fifty, there is some degree of degeneration in most individuals. For this reason, after the age of forty even slight stresses and injuries which are usually forgotten cause

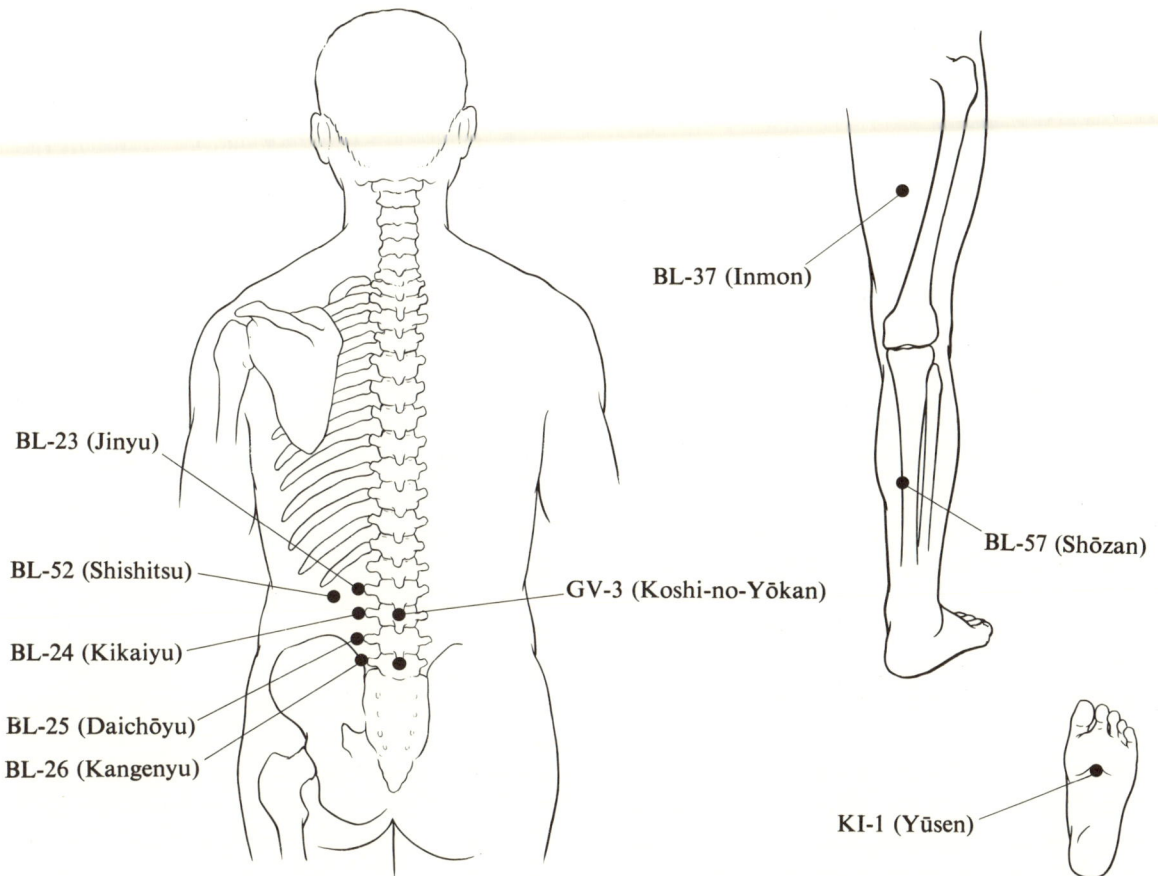

BL-37 (Inmon)

BL-57 (Shōzan)

BL-23 (Jinyu)

BL-52 (Shishitsu)

GV-3 (Koshi-no-Yōkan)

BL-24 (Kikaiyu)

BL-25 (Daichōyu)

BL-26 (Kangenyu)

KI-1 (Yūsen)

damage to the annulus fibrosus and eventually lead to herniated disks. When the annulus fibrosus ruptures, there is usually a sharp pain in the lumbar region, and this is commonly referred to as a "slipped disk." The herniation occurs to one side in the majority of cases, but in some cases there is posterior herniation or bilateral herniation.

Acupuncture points

Gluteal region—Onodera Point (tender point on inferior margin of iliac crest; over superior gluteal nerve)

Lumbar region—BL-23, BL-24, BL-25, BL-26, BL-52, GV-3, GV-4

Posterior leg—BL-37, BL-57

Dorsum of foot—KI-1

Treatment

In the acute phase there is great sensitivity and tenderness between the spinous process of either the fourth and fifth lumbar vertebrae or the fifth lumbar vertebra and first sacral crest. In this case do simple insertions in the sensitive points with the thinnest needles possible. BL-23, BL-25, and BL-52 also tend to be tender, so insert needles in these points when they are tender and provide gentle lifting and thrusting. When pain radiates down the sciatic nerve, needle tender points around BL-37, BL-57, and KI-1. In the acute phase rest is most important. Bathing or otherwise heating the back area is contraindicated, and the back must not be massaged or manipulated.

When the acute phase passes and the pain subsides, warm compresses or ultrasound may be applied to warm the lumbar area and reduce the muscular tension created by the back pain. Needle the tender points on the lower back in the same way as in treatments for the acute condition, but apply slightly stronger stimulation by lifting and thrusting more vigorously and retaining the needles. In some cases it is very effective to apply low frequency electrical stimulation (15 to 20 minutes) by connecting needles inserted adjacent to the spine where the hernia exists and a distal tender point either in the hip or the leg. For the treatment of attendant symptoms of sciatica, refer to the next item.

9. Sciatica

Description

Sciatica is a very common condition and is a clinically significant peripheral nerve disorder for acupuncturists. Since the sciatic nerve is very long and passes relatively close to the skin surface, it is quite susceptible to external injury, cold, and moisture, as well as infectious diseases such as influenza or inflammatory disorders like rheumatoid arthritis. Other conditions which lead to sciatica are the compression of the nerve by a tumor within the pelvic cavity, disorders in the lumbar or sacral spine (e.g., herniated disk), diabetes, syphilis, and arteriosclerosis. Today the majority of cases of sciatica are caused by herniated disks and are treated as the lumbago-sciatica syndrome. The pain appears only on one side in this case. When sciatica is caused by diseases such as syphilis or diabetes mellitus, usually the pain appears on both sides.

One of the characteristics of sciatica which differs from other types of neuralgia is that the pain, rather than being paroxysmal, is comparatively consistent. The pain typically goes down the back of the leg, and usually a burning sensation or deep pain radiates to the calf and sometimes as far as the foot. The pain is most pronounced when changing positions while lying down or when shifting

BL-22 (Sanshōyu)
BL-23 (Jinyu)

BL-52 (Shishitsu)
BL-25 (Daichōyu)
BL-26 (Kangenyu)

BL-53 (Hōkō)
BL-28 (Bōkōyu)
BL-36 (Shōfu)

GB-30 (Kanchō)

BL-37 (Inmon)
BL-40 (Ichū)
BL-56 (Shōkin)
BL-57 (Shōzan)

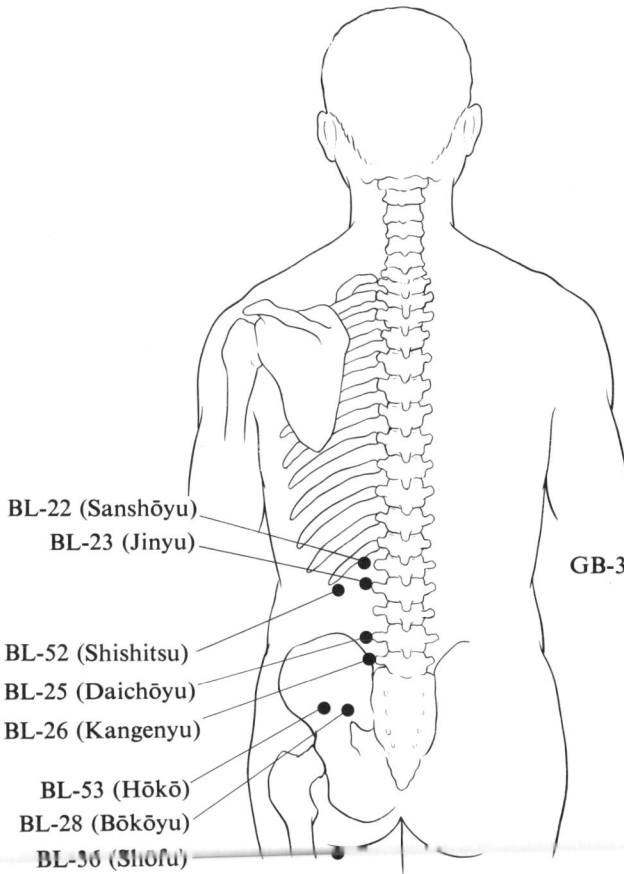

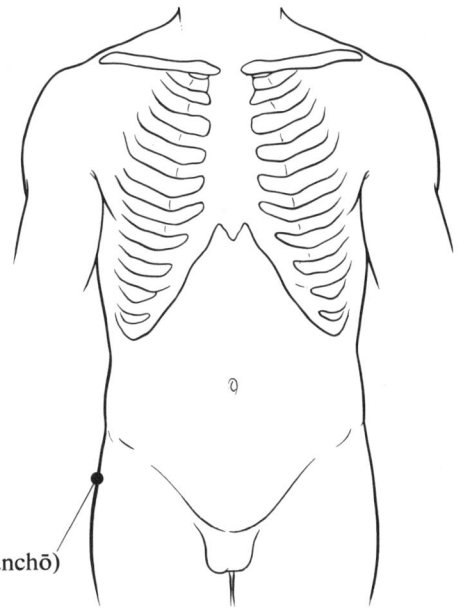

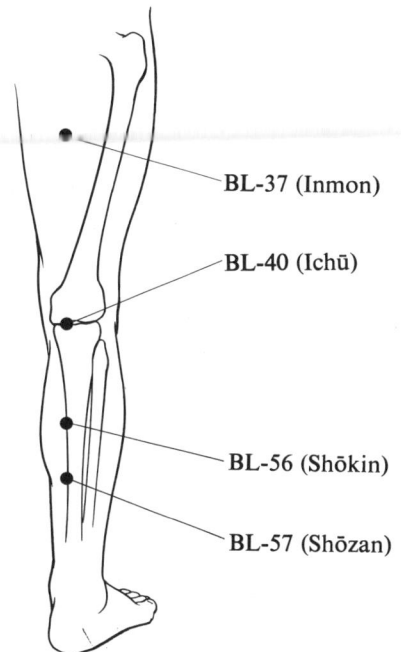

weight from one foot to the other while walking. When the root of the nerve is compressed, the entire path of the sciatic nerve feels pain, but the main tender points are over the sciatic foramen (midsection of the gluteus muscle), popliteal fossa, and the head of the fibula. One way to test for sciatica is to raise the patient's leg (flex the hip joint) in the supine position while holding the knee straight (Lasègue's test). This stretches the posterior aspect of the leg and causes a sharp pain down the back of the leg in cases of sciatica. Sometimes, if the sciatica continues over a long period, there is loss of the Achilles tendon reflex, hypesthesia, and neuromuscular scoliosis.

Acupuncture points

Lumbar region—BL-22, BL-23, BL-25, BL-26, BL-52

Sacral and gluteal region—BL-28, BL-36, BL-53, GB-30

Back of thighs—BL-37, BL-40, BL-56, BL-57

Legs—GB-34, GB-39, ST-36, ST-38, ST-41, SP-6

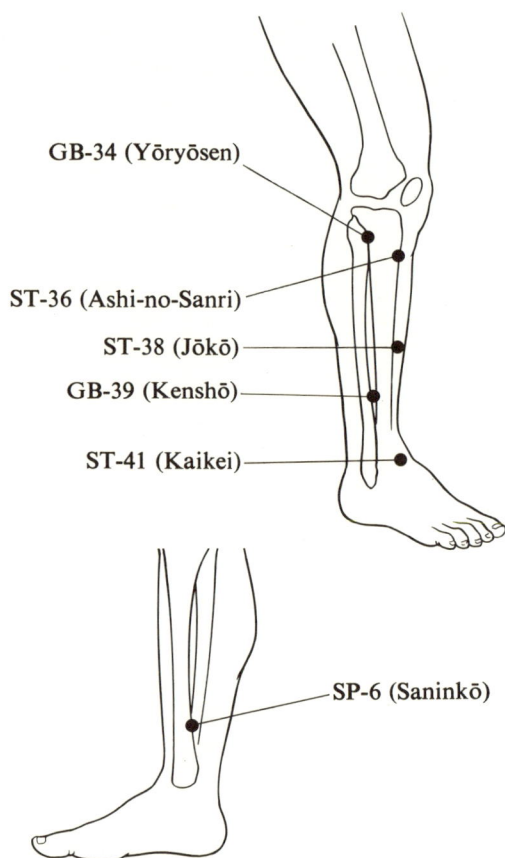

GB-34 (Yōryōsen)

ST-36 (Ashi-no-Sanri)

ST-38 (Jōkō)

GB-39 (Kenshō)

ST-41 (Kaikei)

SP-6 (Saninkō)

Treatment

The sciatic nerve originates from the sacral plexus at the level of the fourth and fifth lumbar and the first and second sacral nerves. It descends through the gluteal region and the posterior thigh where it branches (at the level of BL-37) into the tibial nerve (goes down the posterior side of the lower leg and reaches the sole) and the common peroneal nerve (goes down the lateral side of the lower leg and reaches the dorsum of the foot). The common peroneal nerve divides into the deep peroneal nerve (follows the course of the stomach meridian) and the superficial peroneal nerve (follows the course of the gallbladder meridian). In cases of neuralgia, pain and tenderness appear along the course of the affected nerve, so examine the patient carefully to determine the exact area of sensitivity.

Begin the treatment by applying warm compresses to the lumbar area to reduce the muscular tension. After this start needling from the lumbar region. Insert needles comparatively deeply (up to 5 cm) into BL-22, BL-23, BL-25, BL-26, and BL-52 and apply lifting and thrusting and rotation and retain the needles. Next needle BL-28, BL-36, BL-53, and GB-30 and apply the same manipulation and retain the needles. Then needle the reactive point over the greater sciatic foramen, where the sciatic nerve exits the pelvic cavity. This point is in the center of the gluteal region and pressing it will produce a sharp pain. Use a long needle two to three cun in length and insert deeply until a strong needle sensation is obtained, and then retain the needle. Follow this by needling BL-37 in the middle of the posterior thigh.

The lower leg should be needled according to the location of pain. If the pain radiates down the posterior side of the leg and reaches the sole, needle BL-40 in the center of the popliteal fossa and BL-56 and BL-57 in the center of the gastrocnemius muscle. If the pain radiates down the lateral side of the leg, needle GB-34, GB-39, ST-36, and ST-41. Retain the needles in the lower leg for about ten minutes.

Application of low frequency electrical stimulation is particularly useful for cases of lumbago and sciatica caused by compression of the nerve root due to abnormalities in the lumbar vertebrae. In this case insert comparatively thick needles right next to the problematic vertebrae as well as more distally on the most sensitive point. Connect the electrodes to these needles and stimulate for fifteen to thirty minutes. The polarity can be either way, whichever is more comfortable for the patient, and the intensity should be between one and three Hz where there is slight twitching in the muscles.

Another effective method for sciatica is moxa needling, which combines the effect of acupuncture stimulation with thermal stimulation. Try burning moxa on several needles inserted in the lumbar and gluteal region to determine the effect. After removing all the needles (never retain needles for more than thirty minutes) provide some massage along the course of the affected nerve. Sometimes it is very beneficial to perform Lasègue's test (extend the sciatic nerve) once more after the treatment as a form of exercise therapy. Also it is very useful to teach the patient therapeutic exercises for back pain.

10. Osteoarthritis of the Knee Joint

Description

Many older people complain of knee pain when sitting down and standing up and also when going up or down stairs. This condition is usually osteoarthritis of the knee joint. Just as in osteoarthritis of other joints, osteoarthritis of the knee joint can be brought on by injury, rheumatoid arthritis, and the aging process. It occurs more frequently among overweight individuals, and this points to the exciting cause of continually overloading the knee joint. The initial symptoms of osteoarthritis of the knee joint include chilling and swelling of the knee, scraping sounds upon moving the knee, and motor pain. These symptoms indicate that the bones and ligaments composing the knee joint are beginning to degenerate with age. There is usually increased pain and rigidity in the joint when standing up after sitting. The knee pain subsides after walking for a while, but any fatigue in the legs causes the pain to increase.

The pain in osteoarthritis of the knee joint is mostly felt when moving the joint, but there is pain while at rest in the acute phase when there is inflammation. Many points around the knee are very tender. Also there is substantial restriction in the range of motion and there is reduction in ability to flex and extend the knee as well as to internally and externally rotate the hip. Otherwise, there is abnormal tension in the

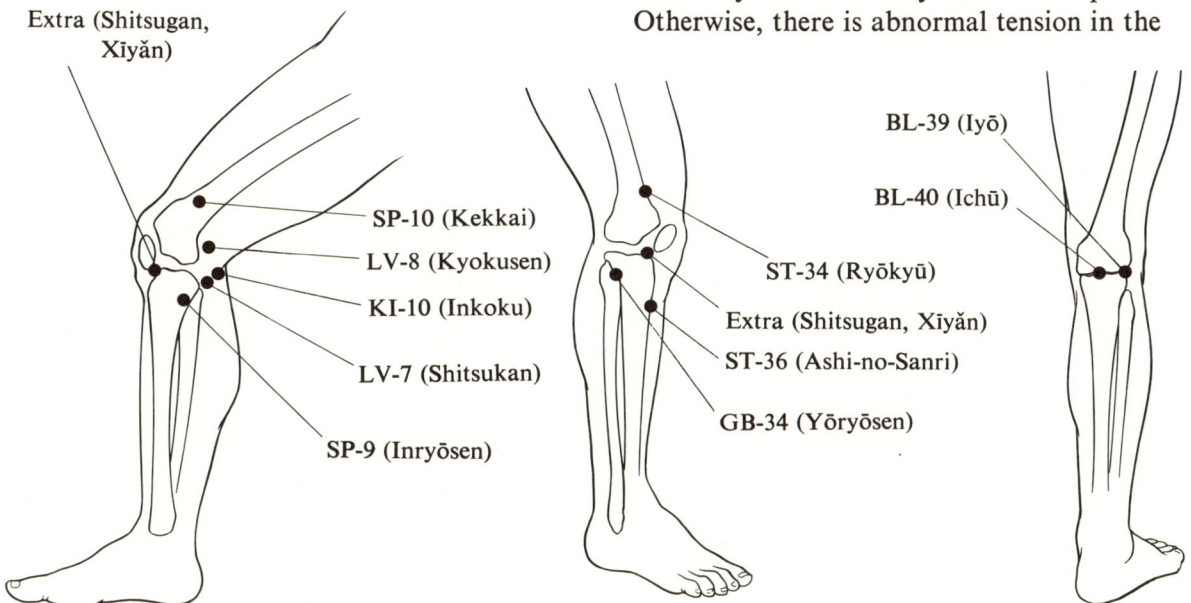

Extra (Shitsugan, Xīyǎn)

SP-10 (Kekkai)
LV-8 (Kyokusen)
KI-10 (Inkoku)
LV-7 (Shitsukan)
SP-9 (Inryōsen)

BL-39 (Iyō)
BL-40 (Ichū)

ST-34 (Ryōkyū)
Extra (Shitsugan, Xīyǎn)
ST-36 (Ashi-no-Sanri)
GB-34 (Yōryōsen)

ST-34 (Ryōkyū)

Extra (Shitsugan, Xīyǎn)

SP-10 (Kekkai)

BL-52 (Shishitsu)

BL-23 (Jinyu)

BL-25 (Daichōyu)

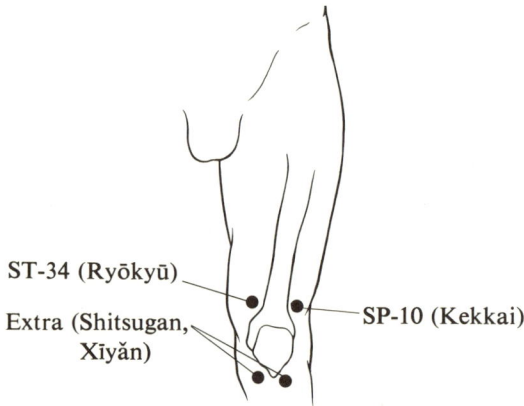

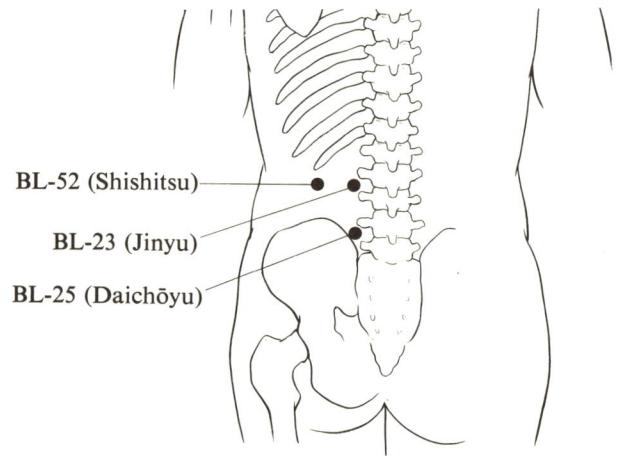

ligaments and surrounding soft tissues, and in severe cases atrophy in the muscles around the joint becomes noticeable.

Acupuncture points

Anterior knee joint—Shitsugan (extra), ST-34, ST-35, ST-36, SP-9, SP-10, GB-34
Posterior knee joint—BL-39, BL-40
Medial knee joint—LV-7, LV-8, KI-10
Lumbar region—BL-23, BL-25, BL-52

Treatment

Before treating osteoarthritis of the knee joint, check to make sure that the knee joint is not warm (inflamed). Then heat the joint with warm compresses to improve circulation. Prior to the treatment place a pillow under the knees to bolster them in a slightly flexed position so that the joints are relaxed. Begin by needling the points around the knees which are the most sensitive. Tenderness can often be found in the acupuncture points listed above as well as in points directly between the femur and the tibia. When inserting needles on either side of the patellar tendon (laterally ST-35 and medially the extra point Shitsugan), point the needles slightly medial and upward to reach the synovial capsule of the knee joint. This should produce a strong needle sensation within the joint. Carefully probe for tender points around the patella, between the femur and the tibia, and at the insertion of the

semitendinosus and semimembranosus muscles. Insert needles into the most sensitive points and retain them after obtaining a needle sensation. Applying infrared light over the needles increases the effect of acupuncture, but do not use infrared light when the knee joints are inflamed.

The pain of osteoarthritis in the knee joint often causes an abnormal posture which can lead to low back pain, excessive tension or atrophy in the quadriceps femoris muscle, and fatigue in the calf muscles. These symptoms must be dealt with accordingly by needling appropriate points. After the treatment, thoroughly massage around the knee joint as well as along the muscles which originate or insert at the knee joint. In the case of chronic osteoarthritis there is articular contracture which severely limits mobility of the joint, so the patient should be advised to undertake exercise therapy including a regimen of gentle active and passive exercises to improve the range of motion.

Moxibustion is also a very effective method for relieving osteoarthritis. Choose a few points around the knee which are particularly sensitive and apply five to seven cones of moxa half the size of a rice grain. Teach the patients how to apply moxa themselves. The pain will be greatly reduced if moxibustion is applied everyday for a few weeks.

11. Chronic Rheumatoid Arthritis

Description

Rheumatism includes rheumatic fever, an acute febrile disease marked by pain and inflammation in the large joints, and also chronic rheumatoid arthritis, a chronic disease in which the smaller joints become painful and inflamed. In both cases, early detection and treatment make all the difference in whether improvement can be expected or not. If rheumatic fever goes untreated, the heart is affected and sometimes there are grave consequences. Chronic rheumatoid arthritis is one of the collagen diseases (collagenosis), and rather than being just a disease of the joints, it is a systemic disease. Rheumatoid arthritis strikes females about three times as often as it does males, and its onset tends to be between the ages of twenty and fifty. The disease usually is first noticed as pain and swelling in the distal joints, and stiffness is felt in these joints particularly upon arising in the morning. These symptoms always occur bilaterally on the same joints on both sides. Other general symptoms include fatigue and lassitude, anorexia, weight loss, tendency to get cold, and a general loss of spirit. The pain either persists or recurs for a period of about three months. The arthritis gradually progresses to affect the larger joints. The affected joints go through a cycle of pain and inflammation and gradually movement becomes more and more restricted and the joint becomes deformed. If the progress of the disease goes unchecked, ankylosis in the affected joints causes contractures and the muscles around the joints weaken and atrophy. In some cases joints become partially dislocated and extreme deformity results. Also many other degenerative changes take place all over the body in the advanced stages of rheumatoid arthritis.

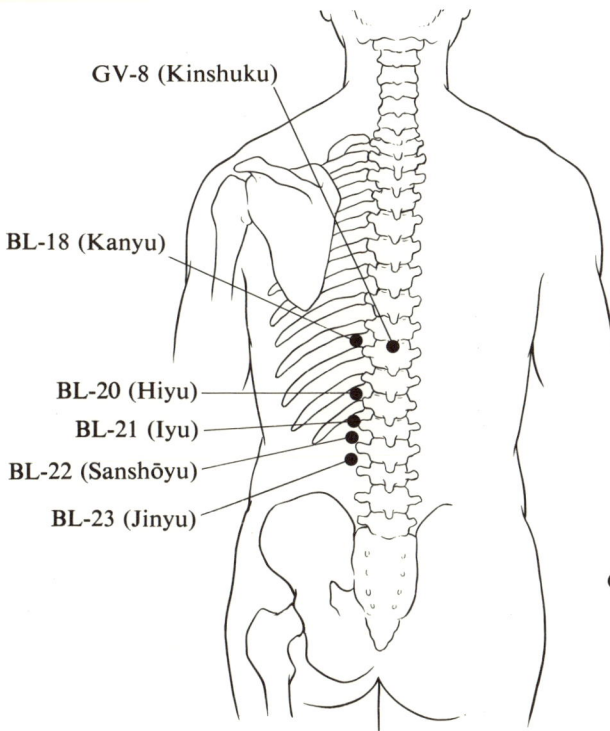

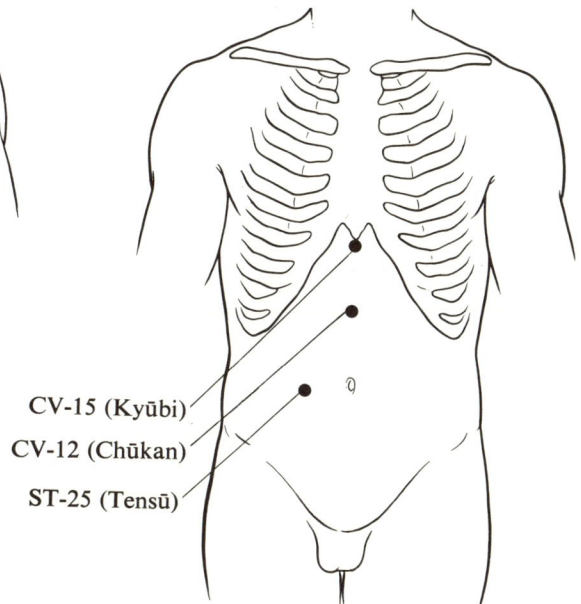

GV-8 (Kinshuku)

BL-18 (Kanyu)

BL-20 (Hiyu)

BL-21 (Iyu)

BL-22 (Sanshōyu)

BL-23 (Jinyu)

CV-15 (Kyūbi)

CV-12 (Chūkan)

ST-25 (Tensū)

LI-15 (Kengū)

LI-11 (Kyokuchi)

SI-8 (Shōkai)

TH-4 (Yōchi)

LI-4 (Gōkoku)

ST-34 (Ryōkyū)

Extra (Shitsugan, Xīyǎn)

ST-36 (Ashi-no-Sanri)

PC-7 (Dairyō)

KI-10 (Inkoku)

Extra (Shitsugan, Xīyǎn)

KI-3 (Taikei)

KI-6 (Shōkai)

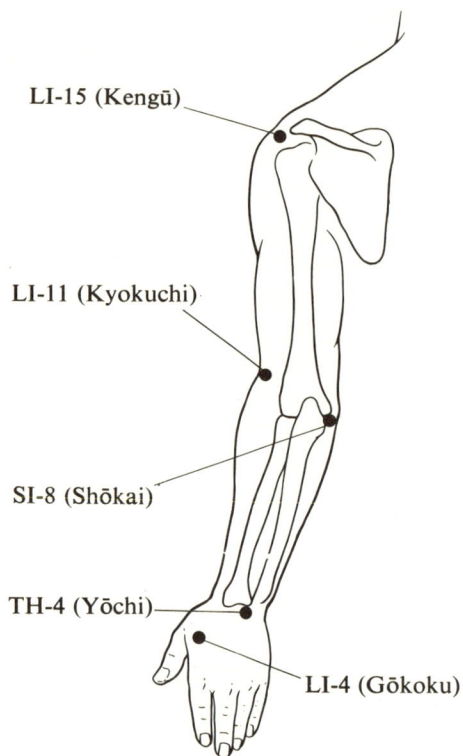

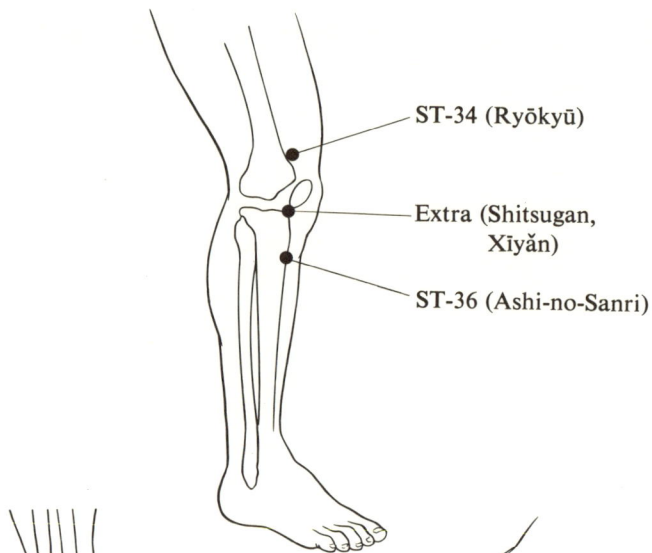

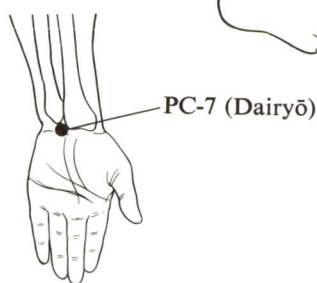

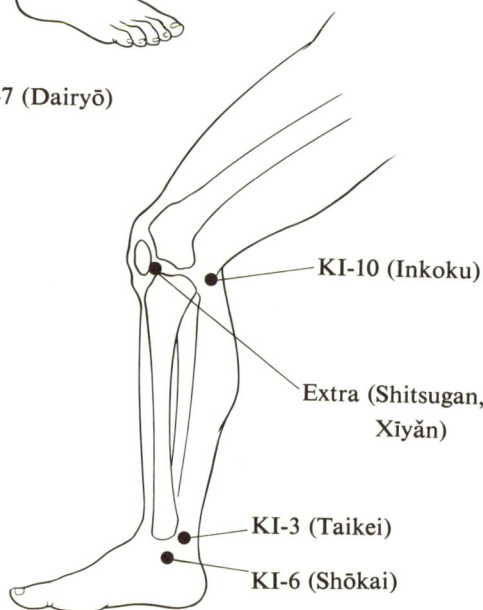

Acupuncture points

Back—BL-18, BL-20, BL-21, BL-22,
BL-23, GV-8
Abdomen—CV-12, CV-15, ST-25
Shoulder—LI-15
Elbows—LI-11, SI-8
Wrists—LI-4, TH-4, PC-7
Knees—ST-34, Shitsugan (extra), ST-36,
KI-10
Ankles—KI-3, KI-6

Treatment

Acupuncture treatments for rheumatoid
arthritis must be provided only after the
patient has seen a physician and is already
receiving necessary medical treatments.
Chronic rheumatoid arthritis is a systemic
and debilitating disease, so there is general
malaise including tendency to tire easily,
anorexia, and insomnia. To improve the
overall physical condition, gently needle
CV-15, CV-12, and ST-25, as well as tender
points and indurations on the back *shu*

points. Points such as ST-36 and LI-4 can
be needled to alleviate digestive problems.

After this the painful joints must be
treated. In chronic rheumatoid arthritis there
is typically an active phase and a remission
phase. In the active phase the joints are
inflamed and feel warm to the touch. Acupuncture is contraindicated during this
period. The joints are not warm during the
remission phase and it is appropriate to
insert needles in tender points around the
affected joints. Retain the needles up to
fifteen minutes. After removing the needles,

massage around the affected joints. This reduces the pain and increases the range of motion. Care must be taken to provide gentle needle stimulation since strong stimulation can cause fatigue in the patient. The best approach when many joints are affected is to perform scatter needling around the site of pain. Placing intradermal needles in sensitive points is another option.

Moxibustion is also effective for chronic rheumatoid arthritis. Moxibustion can be applied to the same points listed above, wherever there is tenderness or induration. Have the patients or their family members apply three to five cones on sensitive points everyday for five days and then rest for two days. This treatment should be continued patiently for several months. As the patient's physical condition improves the sensitive points will change so prescribe different points as the patient makes progress.

Acupuncture cannot restore joints which have contracture and deformity as a result of many years of rheumatoid arthritis, but pain and localized circulatory problems can be reduced or eliminated. In addition, acupuncture can bring relief from complaints of general malaise. In other words, the patient's appetite increases, they have less fatigue, and their feet become warmer due to improved circulation. Chronic rheumatoid arthritis is treated with powerful drugs in Western medicine, so there is a problem with skin rashes occurring as a drug side effect. Acupuncture and moxibustion have a significant effect in reducing and clearing up such skin rashes.

12. Headache

Description

Of all the types of pain, the headache is the most common and familiar type of pain. Headaches are caused by many things and are associated with a wide variety of diseases and conditions. Headaches can be classified roughly as follows:

(1) Headaches due to fever from various diseases
(2) Headaches due to diseases within the cranium (e.g., encephalitis, epidemic meningitis, encephaloma, etc.)
(3) Headaches due to high or low blood pressure (this includes headaches from cerebral arteriosclerosis)
(4) Headaches due to toxins in blood (the accumulation of toxic substances in the blood from gas poisoning, alcoholism, uremia, diabetes, constipation, hepatitis, cholelithiasis, etc.)

(5) Psychogenic headaches (headaches occurring because of psychological tension or anxiety)
(6) Headaches due to disease of the eye, ear, nose, or teeth
(7) Headaches related to environmental

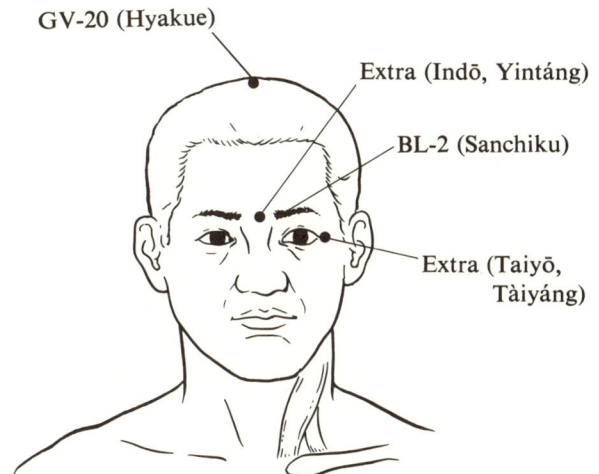

GV-20 (Hyakue)
Extra (Indō, Yintáng)
BL-2 (Sanchiku)
Extra (Taiyō, Tàiyáng)

GB-21 (Kensei)

GB-20 (Fūchi)

SI-13 (Kyokuen)

BL-10 (Tenchū)

GV-21 (Zenchō)

BL-7 (Tsūten)

GV-19 (Gochō)

GB-5 (Kenro)

GB-12 (Kankotsu)

LI-11 (Kyokuchi)

LI-4 (Gōkoku)

BL-60 (Konron)

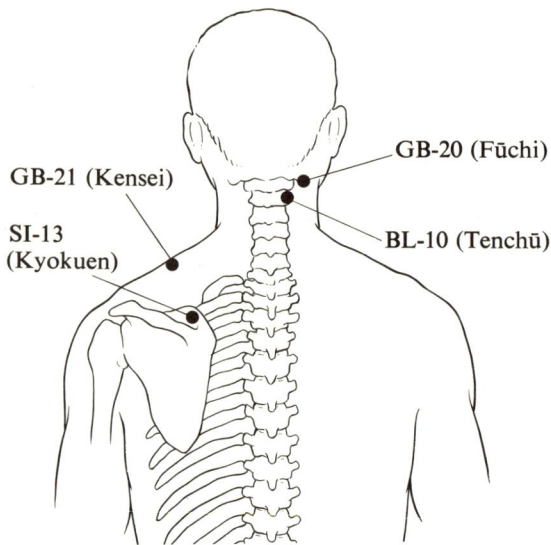

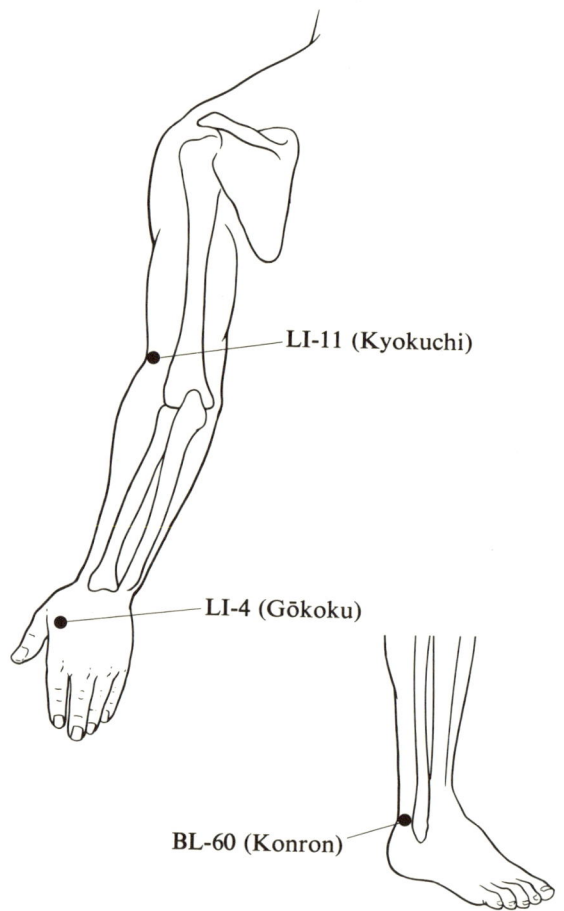

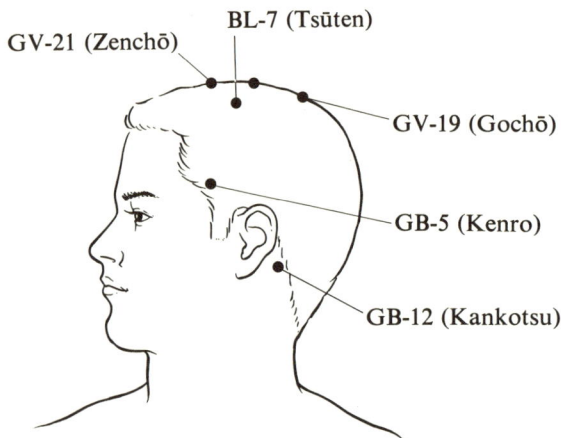

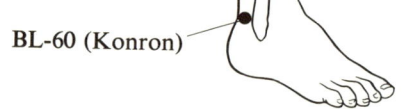

conditions (e.g., winter cold, summer heat, extreme humidity, etc.)

When a headache is slight there is only a feeling of pressure or tension, but strong headaches can be excruciating and cause vomiting. There is often some fluctuation in the intensity of headaches over time. Some headaches are relatively continuous while others are recurrent or paroxysmal. Headaches are also classified by the site of pain such as frontal, temporal, and occipital. Also headaches are sometimes identified as being either general or localized, and superficial or deep.

In case of chronic headaches, the pain is often dull and generalized. Another symptom similar to a headache is a sensation of heaviness over the head as if it were covered with something. In most cases heaviness of the head is related to cerebral hyperemia. Regardless of the nature of the headache, the patient must be examined thoroughly to rule out serious diseases before giving an acupuncture treatment.

Acupuncture points
Cranium—GV-20, GV-21, GV-19, BL-7, GB-5, Taiyang (extra)
Occiput—BL-10, GB-12, GB-20
Face—BL-2, Yintang (extra)
Shoulder—GB-21, SI-13
Arms—LI-4, LI-11
Legs—BL-60

Treatment

The standard points needled for all common headaches are LI-4, GB-20, and Taiyang. When the pain seems to come from the core of the head and extends over the whole head, GV-20 on the vertex must be needled. Insert the needle in GV-20 horizontally about three centimeters with the needle tip pointing anteriorly so that the needle slips between the cranium and the scalp. When a headache is in the anterior half of the cranium, needle GV-20, GV-21, and BL-7 with the needles aimed anteriorly. For dull pain and heaviness in the occipital region, needle GV-20, GV-21, and BL-7 with the needles aimed posteriorly. Also needle GB-12, GB-20, and BL-10 (vertical insertion toward center of head). In cases of a frontal headache or when there are symptoms in the eyes, nose, or ears, also needle BL-2 and Yintang. In cases of a temporal headache needle Taiyang vertically and GB-5 horizontally with the needles pointed posteriorly. When there is also tension in the neck and shoulders, needle GB-21 and SI-13. For headaches related to gastrointestinal disorders (constipation) provide acupuncture on appropriate abdominal and lumbar points as well as on LI-11 and LI-4. Needling BL-60 is sometimes extremely effective in alleviating migraine headaches. Massage is very useful for those patients with symptoms of cerebral hyperemia (heaviness of the head). In addition to the acupuncture treatment, apply finger pressure on the head and massage the neck area (especially the sternocleidomastoid muscle).

13. Vertigo

Description

Among the many types of vertigo, giddiness or dizziness related to low blood pressure and cerebral hypoaemia is common. Dizziness upon standing up occurs when the blood pressure regulating mechanism is not working properly and the blood pressure in the cranium suddenly drops as a person stands up. This condition is called orthostatic hypotensive asthenia. Vertigo is also caused by disturbances in ocular circulation and oxygen supply as well as by low blood sugar due to hypoglycemia. Severe vertigo is also one of the symptoms of epilepsy.

Rotary vertigo is generally caused by a disturbance in the balancing mechanism of

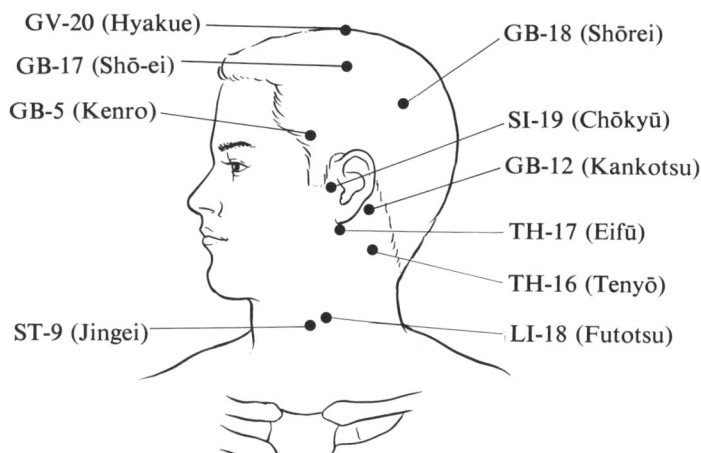

GV-20 (Hyakue)
GB-17 (Shō-ei)
GB-5 (Kenro)
ST-9 (Jingei)

GB-18 (Shōrei)
SI-19 (Chōkyū)
GB-12 (Kankotsu)
TH-17 (Eifū)
TH-16 (Tenyō)
LI-18 (Futotsu)

GB-20 (Fūchi)

GB-21 (Kensei)

BL-10 (Tenchū)

BL-15 (Shinyu)

BL-18 (Kanyu)

BL-20 (Hiyu)

BL-23 (Jinyu)

LI-10 (Te-no-Sanri)

PC-6 (Naikan)

ST-36 (Ashi-no-Sanri)

SP-6 (Saninkō)

LV-3 (Taishō)

CV-15 (Kyūbi)

CV-12 (Chūkan)

ST-27 (Daiko)

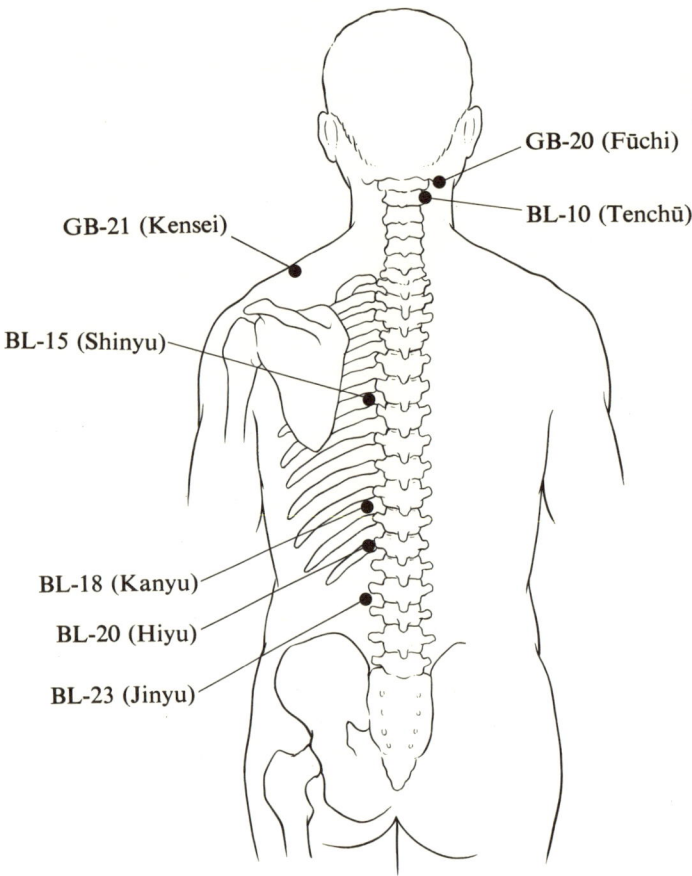

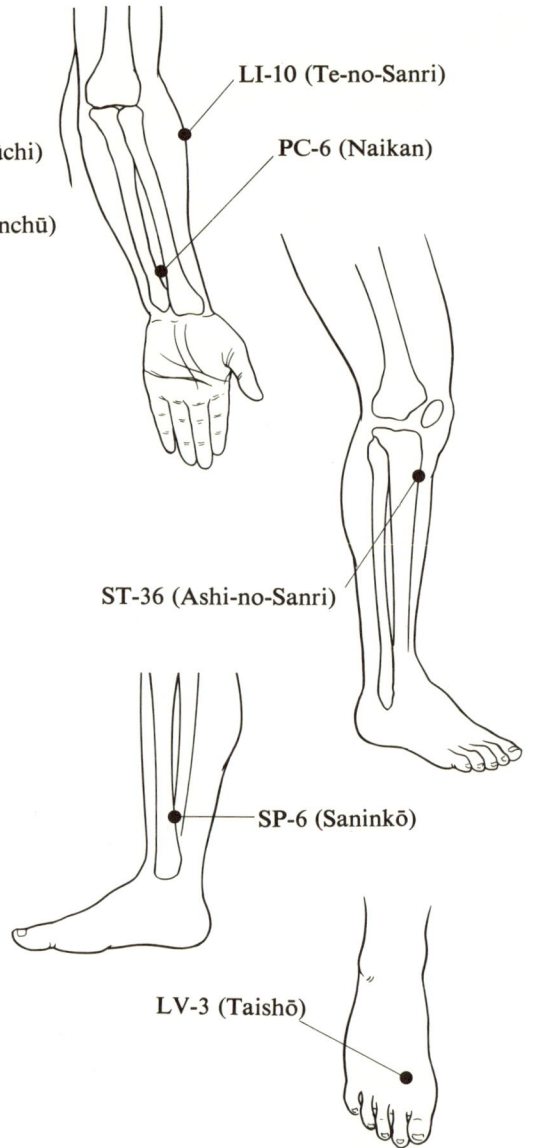

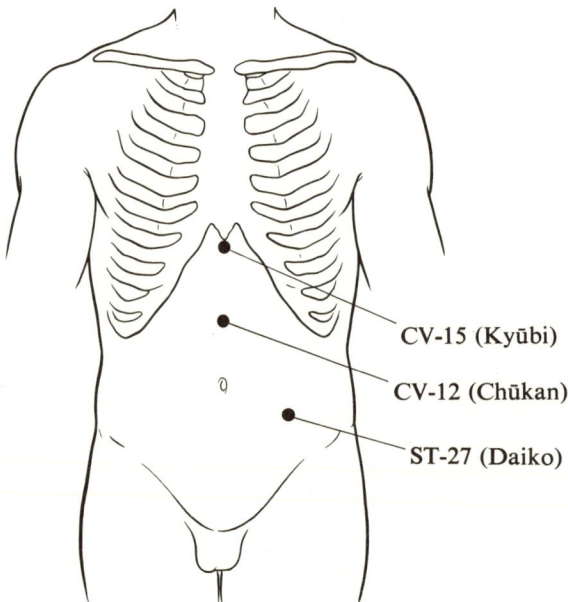

the body, and there is often some dysfunction in the semicircular canals of the inner ear or the cerebellum or in their nervous transmission routes. If this is the case there is usually nausea and vomiting in addition to vertigo. It therefore follows that vertigo is a typical symptom when there are diseases of the middle ear or inner ear, when brain function is impaired by alcohol or drugs, or when circulatory disturbances affect the cerebellum or its transmission route.

Dizziness upon standing, which is due to

cerebral anemia and other conditions of abnormally low blood pressure, can usually be remedied just by quietly resting for a while. Vertigo which goes away by itself does not require treatment, but when strong vertigo persists, a physician must be consulted to determine the cause. In many cases of vertigo no specific cause can be identified, but infrequently it is an early symptom of a serious disease, so a thorough examination is in order.

Acupuncture points
Head—GV-20, GB-5, GB-17, GB-18
Around the ear—SI-19, TH-17
Occiput—BL-10, GB-12, GB-20
Neck—TH-16, ST-9, LI-18
Shoulder—GB-21
Back—BL-15, BL-18, BL-20, BL-23
Abdomen—CV-15, CV-12, ST-27
Arms—LI-10, PC-6
Legs—ST-36, SP-6, LV-3

Treatment
For vertigo associated with hypotension, psychological stress, autonomic dystonia, eyestrain, and climacteric disorders, the acupuncture treatment should concentrate on improving the overall physical condition. Keeping the symptoms other than vertigo in mind, select some of the points listed above and apply comparatively mild stimulation. Treatments are aimed at enhancing the body's self-regulating function and the patient needs to receive regular treatments over a long period of time. Moxibustion is also very effective for the above mentioned condition. For moxibustion select several of the above points and apply three cones of moxa on each point. Teach patients how to apply moxa themselves because they need moxibustion treatments everyday for at least one month.

In cases of rotary vertigo, in addition to overall treatments, points on the head and neck such as SI-19, BL-10, GB-12, GB-20, GB-21, TH-16, TH-17, LI-18, and ST-9 should be needled. In this case insert the needles until a sensation is obtained, then apply lifting and thrusting and twisting to the needles, and then retain the needles for ten to fifteen minutes. This will serve to improve circulation in the cranium and reduce the tension in the neck and shoulders.

Even Ménière's disease, which is representative of conditions of severe vertigo, is also said to be related to psychological stress and autonomic dystonia. Therefore, good results can be expected in the long term by providing the above treatment on a regular basis.

14. Tinnitus

Description
It is estimated that 50 to 80 percent of the patients who visit ear and nose specialists have the complaint of tinnitus. The majority of patients with tinnitus have no other problem except the subjective symptom of ringing in the ears, since to this day there is no way to examine and objectively assess tinnitus. Tinnitus often occurs as one of the symptoms of other physical problems such as anemia, arteriosclerosis, diabetes, circulatory diseases, and endocrine disorders. Tinnitus is most often just one symptom of a systemic disease when it is accompanied by loss of hearing, vertigo, headaches, high blood pressure, or low blood pressure. Simple causes of tinnitus include obstruction of the external auditory canal by ear wax or other material, obstruction of the eustachian tube, otitis media, and diseases of the outer ear

and the middle ear. This type of tinnitus is called conductive tinnitus and the noise in the ears is generally a low buzzing sound and is usually one-sided. Tinnitus caused by otitis interna, poisoning, presbycusis (deafness from aging), Ménière's disease, an auditory nerve tumor, or encephaloma is called sensory tinnitus and the noise in the

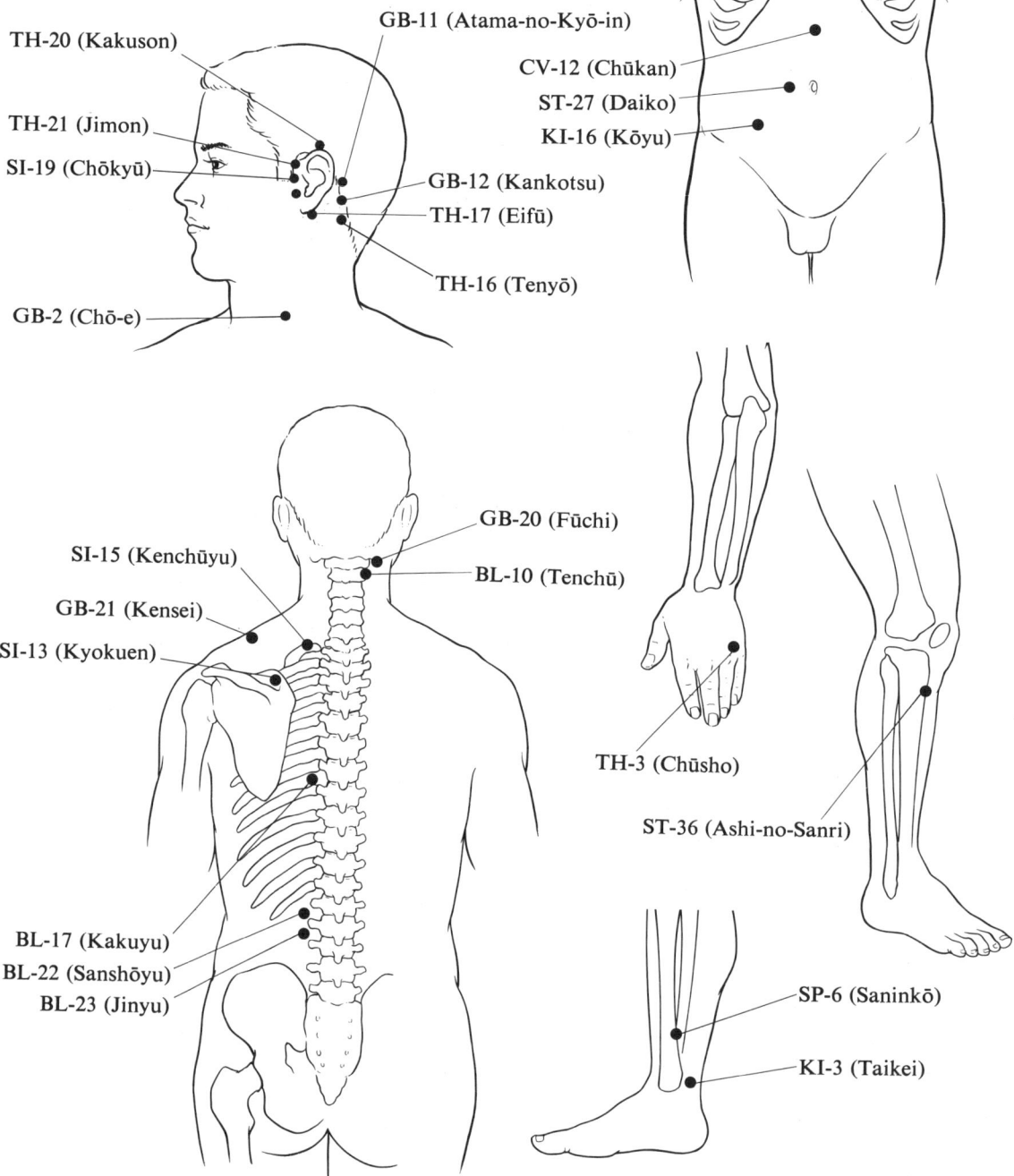

TH-20 (Kakuson)

GB-11 (Atama-no-Kyō-in)

CV-12 (Chūkan)

ST-27 (Daiko)

KI-16 (Kōyu)

TH-21 (Jimon)

SI-19 (Chōkyū)

GB-12 (Kankotsu)

TH-17 (Eifū)

TH-16 (Tenyō)

GB-2 (Chō-e)

SI-15 (Kenchūyu)

GB-21 (Kensei)

SI-13 (Kyokuen)

GB-20 (Fūchi)

BL-10 (Tenchū)

TH-3 (Chūsho)

ST-36 (Ashi-no-Sanri)

BL-17 (Kakuyu)

BL-22 (Sanshōyu)

BL-23 (Jinyu)

SP-6 (Saninkō)

KI-3 (Taikei)

ears is usually a high pitched tone. Tinnitus occurs most often as a secondary symptom to sensory neural deafness, and such sensory tinnitus is very difficult to cure except in special cases. Before treating patients with tinnitus, it is advisable to have them consult a physician to rule out serious or acute diseases.

Acupuncture points

Around the ear—TH-17, TH-20, TH-21, GB-2, GB-11, SI-19

Neck—BL-10, GB-12, GB-20, TH-16, ST-9, adjacent to the spinous process of the fourth cervical vertebra

Shoulders—GB-21, SI-13, SI-15

Back—BL-17, BL-22, BL-23

Abdomen—CV-12, KI-16, ST-27

Hands—TH-3

Legs—ST-36, SP-6, KI-3

Treatment

Tinnitus is best treated by providing local treatments around the ear along with general treatments to improve the overall physical condition. Begin the treatment by needling several points around the ear, especially TH-17, and insert the needle deep enough to cause a needle sensation deep within the ear. Next provide a mild to medium amount of stimulation to BL-10, GB-12, and GB-20 and retain the needles for ten to twenty minutes. Also there is a point in the vicinity of TH-16 which is tender or tight when there is tinnitus, and strong finger pressure on this point often affects the ringing in the ears. When such a reaction is present, insert a needle in this point and apply some lifting and thrusting and twisting.

After inserting the needles, low frequency electrical stimulation can be applied on the points showing an especially strong reaction. Good results can be obtained by applying a frequency of one to three Hz for about fifteen minutes. Another approach that is sometimes useful is to stimulate circulation in the cranium by needling the stellate ganglion or the carotid sinus. The stellate ganglion can be stimulated by needling the point on the anterior border of the sterno-cleidomastoid muscle two to three centimeters above the sternoclavicular joint. Insert the needle quite deeply (about 5 cm) and gently apply lifting and thrusting for about five minutes, being careful to avoid the trachea. The carotid sinus can be stimulated by carefully needling ST-9 to a depth of one to one and a half centimeters until the arterial wall is reached. The head of the needle should move with the pulsing of the artery. Withdraw the needle after thirty seconds.

The more chronic the tinnitus is, the more there tends to be other general complaints such as tension and stiffness in the neck and shoulders, insomnia, chilling of the feet, and constipation. For tension and stiffness in the neck and shoulders, needle BL-10, GB-20, GB-21, SI-13, SI-15, and the point adjacent to the spinous process of the fourth cervical vertebra. For irritability and insomnia, needle KI-16, BL-17, and BL-23, and also massage the back to reduce the tension in the erector spinae muscles. For chilling of the feet, needle tender points in the lower back along with SP-6 and KI-3. In traditional Chinese medicine the ears are under the control of the kidneys, and for patients with an asthenic constitution or weakened condition, kidney points such as BL-23, KI-16, and KI-3 are very useful.

15. Insomnia

Description

There are many types of insomnia, but insomnia can roughly be classified into three kinds: (1) insomnia in which one has difficulty in getting to sleep, (2) insomnia in which the sleep is shallow and one does not feel rested, and (3) insomnia in which one wakes up very early. Sleep is often disturbed when there is overexcitation of the central nervous system due to mental disturbances, psychological strain, or arteriosclerosis. Otherwise, symptoms such as anxiety, tension, pain, itching, coughing, or diarrhea can keep one awake. Most of the insomnia encountered in the acupuncture clinic, however, is a psychosomatic condition where patients think that they are not getting enough sleep. Acupuncture is very effective in such cases of insomnia in which psychological stress or mental and physical fatigue is the primary cause.

Acupuncture points
Head—GV-20, BL-10
Back—BL-17, BL-18, BL-23

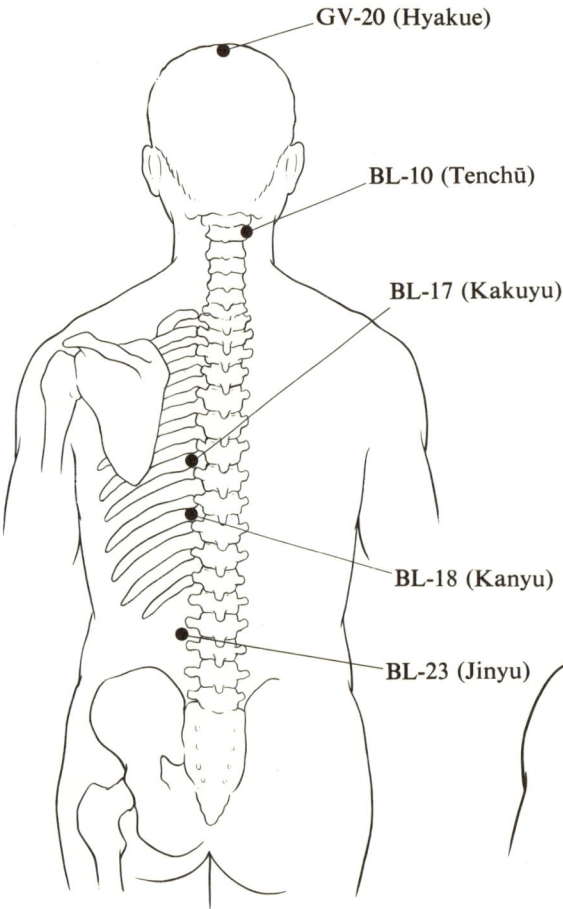

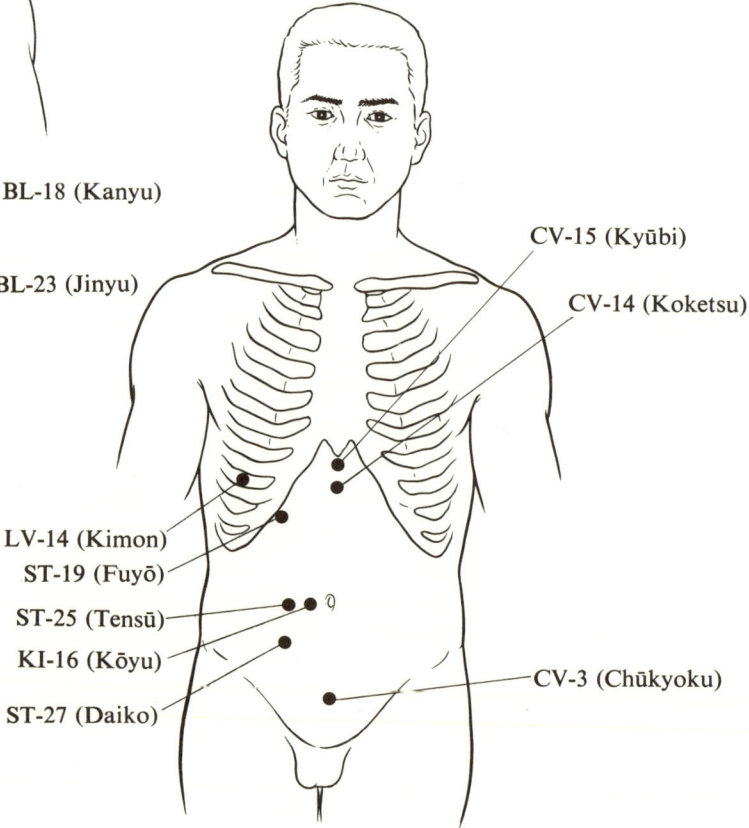

GV-20 (Hyakue)

BL-10 (Tenchū)

BL-17 (Kakuyu)

BL-18 (Kanyu)

BL-23 (Jinyu)

CV-15 (Kyūbi)

CV-14 (Koketsu)

LV-14 (Kimon)
ST-19 (Fuyō)
ST-25 (Tensū)
KI-16 (Kōyu)
ST-27 (Daiko)

CV-3 (Chūkyoku)

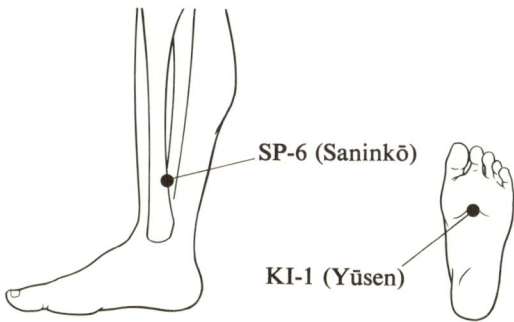

SP-6 (Saninkō)

KI-1 (Yūsen)

Abdomen—CV-3, CV-14, CV-15, ST-19, ST-25, ST-27, LV-14, KI-16

Feet—KI-1, SP-6

Treatment

Many people with insomnia have strong tension around BL-17 in the back, so reactive points around BL-17 and BL-18 should be needled first in such cases to reduce the tension in the middle of the back. After treating the back, needle some points on the abdomen such as CV-14, CV-15, ST-19, and LV-14 to reduce the stifling sensation in the epigastric and hypochondriac region which is very common in those with insomnia. Patients will find it much easier to get to sleep after the tension in the upper back and under the ribs is reduced. In addition, needle GV-20 and BL-10 to calm the nerves and relieve headaches associated with insomnia.

To cure insomnia it is important to bring an improvement to the patient's overall physical condition. Therefore it is important to needle BL-23 and KI-1 to raise the basic level of vitality. Also needle SP-6 to reduce hotness in the face and warm up the feet. Use ST-25 for the purpose of improving the digestive function. ST-27 can be used to alleviate constipation, which is a common complaint along with insomnia. When there is polyuria, CV-3 and BL-23 should be needled. Patients with nervous disorders like insomnia tend to be very sensitive so the needle stimulation should be kept relatively mild.

16. Neck and Shoulder Tension

Description

The common symptom of tension or stiffness in the neck and shoulders ranges from simple cases where simple exercises like rolling the head around and moving the shoulders up and down relieves the tension to more severe cases which lead to dizziness and nausea. Tension in the neck and shoulders is a very widespread phenomenon which is not clearly understood by medical science. The type of neck and shoulder tension for which acupuncture is effective is the type related to mental and physical fatigue such as that from long hours of manual labor or sitting all day in a tense situation like a business conference. The muscular tension in these cases are a product of fatigue from the muscle being held in the shortened or lengthened position for a long time. The muscular tension reduces circulation and leads to the feeling of stiffness.

Another type of neck and shoulder tension is caused by cervicobrachialgia. In this case, in addition to stiffness in the neck and shoulders, there is strong pain. There is also numbness and muscle atrophy in the arms and a patient is more prone to drop things. This type of neck and shoulder stiffness is common to typists and computer terminal operators. Acupuncture is effective for this type of shoulder stiffness also.

Shoulder stiffness also occurs in some organic diseases including lung and heart diseases, liver diseases, stomach diseases, gynecological diseases, and climacteric disorders. Pathology in the pylorus of the

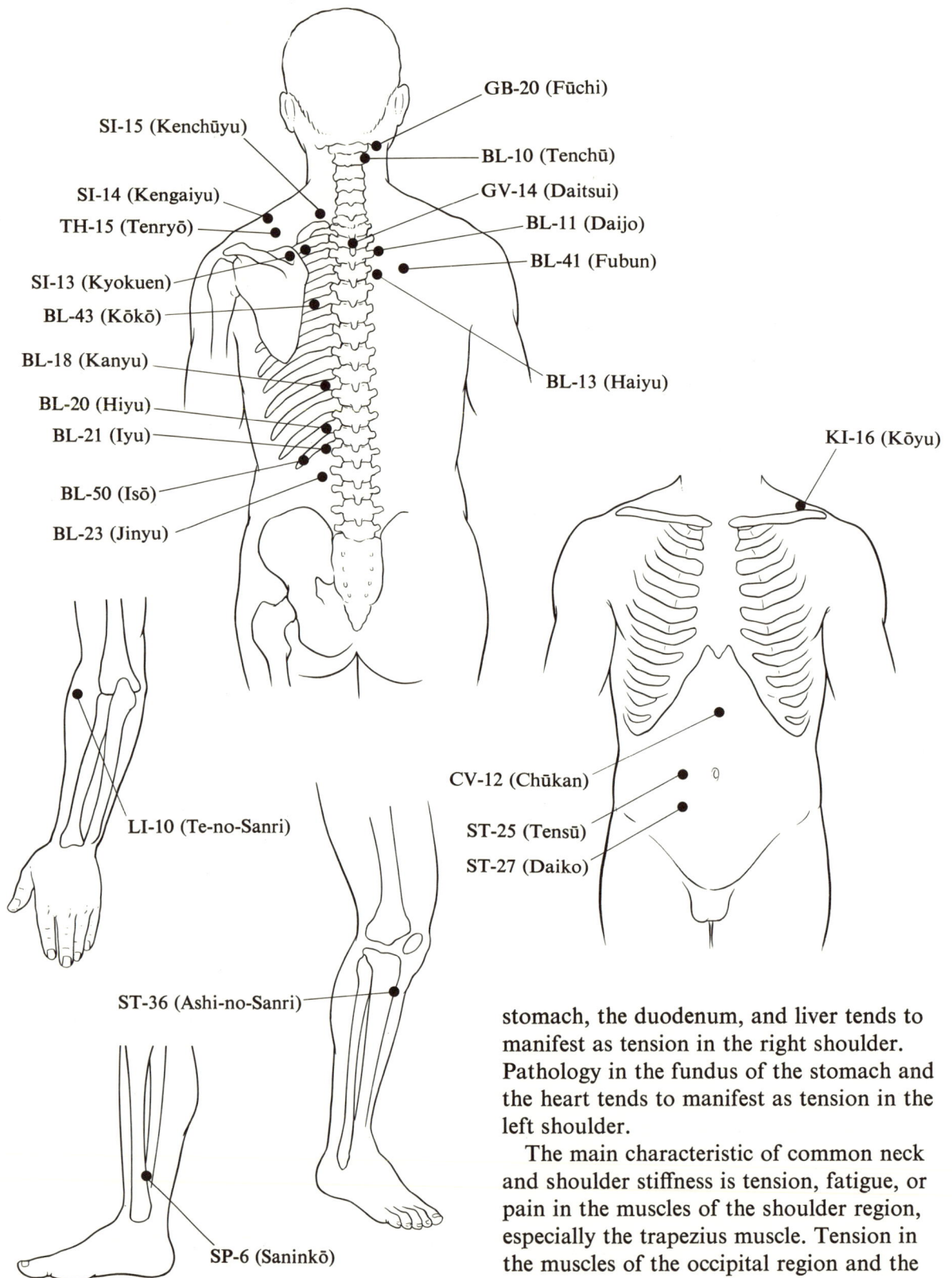

GB-20 (Fūchi)

SI-15 (Kenchūyu)

BL-10 (Tenchū)

SI-14 (Kengaiyu)

GV-14 (Daitsui)

TH-15 (Tenryō)

BL-11 (Daijo)

BL-41 (Fubun)

SI-13 (Kyokuen)

BL-43 (Kōkō)

BL-18 (Kanyu)

BL-13 (Haiyu)

BL-20 (Hiyu)

KI-16 (Kōyu)

BL-21 (Iyu)

BL-50 (Isō)

BL-23 (Jinyu)

LI-10 (Te-no-Sanri)

CV-12 (Chūkan)

ST-25 (Tensū)

ST-27 (Daiko)

ST-36 (Ashi-no-Sanri)

SP-6 (Saninkō)

stomach, the duodenum, and liver tends to manifest as tension in the right shoulder. Pathology in the fundus of the stomach and the heart tends to manifest as tension in the left shoulder.

The main characteristic of common neck and shoulder stiffness is tension, fatigue, or pain in the muscles of the shoulder region, especially the trapezius muscle. Tension in the muscles of the occipital region and the anterior scalenus muscle is also experienced as shoulder stiffness. In general the area that is stiff feels dull and heavy as if the muscle were fatigued, and pressing the muscles causes some pain, but this is usually a tolerable and even pleasant sensation.

Acupuncture points

Neck—BL-10, BL-11, GB-20, GV-14
Shoulder—GB-21, TH-15, SI-13, SI-14, SI-15, BL-13, BL-41, LI-16
Back—BL-18, BL-20, BL-21, BL-43, BL-50
Abdomen—CV-12, ST-25, ST-27
Lumbar region—BL-23
Arms—LI-10
Legs—ST-36, SP-6

Treatment

When there is a structural disorder causing the stiffness and tension, the disorder must be treated first. Since neck and shoulder stiffness is a condition of abnormal tension in the muscles attached to the cervical vertebrae and the shoulder joint, the aim of acupuncture treatments is to reduce the tension in these muscles. First have the patient assume the prone position and carefully examine the neck and shoulder area (especially around BL-10, BL-11, BL-41, GB-20, GB-21, TH-15, SI-13, SI-14, SI-15, and LI-16) for tender points and indurations. Needle those points where it feels good to be pressed, where there is a dull sensation, or where there are indurations. Insert the needles to the point where a mild needle sensation is elicited and lift and thrust and twist the needles briefly and then retain them for about ten minutes.

Another effective approach for neck and shoulder stiffness is to insert needles in the motor points at the origin or insertion of the muscles which are the most tense and to apply low frequency electrical stimulation. Raise the voltage up to the point where the muscles twitch lightly, but do not raise it so high as to cause the patient discomfort. The muscular tension should be greatly relieved after fifteen minutes of electrical stimulation.

Patients who have gastrointestinal problems and are underweight tend to get stiff neck and shoulders as do overweight patients with a reddish complexion and high blood pressure. For these patients, in addition to needling local points to reduce the tension, points for adjusting their overall condition such as improving digestion and reducing blood pressure are also important. Effecting a change in a patient's physical constitution requires treatments over a long period.

Providing a light massage in the neck and shoulder area after removing the needles improves circulation even more and helps make a patient feel relaxed and refreshed.

17. Chronic Bronchitis

Description

The primary type of chronic bronchitis occurs mostly among those with occupations involving exposure to noxious gases or dust (e.g., stone masons, textile workers, etc.) as well as those whose work requires the exaggerated use of their voice, heavy smokers, and those with recurrent infections of the upper respiratory tract. The secondary type of chronic bronchitis occurs when acute bronchitis becomes protracted, or by congestion in pulmonary circulation, or as a complication of lung disease. The main symptoms are coughing, expectoration of phlegm, and labored breathing. There is no fever in chronic bronchitis, and in the early

BL-10 (Tenchū)

BL-12 (Fūmon)

BL-13 (Haiyu)

BL-15 (Shinyu)

BL-17 (Kakuyu)

BL-23 (Jinyu)

BL-52 (Shishitsu)

LI-17 (Tentei)

CV-22 (Tentotsu)

LU-1 (Chūfu)

CV-17 (Danchū)

CV-14 (Koketsu)

CV-12 (Chūkan)

ST-25 (Tensū)

ST-27 (Daiko)

LU-7 (Rekketsu)

ST-36 (Ashi-no-Sanri)

ST-40 (Hōryū)

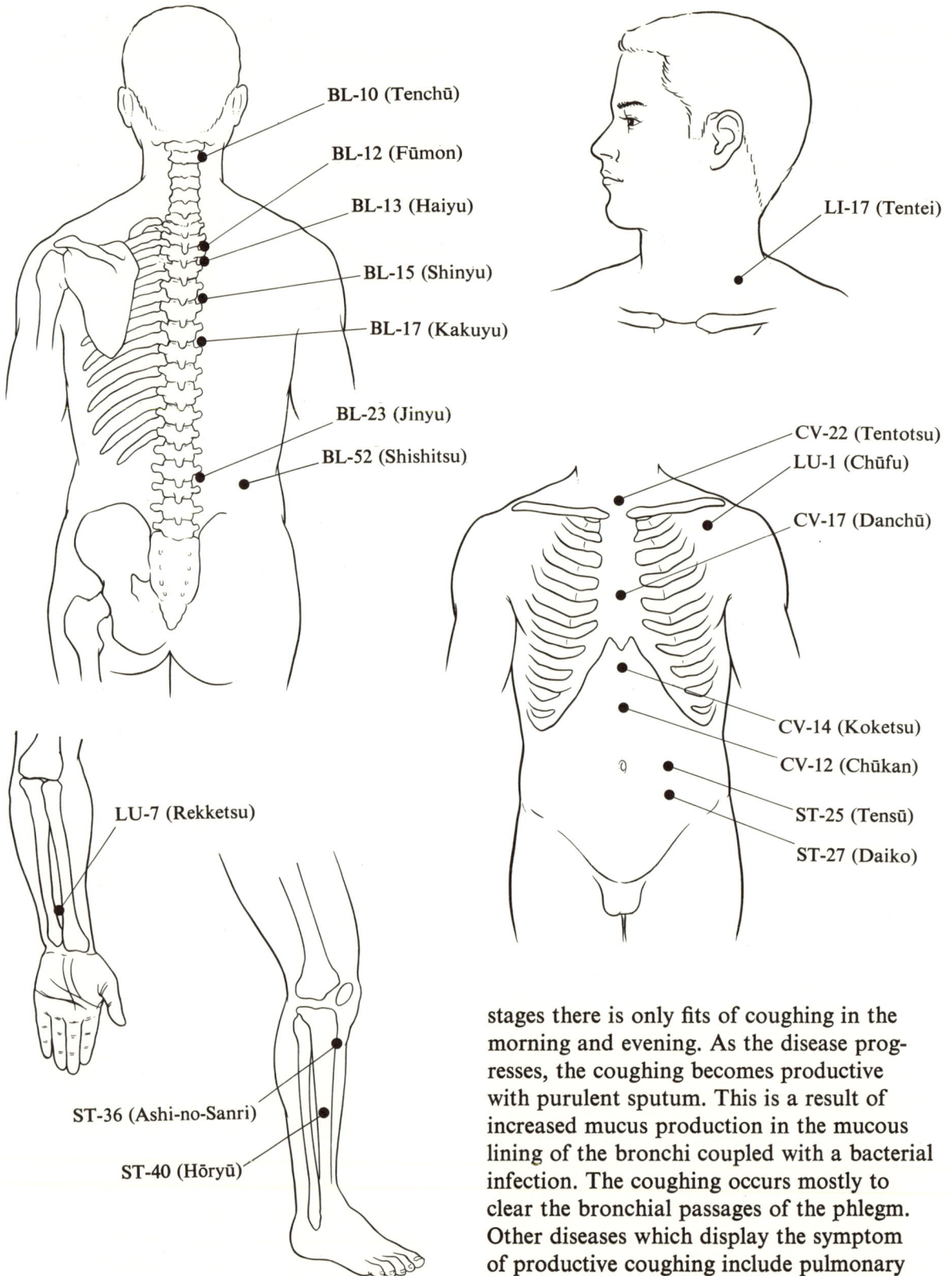

stages there is only fits of coughing in the morning and evening. As the disease progresses, the coughing becomes productive with purulent sputum. This is a result of increased mucus production in the mucous lining of the bronchi coupled with a bacterial infection. The coughing occurs mostly to clear the bronchial passages of the phlegm. Other diseases which display the symptom of productive coughing include pulmonary tuberculosis, emphysema, bronchiectasis, and lung cancer, so a patient must first undergo a thorough medical examination. The treatment for chronic bronchitis in Western medicine primarily consists of administering antibiotics for infections, cough suppressants, anti-inflammatory agents, and inhalation therapy. It is difficult to effect a complete cure for chronic bronchitis. Acupuncture is performed for cases of chronic bronchitis to reduce symptoms of pain and discomfort in the chest, sore throats, coughing, and excessive phlegm. Acupuncture is also effective in improving the patient's overall physical condition and increases appetite and alleviates general symptoms such as headaches and heaviness of the head.

Acupuncture points

    Neck—BL-10, LI-17
    Back—BL-12, BL-13, BL-15, BL-17, BL-23, BL-52
    Chest—CV-14, CV-17, CV-22, LU-1
    Abdomen—CV-12, ST-25, ST-27
    Arms—LU-7
    Legs—ST-36, ST-40

Treatment

Acupuncture treatments of chronic bronchitis must focus on improving the function of the lungs by stimulating the lung meridian. For this reason be sure to needle BL-13 (the back *shu* point of the lung meridian) and LU-1 (the front *mu* point of the lung meridian) as well as BL-12 and LU-7 (the *luo* point of the lung meridian). When there is excessive coughing and phlegm, needle CV-22, ST-36, and ST-40. Insert the needle in CV-22 by having the patient extend his neck in the supine position and direct the needle downward just behind the manubrium of the sternum. Insert the needle no deeper than three centimeters and gently lift and thrust and twist the needle. A good effect can be expected when a needling sensation is obtained inside the chest. Also needle BL-15, BL-17, and CV-17 when there is a sense of oppression in the chest. When there is a stifling sensation in the epigastric region, needle CV-14. For painful and sore throats, needle LI-17, on either side of the laryngeal prominence. If there is heaviness of the head or headaches, needle BL-10. If there is anorexia or gastrointestinal problems, also needle CV-12, ST-25, and ST-27. The treatment is more effective when BL-23 and BL-52 are included to raise the level of vitality. Retain the needles in the above points for up to ten minutes. It is also useful to apply an infrared lamp over the retained needles on the back and abdomen.

18. Bronchial Asthma

Description

Bronchial asthma is a fairly common condition and is one of the most widespread allergic conditions. Bronchial asthma occurs in those who have a predisposition to asthma when they are exposed to allergens. The allergic reaction of asthma often occurs with allergens of animal protein such as eggs, beef, pork, fish, or by certain vegetables, odors, dust, or pollen. It can also be caused by the climate or extremes of cold and heat. In 10 to 20 percent of asthmatics, the allergen or exciting cause is unclear, and it is thought that there is some family tendency, autonomic dysfunction, or endocrine disorder.

During an asthma attack, excitation of the parasympathetic nervous system causes a sudden spasmodic contraction of the smooth muscles of the bronchial wall, and

GV-14 (Daitsui)

Dingchuan (extra)

BL-13 (Haiyu)

BL-15 (Shinyu)

BL-23 (Jinyu)

BL-52 (Shishitsu)

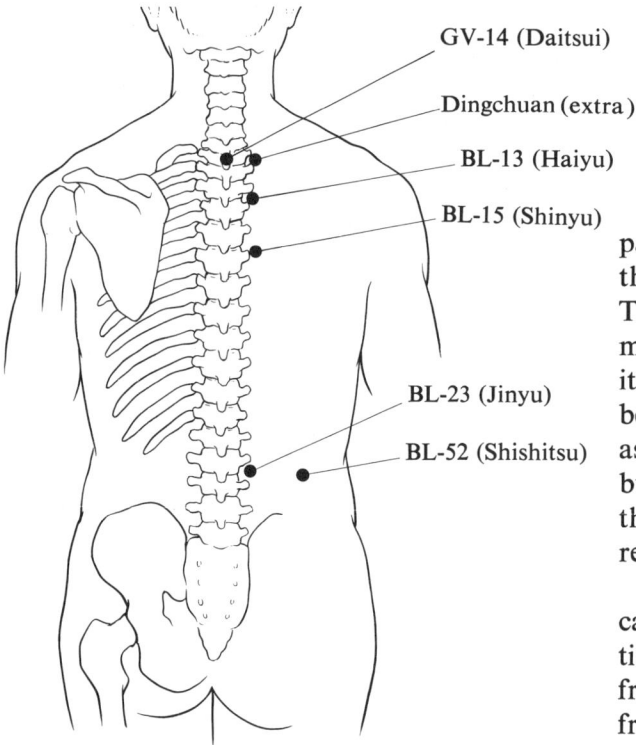

pale, and along with labored breathing, there is a characteristic wheezing sound. The asthma attack usually lasts from thirty minutes to several hours, but in rare cases it continues for several days. Asthma which begins in childhood quite often becomes asymptomatic as a person reaches adulthood, but those cases that begin or continue through adolescence quite often persist with recurrent attacks.

In addition to bronchial asthma, there is cardiac asthma and uremic asthma. A practitioner must differentiate bronchial asthma from these other types of asthma as well as from other lung diseases such as bronchitis or pulmonary tuberculosis. The main distinguishing features of bronchial asthma is

this obstructs one's breathing, especially expiration. Also the mucous lining of the bronchial tubes become inflamed and there is a marked increase in mucoid secretions. During an attack the patient's face turns

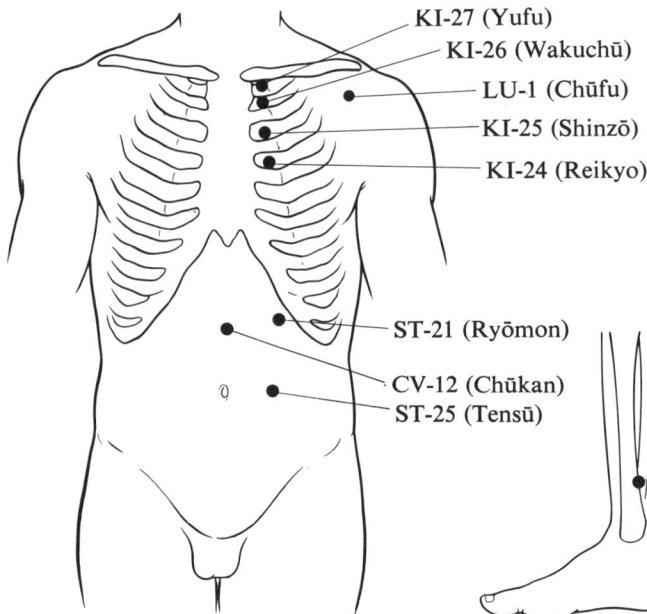

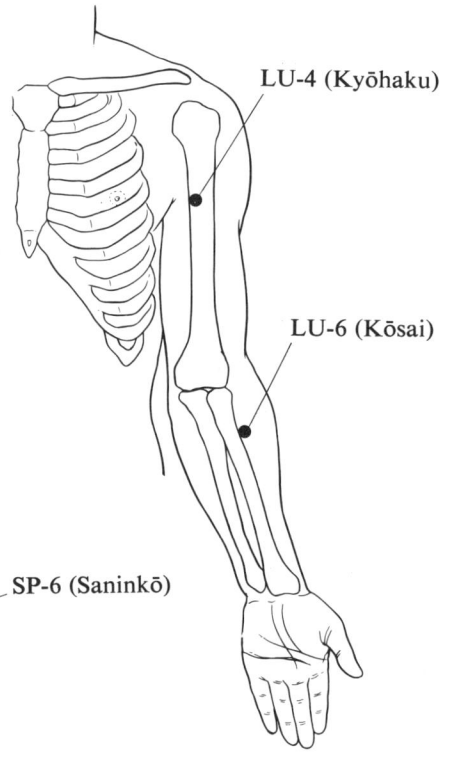

KI-27 (Yufu)

KI-26 (Wakuchū)

LU-1 (Chūfu)

KI-25 (Shinzō)

KI-24 (Reikyo)

LU-4 (Kyōhaku)

LU-6 (Kōsai)

ST-21 (Ryōmon)

CV-12 (Chūkan)

ST-25 (Tensū)

SP-6 (Saninkō)

paroxysmal attacks and the characteristic wheezing sound. Also asthma is easy to distinguish because of a family tendency or the allergic constitution of the patient with a tendency to get eczema or hives.

Acupuncture points

Back—BL-13, BL-15, BL-23, BL-52, GV-14, Chizen (extra)
Torso—LU-1, CV-12, ST-21, ST-25, KI-24, KI-25, KI-26, KI-27
Arms—LU-4, LU-6
Legs—SP-6

Treatment

Acupuncture treatments can be performed during an asthma attack to relieve the acute symptoms of respiratory distress. In this case shallowly needle the kidney points KI-24, KI-25, KI-26, and KI-27. Follow this by inserting a needle in GV-14, directly under the spinous process of the seventh cervical vertebra. Also needle the extra point Chizen, half a cun lateral to GV-14, along with BL-13 and BL-15. These needles should be inserted obliquely with the tips pointed medially to a depth of up to three centimeters.

Patients with asthma develop abnormal tension in the rectus abdominis and erector spinae muscles due to the wheezing and coughing during attacks. Before giving an acupuncture treatment between asthma attacks it is useful to apply warm compresses on the tense areas of the back and abdomen to relieve muscular tension. For the acupuncture treatment, in addition to the above mentioned points, gently needle BL-23 and BL-52 in the lumbar region, CV-12, ST-21, and ST-25 on the abdomen for the purpose of improving the overall physical condition. Also provide comparatively strong stimulation at LU-4 and LU-6 on the arm. SP-6 on the leg can be needled for the purpose of reducing chilling of the legs and feet.

Moxibustion can be applied on GV-14 and Chizenn regularly as a preventive measure. Apply three cones half the size of a rice grain on each point. The majority of patients with bronchial asthma have an allergic constitution, so in addition to alleviating the symptoms with acupuncture during an attack, they must be encouraged to receive acupuncture treatments over a long period to improve their physical constitution. In cases of childhood asthma, the same treatment as adults may be applied but with less stimulation. For babies and small children it is usually sufficient to provide light stimulation on the skin with roller needles or plum blossom needles. Lightly stimulate the skin along the lung meridian on the arm and along the spleen and kidney meridians on the leg until the skin begins to turn red. Providing this cutaneous stimulation on a daily basis is very effective against asthma in young children.

19. Hypertension

Description

A person is said to have hypertension, or high blood pressure, when the systolic pressure exceeds 160 mmHg or the diastolic pressure exceeds 95 mmHg for an extended period. Hypertension for no discernible cause is known as essential hypertension and this accounts for 80 to 90 percent of all hypertensive patients. Hypertension which results from other pathology is known as secondary hypertension and the majority of this is due to kidney disease. In the early stages of essential hypertension, the amount of vascular tension in all the arterioles throughout the body increases (functional disorder), but there is no structural change. When this type of hypertension persists for a number of years, however, arteriosclerosis (hardening of the arteries) begins to occur in the arterioles. Hypertension is often a constitutional problem with high familial incidence, and the real cause is still unclear.

The symptoms of hypertension vary widely in their subjective and objective manifestations, but there are very few symptoms in the incipient stage for the first few years. Over the years various symptoms begin to

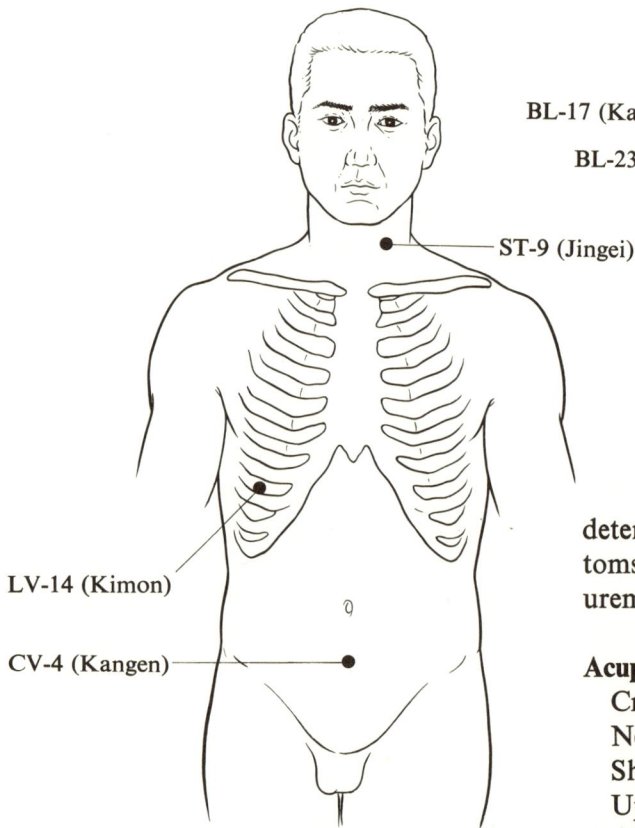

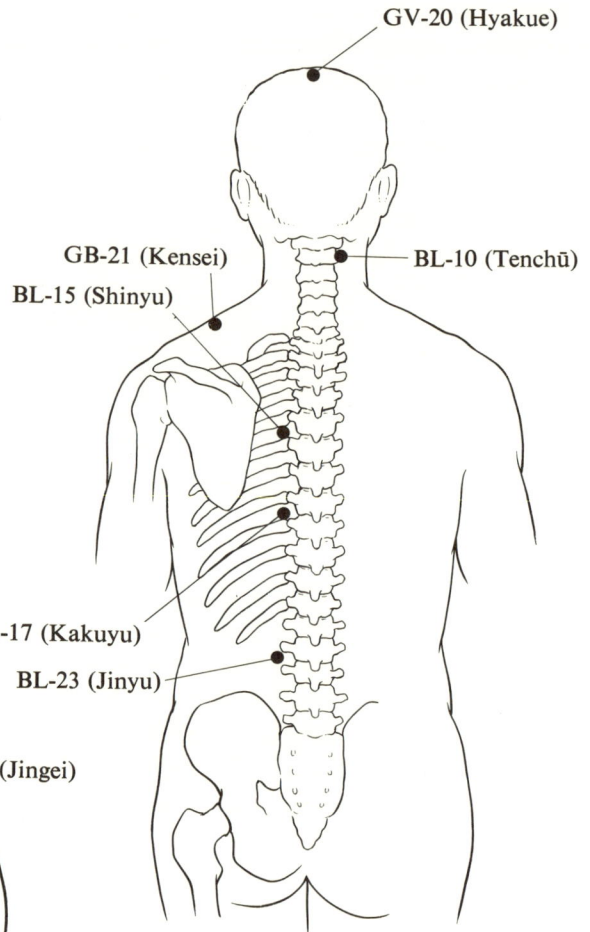

GV-20 (Hyakue)

GB-21 (Kensei)

BL-15 (Shinyu)

BL-10 (Tenchū)

BL-17 (Kakuyu)

BL-23 (Jinyu)

ST-9 (Jingei)

LV-14 (Kimon)

CV-4 (Kangen)

deterioration of vision. The terminal symptoms are apoplexy, angina pectoris, or uremia.

Acupuncture points
Cranium—GV-20
Neck—BL-10, ST-9
Shoulder—GB-21
Upper back—BL-15, BL-17
Abdomen—LV-14, CV-4
Lumbar region—BL-23
Legs—SP-6, GB-39, KI-1

Treatment
There are no acupuncture points effective for keeping the blood pressure down, so the

appear. They begin with headaches, heaviness of the head, dizziness, and tinnitus, and gradually progress to palpitations, shortness of breath, nocturnal enuresis, and occasionally hemorrhage at the base of the brain and

SP-6 (Saninkō)

GB-39 (Kenshō)

KI-1 (Yūsen)

is the strongest. At the bifurcation of the common carotid artery there is the carotid sinus that contains a pressure receptor which slows down the heart rate and serves to reduce blood pressure. The carotid sinus can be stimulated by carefully inserting a needle in this point one to one and a half centimeters until the arterial wall is reached. The needle should move with the pulsing of the artery. The needle must not be retained for more than a minute when a needle is inserted in ST-9 to reach the carotid sinus. Also insert needles in KI-1 to a depth of one to one and a half centimeters and retain the needles for up to five minutes.

For hypertensive patients with headaches and neck and shoulder tension, in addition to the above points, needle GV-20, BL-10, and GB-21. For those with insomnia, also use BL-17 and LV-14. For those experiencing fatigue and lassitude, also use BL-23 and CV-4. For those with chilling of the feet, also use SP-9 and GB-39. For those with strong palpitations, also use BL-15. It takes repeated treatments over a long period to control hypertension. Care must be taken in each session to keep the total amount of stimulation at a moderate level.

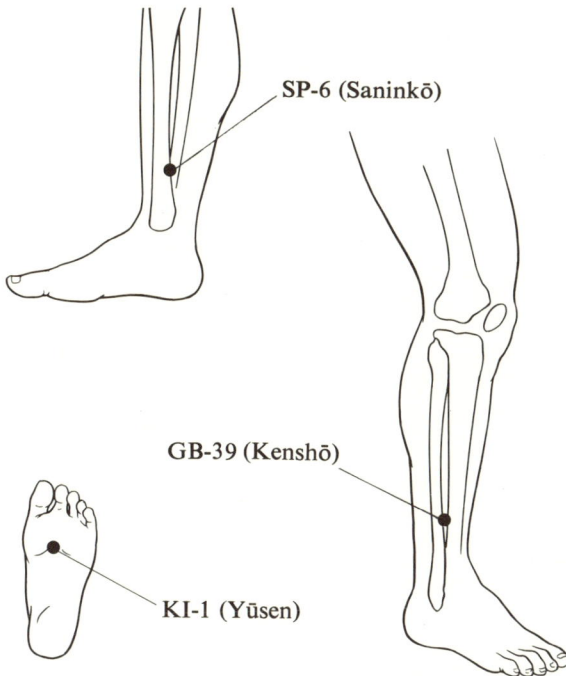

aim of the treatment should be to relieve the general symptoms one by one. Begin the treatment by needling ST-9 and KI-1, points which are known to reduce blood pressure. ST-9 is located on the medial border of the sternocleidomastoid muscle over the carotid artery where the pulsation

20. Hypotension

Description

Hypotension is a condition of lower than normal blood pressure, and although there are several opinions regarding what exactly constitutes hypotension, the general consensus is a systolic pressure of under 100 mmHg (age must be taken into consideration). As causes of hypotension, there are three possibilities: a reduction in the heart's contractile strength or stroke pressure, a reduction in the amount of blood in circulation, and a reduction in resistance of peripheral vessels (vascular resistance). Some

patients become worried when they learn that they have hypotension, but actually there is no need for concern when there are no special symptoms. It is even said that people with low blood pressure tend to live longer.

Hypotension can be roughly classified into three types. Essential hypotension is hypotension which occurs for no definable cause. Secondary hypotension is hypotension for which the cause is clear, such as severe hemorrhage or anemia. Orthostatic hypotension is a condition where dizziness

GV-20 (Hyakue)

GB-21 (Kensei)

BL-10 (Tenchū)

BL-15 (Shinyu)

BL-44 (Shindō)

BL-23 (Jinyu)

CV-12 (Chūkan)

KI-16 (Kōyu)

ST-27 (Daiko)

LI-11 (Kyokuchi)

LI-4 (Gōkoku)

SP-9 (Inryōsen)

SP-6 (Saninkō)

KI-3 (Taikei)

KI-6 (Shōkai)

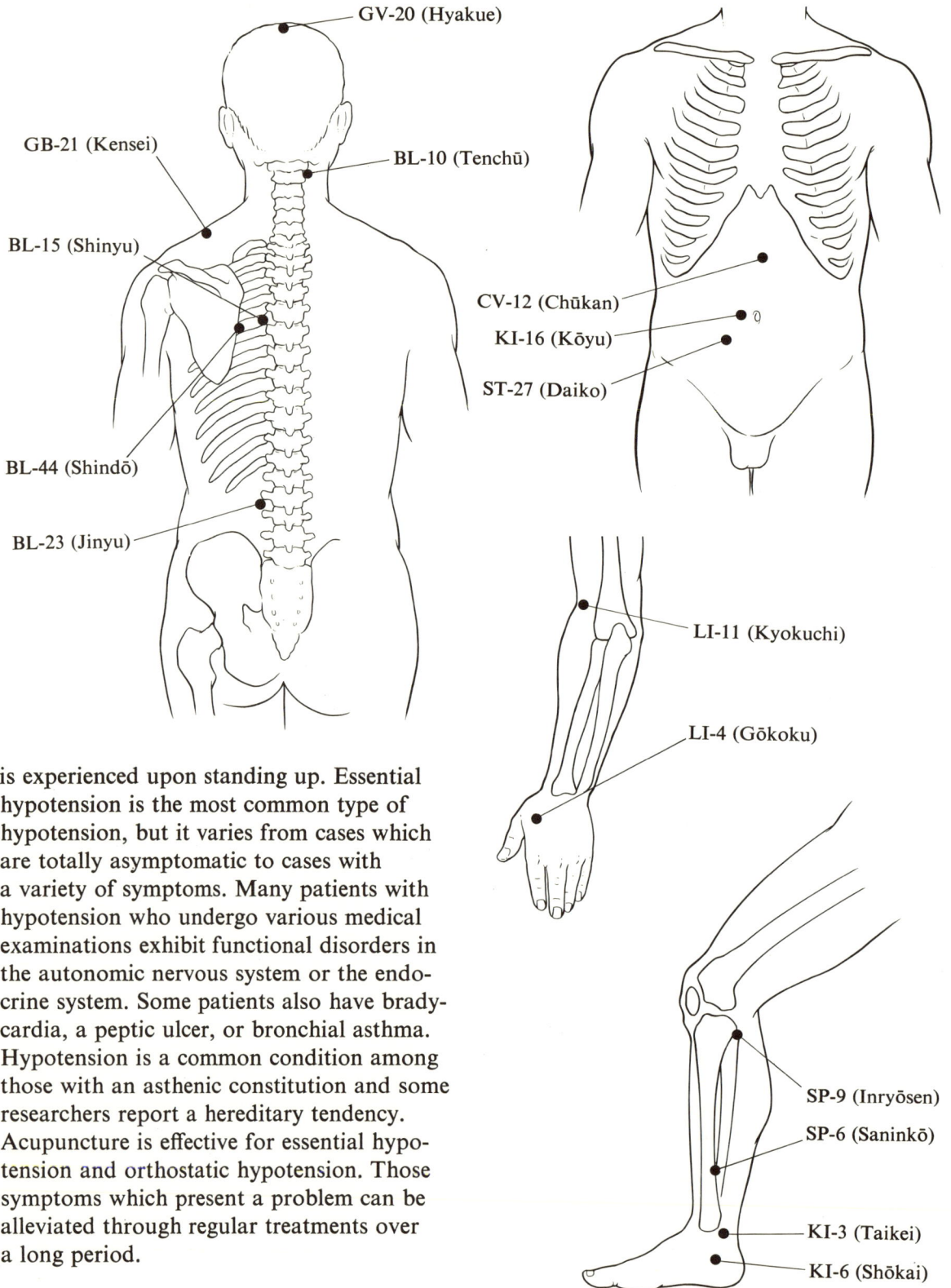

is experienced upon standing up. Essential hypotension is the most common type of hypotension, but it varies from cases which are totally asymptomatic to cases with a variety of symptoms. Many patients with hypotension who undergo various medical examinations exhibit functional disorders in the autonomic nervous system or the endocrine system. Some patients also have bradycardia, a peptic ulcer, or bronchial asthma. Hypotension is a common condition among those with an asthenic constitution and some researchers report a hereditary tendency. Acupuncture is effective for essential hypotension and orthostatic hypotension. Those symptoms which present a problem can be alleviated through regular treatments over a long period.

Acupuncture points

Cranium—GV-20
Neck—BL-10
Shoulder—GB-21
Back—BL-15, BL-23, BL-44
Abdomen—CV-12, KI-16, ST-27
Arms—LI-11, LI-4
Legs—SP-6, SP-9, KI-3, KI-6

Treatment

In cases of secondary hypotension, the causative factor must be treated medically and acupuncture can be provided in addition. When a patient's head feels hazy, insert a needle horizontally in GV-20 and retain. After this, needle BL-10 and GB-21 and reduce the muscular tension there by gentle lifting and thrusting and then retain the needles briefly. When there is chilling of the extremities, either massage or acupuncture can be performed. In the case of acupuncture, provide light stimulation to LI-11, LI-4, SP-6, and SP-9. When a patient feels dull and listless, provide light needle stimulation to CV-12, KI-16, and ST-27 on the abdomen, BL-15, BL-23, and BL-44 on the back, and KI-3 and KI-6 on the foot. Patients with hypotension have a deficient condition so light stimulation is appropriate.

There are patients with essential hypotension who have a variety of symptoms which fluctuate from day to day along with changes in the weather and their temperament. This is known as complaints of general malaise, and acupuncture is usually quite effective in these cases. The treatment should be aimed at regulating the function of the autonomic nervous system, and the same points listed above can be used. The bladder points along the spine are especially useful for regulating the autonomic nervous system since they are close to the sympathetic nerve trunk. Also CV-12 in the upper abdomen is useful because it is directly over the solar plexus, a sympathetic ganglion controlling the function of abdominal organs. Needle these points with care, making sure not to overstimulate. Treating hypotension requires time, so it is necessary for the patient to receive regular treatments over a long period.

21. Pyrosis and Eructation

Description

Pyrosis is commonly known as heartburn and indicates a burning discomfort which goes up the esophagus from the epigastric region to the chest. Often pyrosis is accompanied by eructation. Eructation is belching, or releasing gas in the stomach through the mouth. Even healthy persons, if they have a habit of gulping in air while they eat, get a great deal of air into the stomach. Thus belching a few times after a meal is not unusual, but excessive and continuous belching is a sign of gallbladder diseases, gastric neurosis, or gastroasthenia. Among the various types of eructation, the kind without any odor is relatively normal; usually air which collected in the stomach is being released spontaneously. Eructation with a foul odor or a bitter or sour smell requires some attention. If patients also experience other symptoms such as nausea or abdominal pain, it is best to have them undergo a comprehensive medical examination before treating them with acupuncture.

When pyrosis is experienced continuously with no relation to meals or the time of day, chronic gastritis, peptic ulcers, or duodenal ulcers may be suspected, and it is even possible that pyrosis is being caused by stomach cancer or heart disease. On the other hand, there are many cases where pyrosis is experienced when there is no

CV-22 (Tentotsu)

CV-14 (Koketsu)

LV-14 (Kimon)

CV-12 (Chūkan)

ST-25 (Tensū)

BL-19 (Tanyu)

BL-20 (Hiyu)

BL-21 (Iyu)

PC-6 (Naikan)

ST-36 (Ashi-no-Sanri)

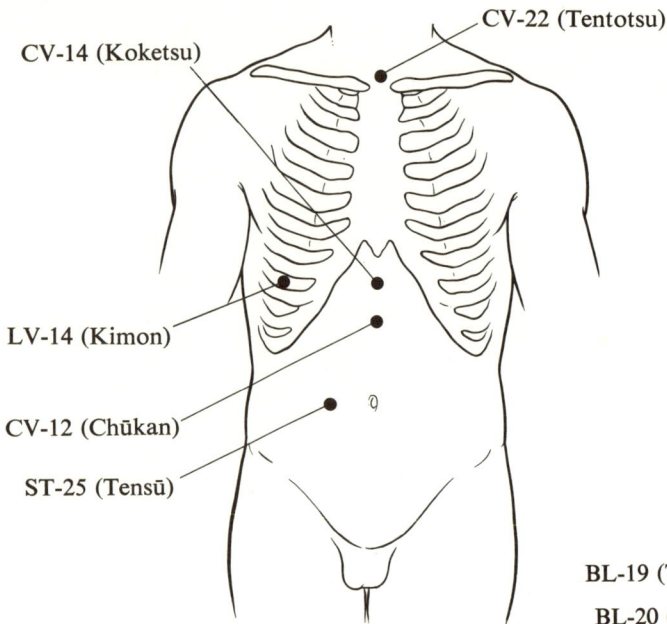

pathology. There are many so-called psycho-somatic cases in which the symptom goes away as soon as the person calms down.

Acupuncture points

Throat—CV-22
Abdomen—CV-12, CV-14, LV-14, ST-25
Back—BL-19, BL-20, BL-21
Arms—PC-6
Legs—ST-36

Treatment

Both pyrosis and eructation should be treated by needling points along the stomach, liver, and conception vessel meridians. Begin by inserting a needle obliquely downward in CV-22 just behind the manubrium of the sternum. Follow this by needling CV-14, CV-12, LV-14, and ST-25 on the abdomen. Always needle ST-36 to regulate the gastro-intestinal function and improve the overall physical condition. Also needle PC-6, a point effective for controlling eructation and nausea. Retain the needles for about ten minutes. After removing the needles, have the patient assume the prone position to needle BL-19, BL-20, and BL-21 on the back.

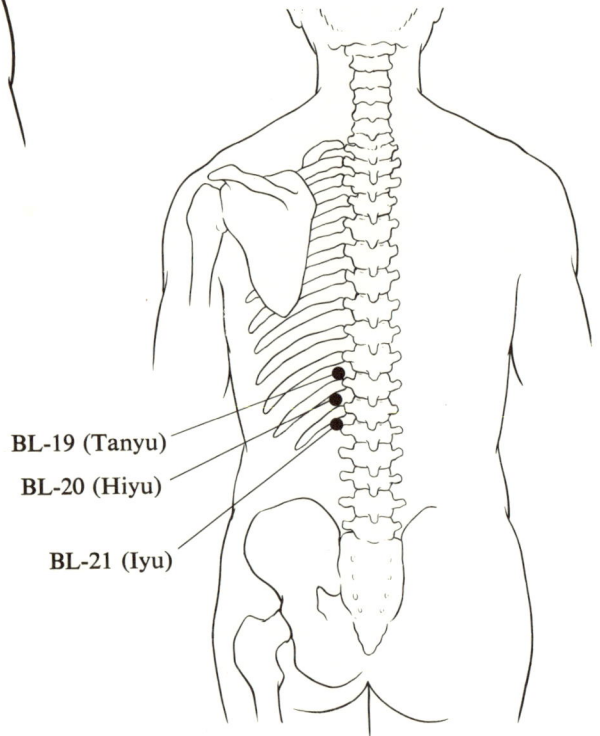

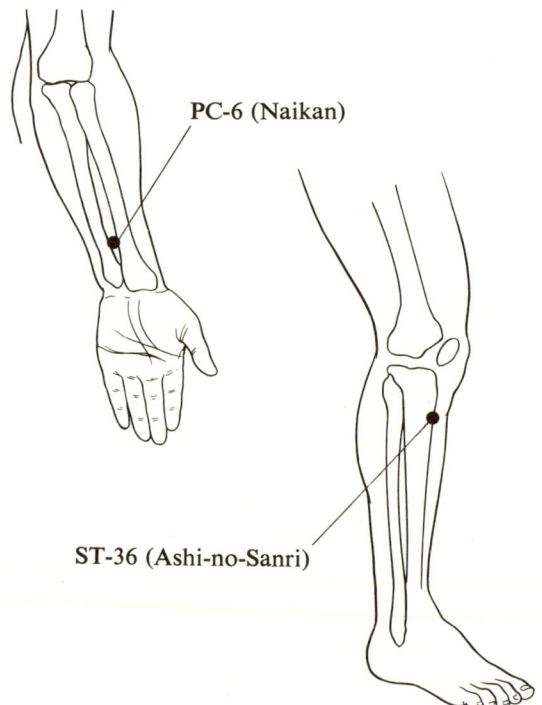

22. Nausea and Vomiting

Description

Nausea and vomiting are very common symptoms which often accompany serious illnesses so a practitioner must exercise caution when treating these symptoms. Nausea and vomiting constitute a sequence of physiological responses. Nausea is generally considered to come before vomiting, and the secretion of stomach acids increases and one's stomach seems to turn. Vomiting is a reflexive protective mechanism of the body by which rotten food and poisons in the stomach are expelled to keep the body from harm. Normally when a person vomits, his face turns pale and there is extreme discomfort, but for those who vomit habitually, there does not seem to be so much discomfort. It is unusual but yet possible to vomit suddenly without any nausea. The vomiting center is located in the medulla oblongata and is close to the dorsal nucleus of the vagus nerve. The vomiting center reacts to various stimuli and sets off an organized series of impulses to the muscle groups involved in vomiting. The irritant or the cause of vomiting varies widely from ingestion of rotten foods and poisonous substances to irritation of the stomach lining by diseases like gastritis or peptic ulcers. Otherwise nausea and vomiting is caused by mechanical stimulation near the pharynx, diseases of organs in the pelvic cavity (appendicitis, peritonitis, gallstone, intestinal obstruction, and disorders of female reproductive organs), abnormal signals from the semicircular canals (seasickness), strong headaches and diseases causing a rise in intracranial pressure (brain tumors, cerebral

hemorrhage, etc.), and cerebral hypoxia. Generally nausea is related to stomach problems or gastrointestinal disorders, but since it is a symptom occurring in so many conditions, a practitioner must carefully ascertain the cause before providing treatment. First the disease or condition causing the nausea and vomiting must be determined and treated. The vomiting reflex must not be controlled when caused by the ingestion of harmful substances, since it is the normal and necessary response for survival. Generally patients who are vomiting must be kept still and warm. Physicians should be consulted when there is a high fever and severe abdominal pain. Acupuncture therapy consists of controlling the vomiting and related symptoms by stimulating a combination of points for general recovery.

Acupuncture points
Throat—CV-22
Abdomen—CV-12, ST-25, LV-14

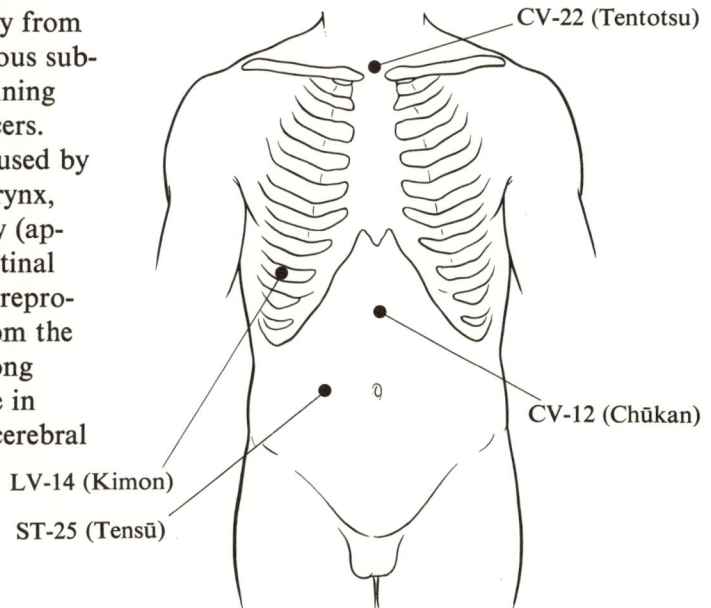

CV-22 (Tentotsu)
CV-12 (Chūkan)
LV-14 (Kimon)
ST-25 (Tensū)

Neck—BL-10
Back—BL-18, BL-19, BL-20, BL-21
Arms—PC-6
Legs—ST-36

Treatment

In the acute phase when there is strong nausea or vomiting, ST-36 and PC-6 are needled for symptomatic relief. Insert the needles vertically up to three centimeters and apply lifting and thrusting and rotation

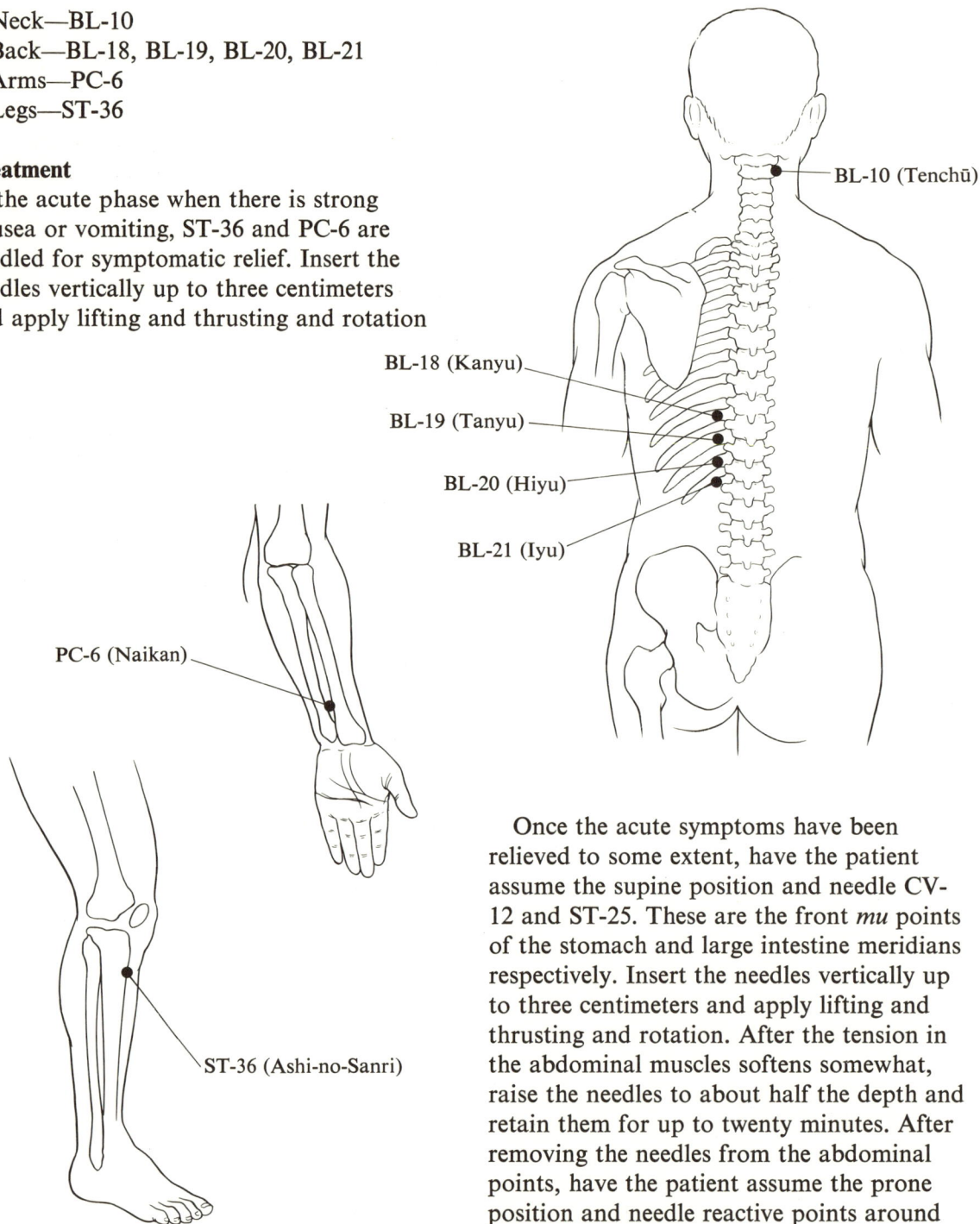

BL-10 (Tenchū)

BL-18 (Kanyu)

BL-19 (Tanyu)

BL-20 (Hiyu)

BL-21 (Iyu)

PC-6 (Naikan)

ST-36 (Ashi-no-Sanri)

to provide comparatively strong stimulation. Applying low frequency electrical stimulation through the above points is also an effective approach.

Once the acute symptoms have been relieved to some extent, have the patient assume the supine position and needle CV-12 and ST-25. These are the front *mu* points of the stomach and large intestine meridians respectively. Insert the needles vertically up to three centimeters and apply lifting and thrusting and rotation. After the tension in the abdominal muscles softens somewhat, raise the needles to about half the depth and retain them for up to twenty minutes. After removing the needles from the abdominal points, have the patient assume the prone position and needle reactive points around BL-20 and BL-21.

If the patient has a deficient condition or a chronic problem, the application of an infrared lamp or moxa needling is indicated. If the nausea and vomiting is associated with liver or gallbladder diseases, needle LV-14 obliquely, aiming the needle up toward the patient's head. Then follow this with stimulation of the back *shu* points of the liver and gallbladder, BL-18 and BL-19. If nausea is a constant problem associated with a deficient condition, the regular application of direct or warming moxibustion on CV-12 and ST-36 is very beneficial.

23. Constipation

Description

Constipation is a condition in which the frequency or quantity of bowel movements is less than normal, and sometimes this causes some physical discomfort. Since brief periods of constipation is not clinically significant, the following discussion deals with chronic constipation. Chronic constipation includes symptomatic constipation, which is a result of other pathology, and habitual constipation, which occurs for no discernible cause. Symptomatic constipation occurs from a variety of causes including obstruction in the lower digestive tract, pressure exerted on the rectum by adjacent organs, adhesions in the peritoneum, and a decrease in peristaltic activity. Obstruction in the digestive tract occurs in cases of rectal cancer and cicatricial stenosis of the rectum (narrowing by scar tissue). Adhesions in the peritoneum occurs with peritonitis or appendicitis. A decrease in peristalsis is seen with chronic enteritis, disorders of the visceral nerves, and in extremely weak patients. In cases of habitual constipation, although there is no apparent cause, the peristaltic action of the intestines is inhibited and insufficient.

Habitual constipation accounts for more than half of all cases of chronic constipation. It is seen most often in women, and this type of constipation is deeply connected with a person's life-style and general environment. Habitual constipation is divided into two basic types: atonic constipation and spastic constipation. The majority of habitual constipation is atonic constipation. The major causes of atonic constipation are deficiency in dietary fiber, lack of exercise, a habit of holding off going to the toilet, and a decrease in muscle tone in the abdominal organs (e.g., mothers who have had many children). Spastic constipation is a spasmodic condition of the intestines which is seen mostly in hypersensitive and nervous

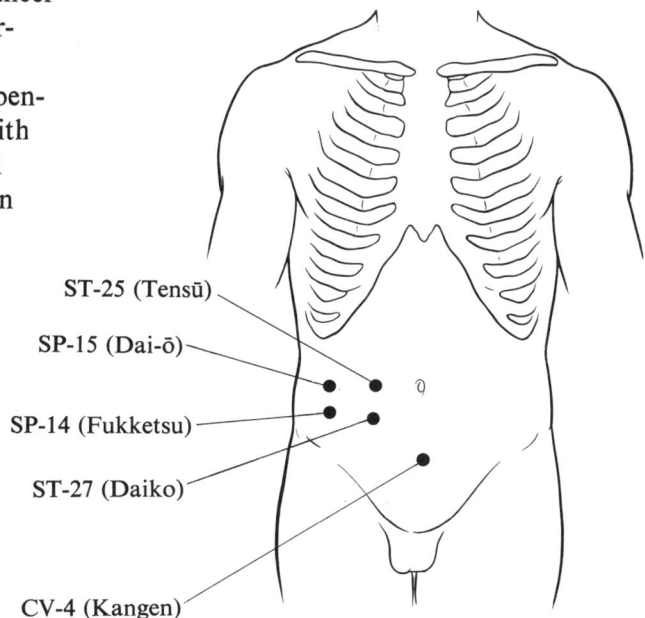

ST-25 (Tensū)
SP-15 (Dai-ō)
SP-14 (Fukketsu)
ST-27 (Daiko)
CV-4 (Kangen)

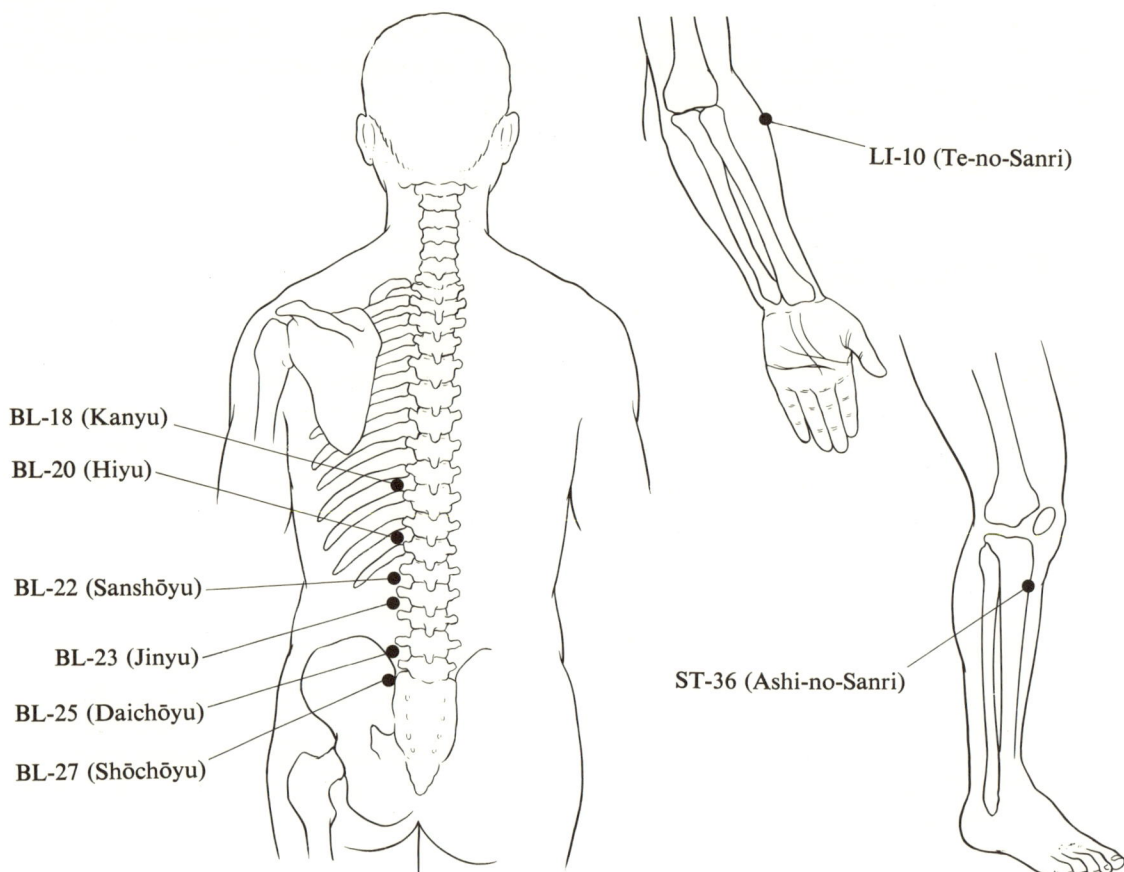

BL-18 (Kanyu)

BL-20 (Hiyu)

BL-22 (Sanshōyu)

BL-23 (Jinyu)

BL-25 (Daichōyu)

BL-27 (Shōchōyu)

LI-10 (Te-no-Sanri)

ST-36 (Ashi-no-Sanri)

individuals. Spasms in the intestines break up the stools so that they come out as little balls or thin pieces. This type of constipation is usually accompanied by many other symptoms such as abdominal distension and pain, headaches, heaviness of the head, anorexia, hotness of the head, dizziness, nausea, insomnia, and anxiety attacks. Modifying the diet is important for controlling chronic constipation. In the case of atonic constipation, a patient must eat foods with a higher fiber content and take more fluids. In the case of spastic constipation, a patient should eat foods which are readily digested and take time to chew well. In general, patients with constipation must get adequate exercise, recreation, and relaxation and strive toward a more balanced life-style.

Acupuncture points
Abdomen—ST-25, ST-27, SP-14, SP-15, CV-4
Back—BL-18, BL-20, BL-22, BL-23, BL-25, BL-27
Arms—LI-10
Legs—ST-36

Treatment
Patients with constipation generally tend to have tenderness and indurations around ST-27 and SP-14 on the left side. Also often there is a reaction along the *dai* channel (belt line) on the left side as well as at BL-23 on the left side.

The objective of acupuncture treatments is to raise the tone of the abdominal muscles and the smooth muscles of the intestines and to increase the peristaltic action of the intestines. For spastic constipation due to psychological factors, first apply warm compresses to the lumbar area to relieve tension before providing acupuncture. Use thin needles on those with a sensitive or nervous disposition and apply only a small amount of stimulation. Begin treatments for constipation by needling points in the lumbar area such as BL-23, BL-25, and BL-27. Insert the needles deeply (about three centimeters) and provide comparatively strong stimulation. After this, needle ST-25, ST-27, SP-14, SP-15, and CV-4. Insert the needles gently in these points on the abdomen until a mild sensation is produced, and then retain them and apply additional mild needle stimulation such as fine vibration. Also needle LI-10 and ST-36

since these are important points regulating gastrointestinal function. For the other symptoms accompanying constipation, needle the appropriate points for each symptom and seek to improve the patient's overall physical condition. After removing all the needles, massage the abdomen to improve the function of the intestines. Give a gentle but deep massage over the course of the colon, starting over the area of the cecum and ending at the beginning of the sigmoid colon. A deep massage over the colon serves to break up the stagnation and facilitate the movement of the intestinal contents toward the rectum.

24. Diarrhea

Description
Diarrhea is an increase in the liquid content of the stools which produces loose or fluid stools. When the stools are loose, they are called soft stools and when the stools are fluid they are called waterlike stools. Among the causes of diarrhea is the increased peristaltic action in the intestines especially that of the colon, which makes the intestinal contents pass through without thorough absorption of moisture. Sometimes there are abnormalities in the mucous lining of the intestines which prevents the normal absorption of moisture or increases the excretion

of moisture. In some cases diarrhea is caused by a combination of the above factors.

Diarrhea can be divided into acute and chronic diarrhea according to the accom-

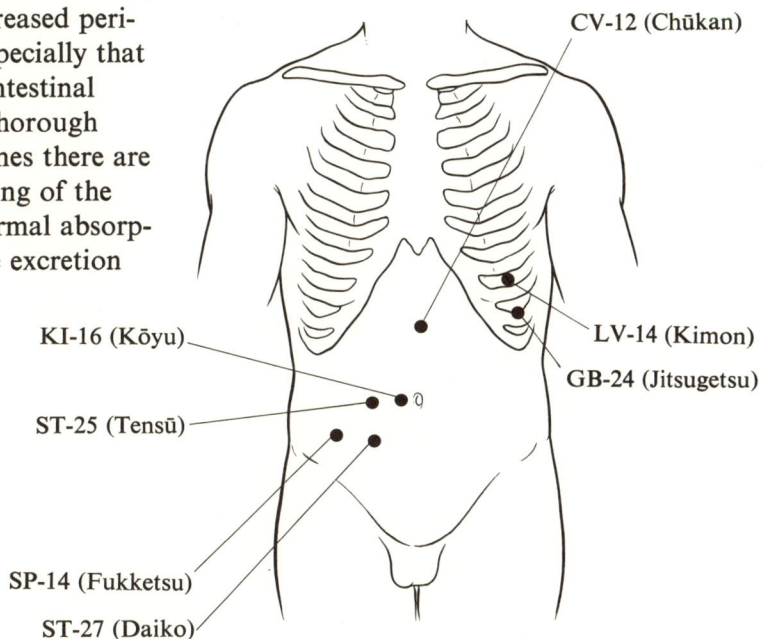

CV-12 (Chūkan)
LV-14 (Kimon)
GB-24 (Jitsugetsu)
KI-16 (Kōyu)
ST-25 (Tensū)
SP-14 (Fukketsu)
ST-27 (Daiko)

panying symptoms. Generally acute diarrhea is caused by enterocolitis, and it is often accompanied by fever, abdominal pain, and vomiting. These symptoms are usually absent in chronic diarrhea, but often there is anorexia and other digestive complaints. Diarrhea is a defense mechanism of the body by which the absorption of harmful substances is prevented when toxic or irritating substances are ingested. For example, inflammation occurs when the body becomes infected by microorganisms and the visceral organs are stimulated. Thus peristaltic action increases and the absorption through the intestinal lining is inhibited. Furthermore, excretion from the intestinal lining increases. This produces diarrhea and the pathogenic organisms and toxins are expelled from the body. Diarrhea is an indispensable mechanism for survival.

When treating diarrhea, it is important that the practitioner determine the cause and be aware of cases which require referral to physicians. Once the cause is determined the treatment must address the basic cause. In addition measures must be taken to deal with dehydration and nutritional needs. The type of diarrhea normally treated with acupuncture is the chronic variety in which the symptoms are less severe and the cause is not very clear. In most cases it is related to nervous conditions and stress.

Acupuncture points
Abdomen—ST-25, ST-27, SP-14, KI-16,
    CV-12, LV-14, GB-24
Back—BL-18, BL-19, BL-22, BL-23,
    BL-25, BL-27
Arms—PC-6
Legs—ST-36, SP-6

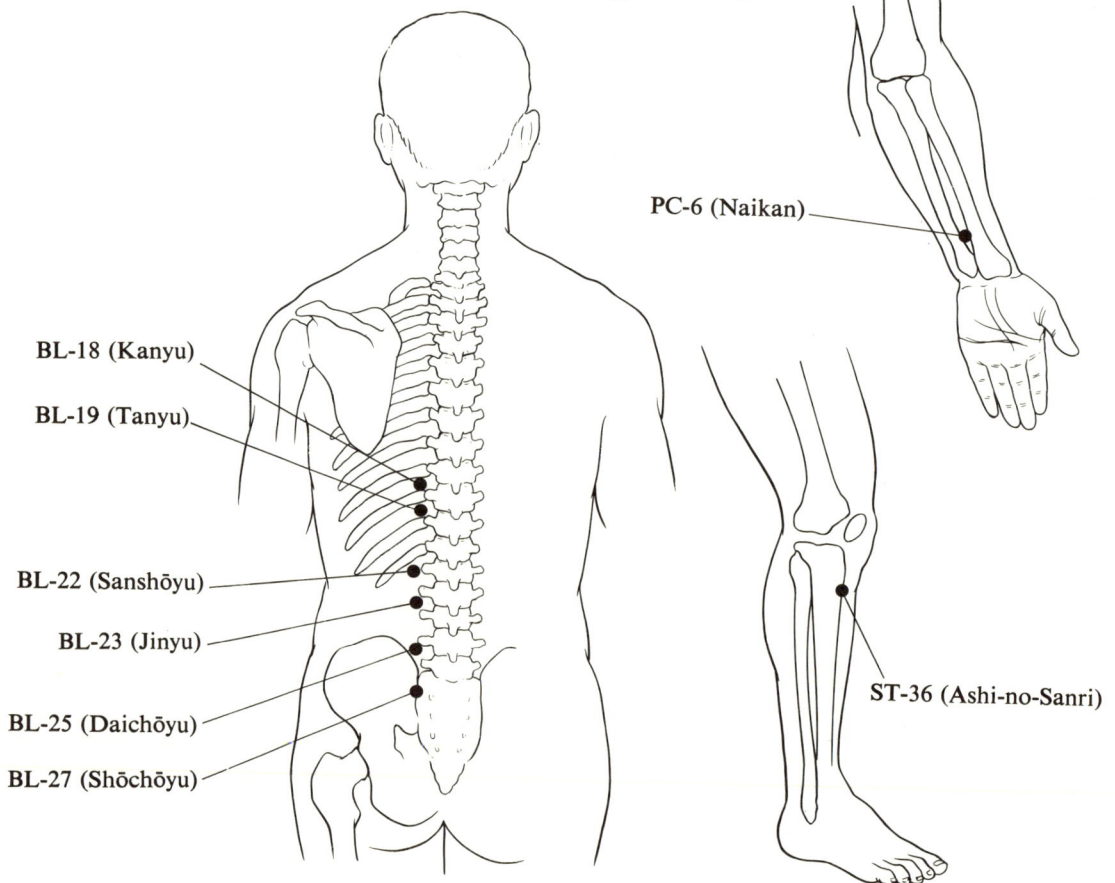

PC-6 (Naikan)

BL-18 (Kanyu)

BL-19 (Tanyu)

BL-22 (Sanshōyu)

BL-23 (Jinyu)

BL-25 (Daichōyu)

BL-27 (Shōchōyu)

ST-36 (Ashi-no-Sanri)

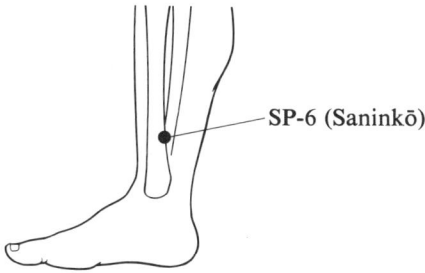

SP-6 (Saninkō)

Treatment

Diarrhea is a gastrointestinal problem so acupuncture points of the stomach and spleen meridians should be selected for the treatment. The main points to needle are ST-25, ST-36, and SP-14. Insert the needles vertically and apply slow lifting and thrusting and twisting. It is beneficial in some cases (e.g., conditions of internal cold) to apply the moxa needle technique. In addition BL-22, BL-25, BL-27, CV-12, and ST-27 are also useful for regulating the function of the intestines.

For diarrhea which occurs as a result of liver and gallbladder disorders, also needle BL-18, BL-19, LV-14, and GB-24 to improve the function of the liver and gallbladder. For thin individuals with lack of muscle tone in their lower abdomen, also needle BL-23 on the back and KI-16 on the abdomen.

Moxibustion is often very effective for diarrhea. The best points to use are BL-22, BL-25, BL-27, CV-12, ST-25, and ST-36. Select a few of the above points which show a reaction and apply up to five small moxa cones (half the size of a rice grain) on each point. Those who are thin and lack tone in their lower abdomen should also receive moxa on BL-23 and KI-16. Applying moxibustion on SP-6 is useful for those patients who experience chilling of their feet. When a patient experiences chilling in the abdomen, garlic moxibustion or warming moxibustion on abdominal points is very useful. Patients with diarrhea due to deficiencies or internal cold need to receive moxibustion treatments over a long period for lasting improvement.

25. Chronic Gastritis

Description

Gastritis is a general term covering all types of inflammation in the mucous lining of the stomach. There are a large number of patients with gastritis in Japan, and fully one-third of all stomach disorders are said to be gastritis. Gastritis is one of the three major stomach diseases in Japan along with peptic ulcers and stomach cancer. The external causes of gastritis include immoderation in eating, drug side effects, accidental ingestion of corrosive substances, and various infectious diseases. The internal causes of gastritis include circulatory problems, diseases of the liver, gallbladder, and pancreas, malnutrition, and emotional disturbances.

Gastritis is classified into acute and chronic types. Chronic gastritis often occurs by the internal causes listed above, but also it can be a protracted case of acute gastritis initially caused by external causes. Gastritis is classified into several categories according to the histological changes of the stomach lining. In atrophic gastritis the normally wrinkled mucous lining of the stomach becomes smooth and the lining becomes thin. (This is thought to be precancerous condition). In hypertrophic gastritis the mucous lining thickens and the stomach lining becomes extremely convoluted. In superficial gastritis mucoid excretion of the stomach increases and there is subepithelial edema and vasodilatation in the capillaries.

Mild cases of chronic gastritis are often

CV-14 (Koketsu)

CV-12 (Chūkan)

ST-21 (Ryōmon)

ST-25 (Tensū)

KI-16 (Kōyu)

BL-17 (Kakuyu)

BL-19 (Tanyu)

BL-20 (Hiyu)

BL-21 (Iyu)

BL-23 (Jinyu)

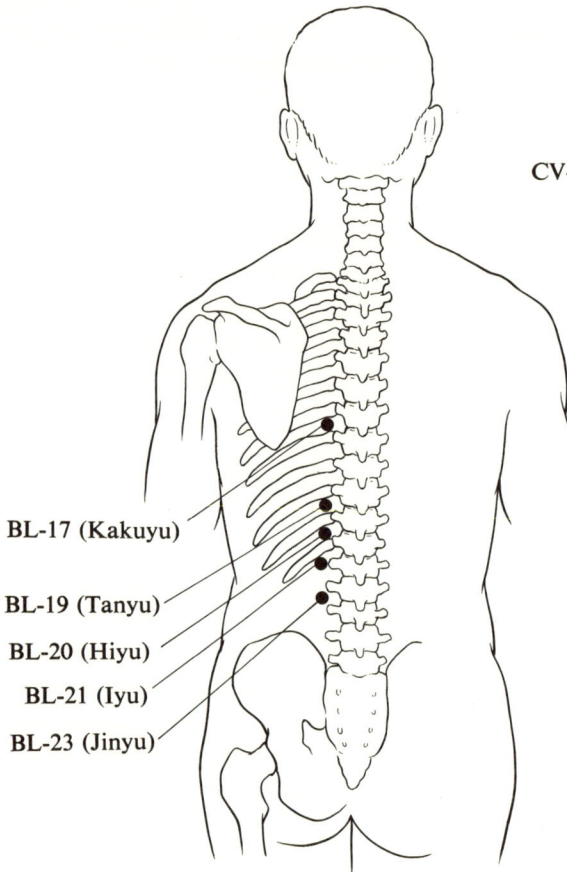

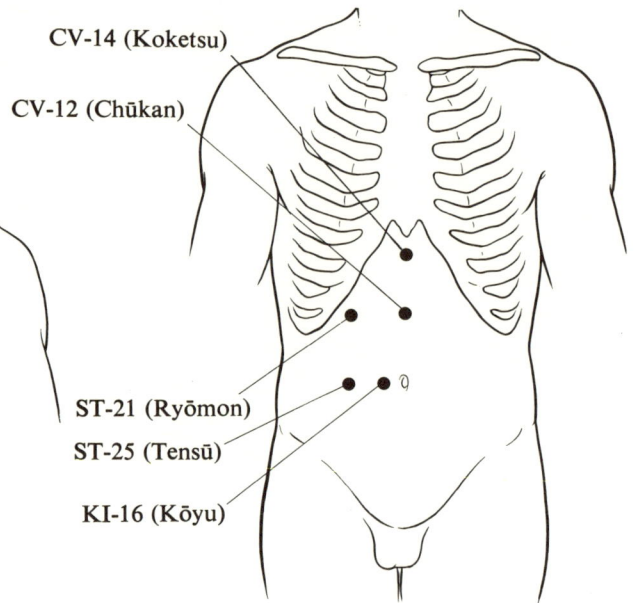

practically asymptomatic. The general symptoms of advanced chronic gastritis are light stomachaches and distension of the stomach after meals, abdominal distension, nausea, vomiting, constipation, and anorexia. The symptoms are light and transitory in the early stages, but as the condition progresses, a patient often begins to lose weight. In

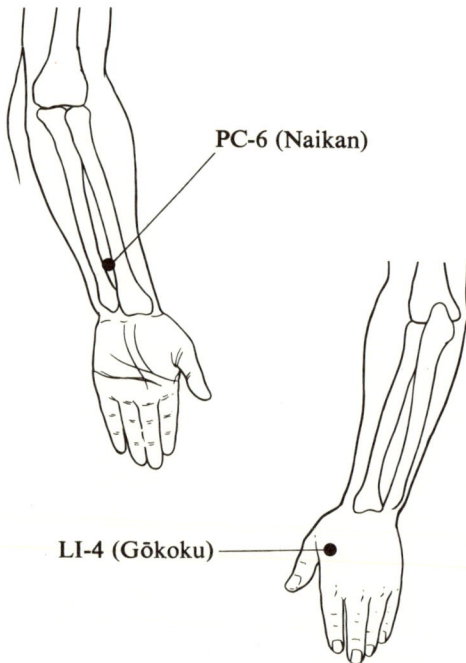

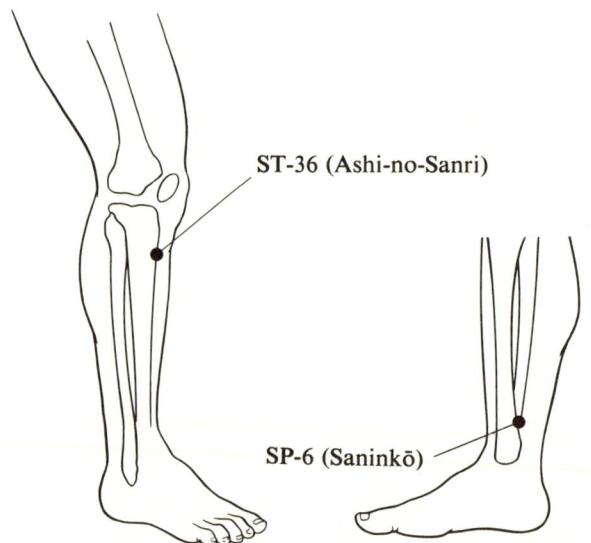

PC-6 (Naikan)

ST-36 (Ashi-no-Sanri)

LI-4 (Gōkoku)

SP-6 (Saninkō)

addition a patient will begin to experience a decline in stamina, a tendency to become fatigued easily, anemic symptoms, and a general lack of motivation. People do not die from gastritis, but often gastritis is a symptom of incipient peptic ulcers. Also gastritis can cause disturbances in the secretion of digestive enzymes and therefore can lead to many other problems. Just as colds are known as the source of all diseases in Japan, gastritis can be called the beginning of all stomach diseases.

Acupuncture points

Back—BL-17, BL-19, BL-20, BL-21, BL-23
Abdomen—CV-12, CV-14, KI-16, ST-21, ST-25
Arms—PC-6, LI-4
Legs—ST-36, SP-6

Treatment

Patients with chronic gastritis almost always have tension and stiffness in the middle of their back. In order to relieve this tension, probe around BL-17, BL-19, BL-20, and BL-21 and insert needles in tender points and indurations. Retain these needles in the back for ten to twenty minutes. Also, in order to strengthen the patient's constitution, insert a needle vertically in BL-23 and retain for the same amount of time. On the abdomen, in order to relieve the oppressive sensation in the epigastrium and distension of the stomach, needle CV-12 and CV-14 along with KI-16 and ST-25. Provide only as much needle stimulation at these points as is comfortable for the patient and then retain the needles for ten to twenty minutes. It is very useful to apply an infrared lamp or some other thermal stimulation on the abdomen while retaining the needles. Acupuncture points on the limbs such as PC-6, LI-4, and ST-36 should also be needled to regulate the function of the stomach. Insert needles in these points vertically and apply lifting and thrusting and twisting until a mild needle sensation is obtained. When the patient complains of strong abdominal pain, begin the treatment by needling ST-36, PC-6 and CV-12 to reduce the pain, and then needle other points after the pain has subsided. If the patient experiences chilling in the legs, also needle SP-6.

Moxibustion is very useful for treating chronic gastritis. The best points to use are BL-19, BL-20, and BL-21 on the back, CV-12, CV-14, and ST-25 on the abdomen, and ST-36 on the legs. The patient should be instructed how to apply moxibustion on CV-12 and ST-36 so that they can apply it everyday. A few additional points for moxa can be taught according to their symptoms.

26. Hemorrhoids

Description

Hemorrhoids are generally varicosities in the veins in the vicinity of the anal sphincter muscles. There are basically three types of hemorrhoids: so-called piles (hemorrhoidal nodules), bleeding hemorrhoids, and anorectal fistulas. The lining of the anus has a complex network of veins and, when there is some hindrance in venous return, parts of the anus begin to protrude and form nodules (varicosities). These nodules are generally termed hemorrhoids. When a fissure forms in the lining of the anus and there is bleeding, this is known as bleeding hemorrhoids. Such hemorrhoids can become chronic and turn into ulcerous sores. In a more advanced condition of hemorrhoids known as anorectal fistula, bacteria enter lesions between the anus and the rectum and infect the intestinal lining. Puss accumulates and then is released through another lesion in the lining. Eventually a maze of holes and tunnels form in the anal canal as this process continues.

Among the three types of hemorrhoids mentioned, anorectal fistulas involve a bacterial infection, so a specialist must be consulted. Even for simple types of hemorrhoids, like bleeding hemorrhoids, surgery may become necessary in more serious cases. Nevertheless, acupuncture is very useful in controlling hemorrhoids so that it does not become serious.

Acupuncture points
  Cranium—GV-20
  Lumbar region—BL-23, BL-25

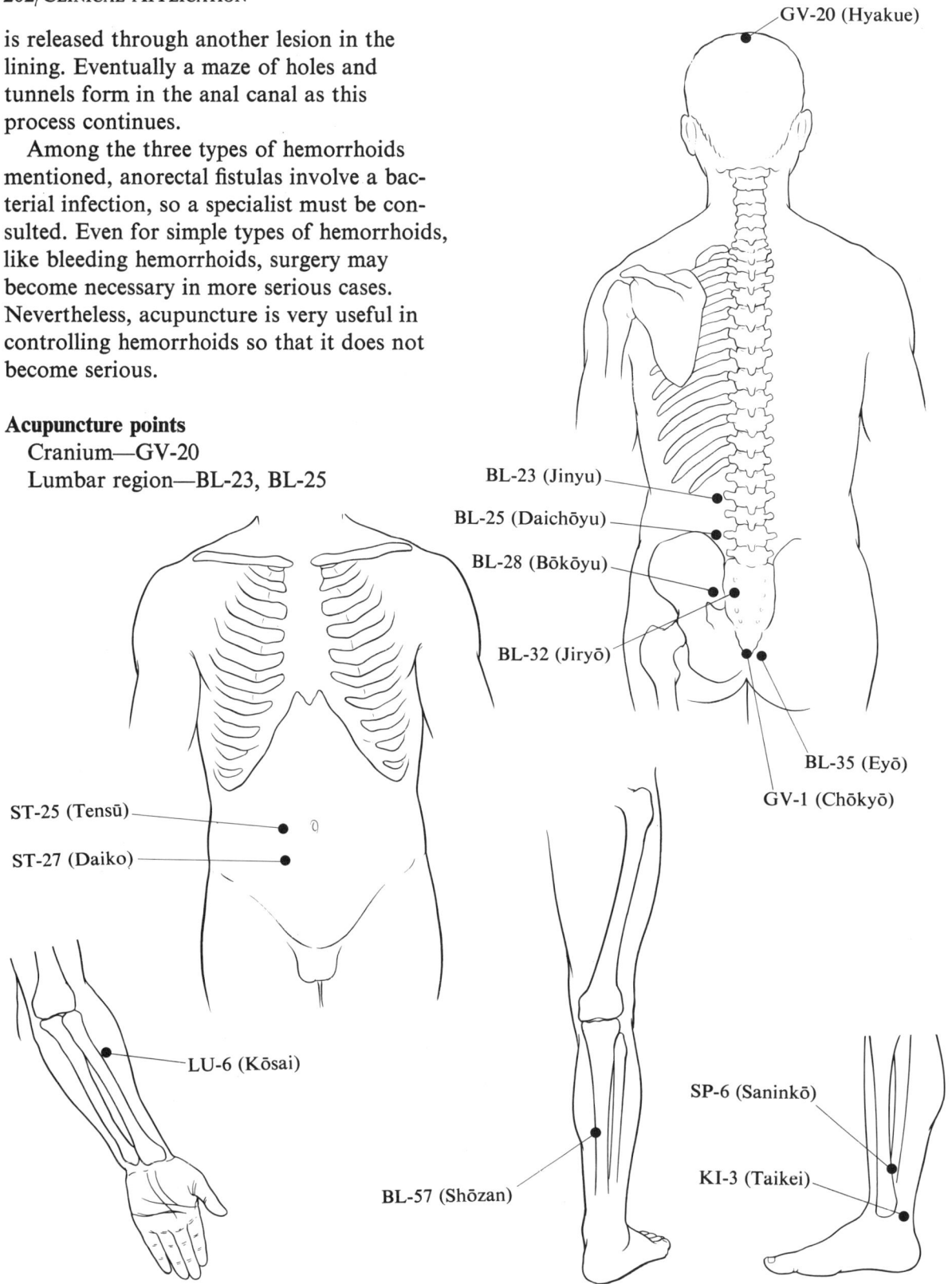

GV-20 (Hyakue)

BL-23 (Jinyu)
BL-25 (Daichōyu)
BL-28 (Bōkōyu)
BL-32 (Jiryō)
BL-35 (Eyō)
GV-1 (Chōkyō)

ST-25 (Tensū)
ST-27 (Daiko)

LU-6 (Kōsai)

SP-6 (Saninkō)
KI-3 (Taikei)

BL-57 (Shōzan)

Sacral region—BL-28, BL-32, BL-35,
  GV-1
Abdomen—ST-25, ST-27
Arms—LU-6
Legs—BL-57, SP-6, KI-3

Treatment

Start the treatment by inserting and retaining needles for ten to twenty minutes in BL-32, BL-57, GV-1, and GV-20. BL-32 and BL-57 should be needled for problems in and around the anus because these points belong to the bladder meridian which encircles the anus. GV-1 is located just posterior to the anus and GV-20 is related to the anus by being the opposite point on the governor vessel meridian.

In almost all cases of hemorrhoids there are other symptoms such as constipation and low back pain. For constipation needle ST-25 and ST-27 on the abdomen, and for low back pain needle BL-23 and BL-25 in the lower back. Retain needles in these points for about ten minutes. When patients experience fatigue or chilling in the lower limbs, also needle SP-6 and KI-3.

Moxibustion is also very effective for hemorrhoids. Aside from the above mentioned points, apply moxibustion on BL-35 (just lateral to GV-1) and LU-6. Acupuncture and moxibustion treatments for hemorrhoids must be applied every other day in the beginning for greatest effectiveness.

27. Chronic Hepatitis

Description

Chronic hepatitis occurs when acute hepatitis does not cure completely and becomes chronic. There are, however, some cases of hepatitis in which there is no chronic phase and the disease has chronic manifestations from the start. Approximately 10 percent of cases of acute (viral) hepatitis become chronic hepatitis. In many cases of chronic hepatitis there are very few subjective symptoms, but the most common ones include lassitude, tendency to fatigue easily, loss of weight, nausea and vomiting, loss of appetite, and feeling of distension in the abdomen. Other less frequently experienced symptoms are headaches, insomnia, itching, and loss of tolerance to alcohol. The serious symptoms of jaundice, fever, and edema are unusual for chronic hepatitis. It is estimated that about 10 percent of all cases of chronic

hepatitis progress into cirrhosis of the liver, but in the majority of cases, appropriate

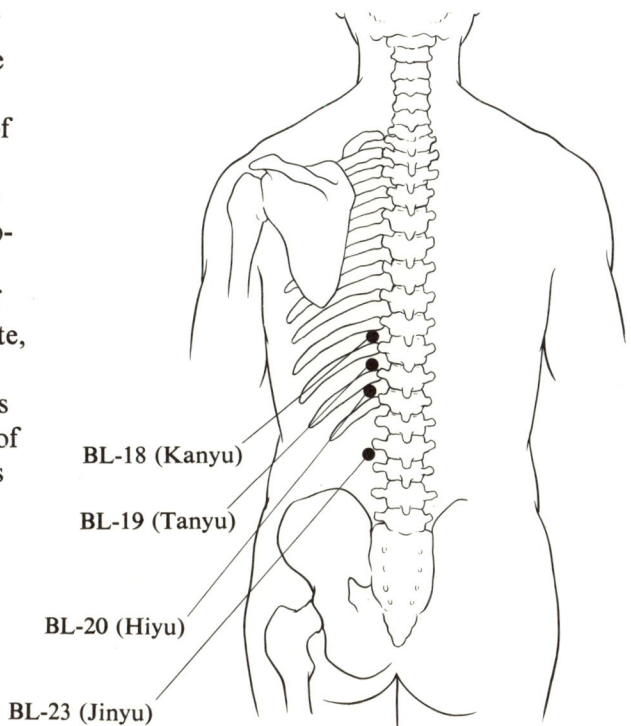

BL-18 (Kanyu)

BL-19 (Tanyu)

BL-20 (Hiyu)

BL-23 (Jinyu)

treatment normalizes liver function and the patient recovers completely.

Dietary therapy and rest are fundamental to the treatment of chronic hepatitis. It is important that patients get good nutrition, and their diet must include high quality proteins and ample calories. Generally there is no need to limit the amount of fat intake. The issue, more than the quantity, is the quality of the diet, so eating a balanced diet is most important. The consumption of alcoholic beverages must be strictly forbidden. The main aim of acupuncture therapy is to increase resistance and raise the patient's level of vitality. The general symptoms of chronic hepatitis such as lassitude and lack of appetite are alleviated in this process.

Acupuncture points
Back—BL-18, BL-19, BL-20, BL-23
Abdomen—LV-13, LV-14, GB-24, KI-16, CV-12, CV-14, ST-27
Legs—LV-3, LV-6

Treatment
The main points to be used are BL-18, BL-19, and BL-20, which are the back *shu* points of the liver, gallbladder, and spleen meridians respectively. On the abdomen needle LV-14, GB-24, and LV-13, which are the corresponding front *mu* points of the above mentioned meridians. After inserting the needle, appropriate stimulation should be applied by lifting and thrusting and twisting, but care must be taken to keep the level of

stimulation moderate. The needles may be retained from ten to twenty minutes at the above points. In cases of extreme lassitude and fatigue in the lower back and lower limbs, also needle BL-23 and KI-16, the *shu* point and *mu* point of the kidney meridian. When there is a sense of oppression in the epigastrium, also needle CV-14, and for lack of appetite, additionally needle CV-12. If the patient complains of constipation, also needle ST-27. Additional points which are highly effective for chronic hepatitis are the distal liver points LV-3 and LV-6.

Moxibustion therapy at home is a very effective approach for chronic hepatitis. A family member of the patient should be taught how to apply moxibustion on BL-18, BL-19, and BL-20 on the back, and LV-13, LV-14, and GB-24 on the abdomen. Moxa cones the size of a rice grain should be

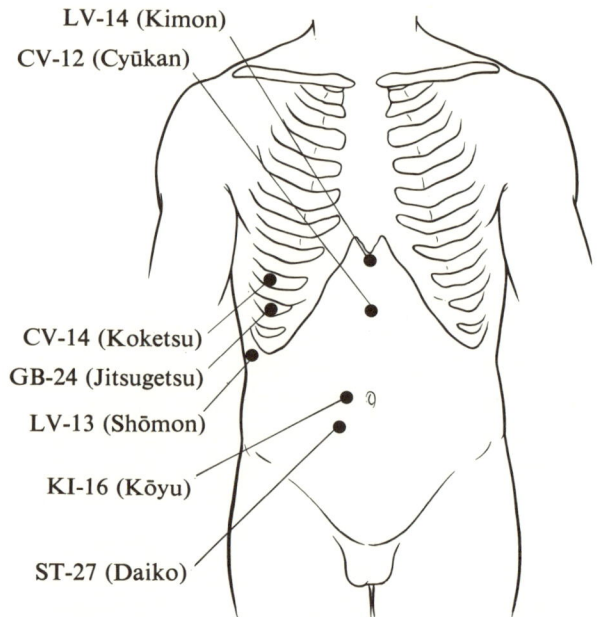

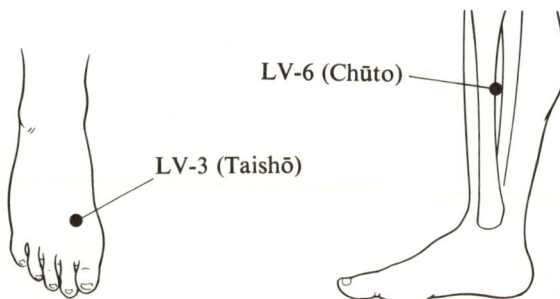

LV-14 (Kimon)
CV-12 (Cyūkan)
CV-14 (Koketsu)
GB-24 (Jitsugetsu)
LV-13 (Shōmon)
KI-16 (Kōyu)
ST-27 (Daiko)

LV-6 (Chūto)
LV-3 (Taishō)

applied three to five times consecutively on each point once a day. This treatment should be provided for three weeks straight and then stopped for a week. Adhering to this regimen for several months will bring steady improvement.

28. Eczema and Urticaria

Description

The medical definition of eczema is quite broad, but the main characteristics of eczema is that it is non-contagious, involves itching, and is composed of a variety of skin eruptions. At present the term dermatitis is often used instead of eczema. Specific names such as contact dermatitis, atopic dermatitis, and autosensitive dermatitis have been assigned to those eczematous skin conditions for which the causes have been determined. Apart from its causes, eczema (dermatitis) is sometimes classified by clinical conditions into acute eczema and chronic eczema. In acute eczema a localized skin area reddens and itches, and after a while eruptions, blisters, and pustules form in the area. Later there is scaling and crusting over the affected area. The formation of many kinds of eruptions in the same area is one of the primary characteristics of eczema. In chronic eczema, either the acute condition progresses to become chronic, or the skin problem starts out as chronic eczema from the beginning. The main feature of chronic eczema is thickening and browning of the skin. The affected skin is dry, rough, and wrinkled

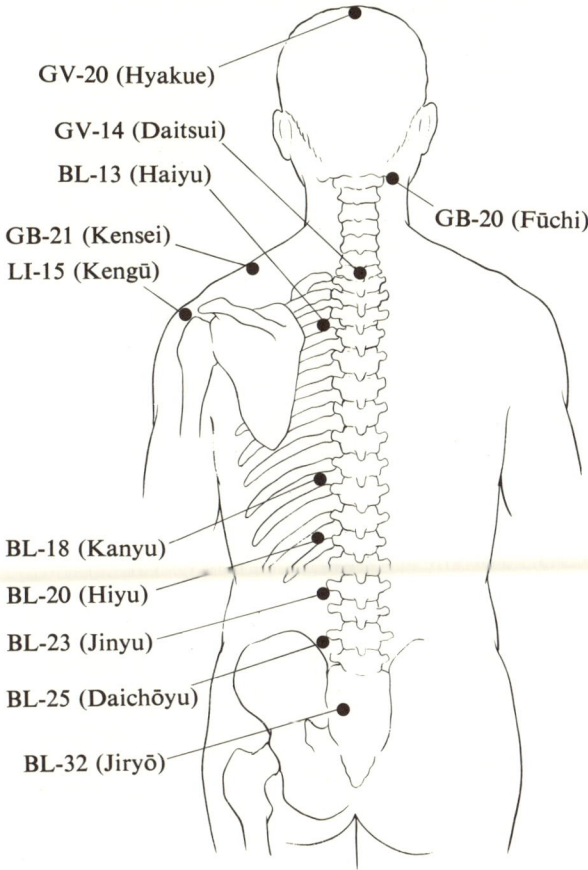

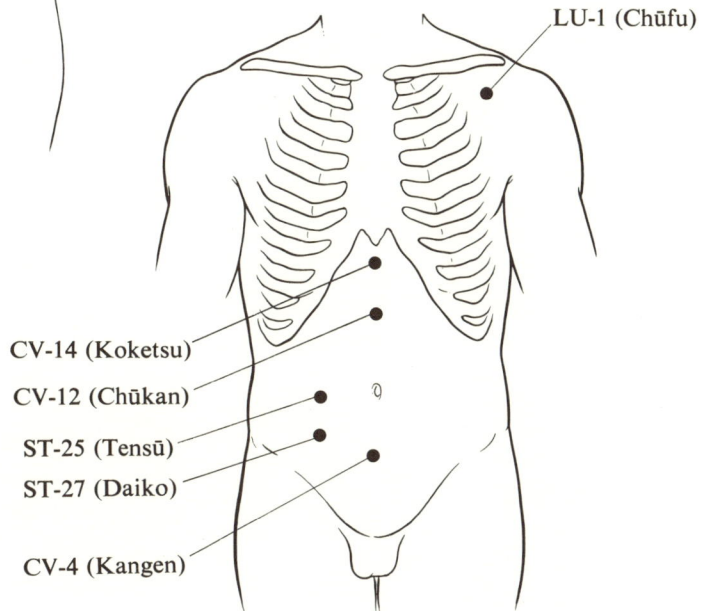

GV-20 (Hyakue)

GV-14 (Daitsui)

BL-13 (Haiyu)

GB-21 (Kensei)

LI-15 (Kengū)

GB-20 (Fūchi)

BL-18 (Kanyu)

BL-20 (Hiyu)

BL-23 (Jinyu)

BL-25 (Daichōyu)

BL-32 (Jiryō)

LU-1 (Chūfu)

CV-14 (Koketsu)

CV-12 (Chūkan)

ST-25 (Tensū)

ST-27 (Daiko)

CV-4 (Kangen)

LU-6 (Kōsai)

LI-10 (Te-no-Sanri)

LI-4 (Gōkoku)

SP-9 (Inryōsen)

SP-6 (Saninkō)

KI-3 (Taikei)

ST-36 (Ashi-no-Sanri)

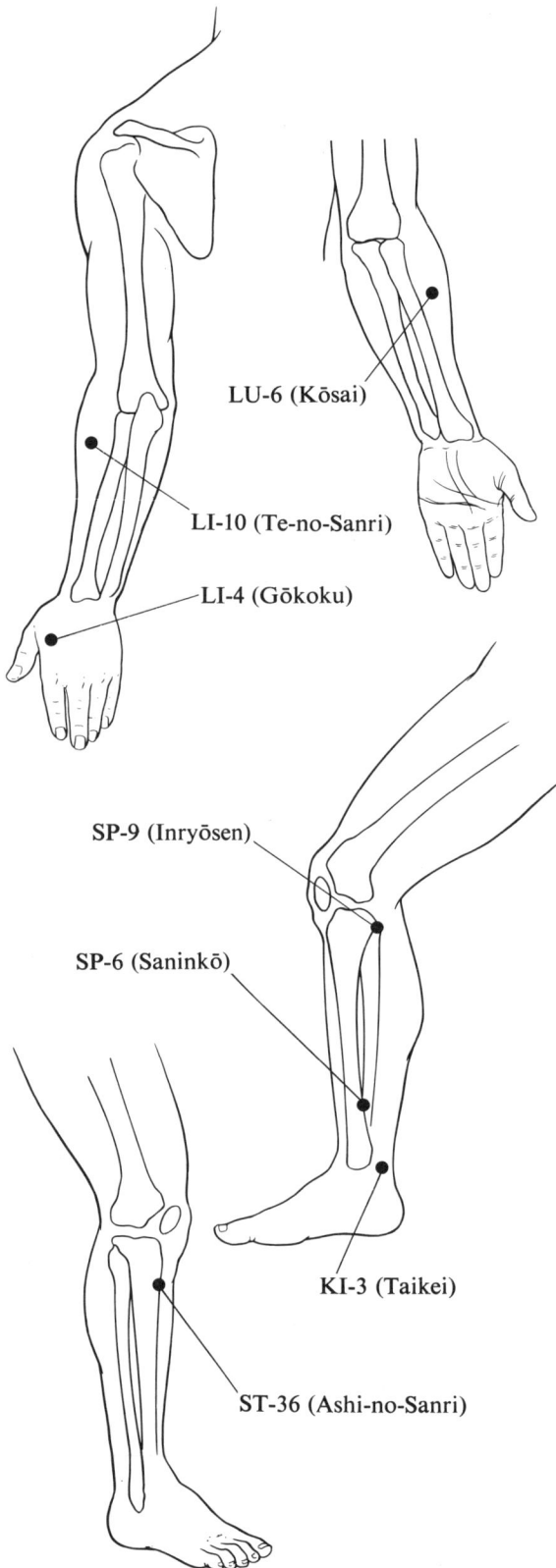

like elephant skin. There is some itching, but not as much as in acute eczema.

Urticaria is an eruptive skin rash also known as nettle rash or hives. In urticaria a localized area breaks out suddenly and itches badly. Often the adjacent areas scratched also break out and the redness and eruptions spread. The affected area changes with time since scratching causes it to spread. However, the eruptions always disappear without a trace in several hours. In most cases the urticaria comes and goes over a period of several days, but usually it is gone completely in a few weeks. In rare cases known as chronic urticaria, the outbreaks of urticaria continue for many months despite treatment. Generally urticaria is caused by an allergic condition, but in some cases there is another factor of exposure to toxins. Urticaria usually begins with exposure of an allergic individual to various irritants such as allergenic food (e.g., shrimp, eggs, and fish) and drugs, and also by incidences of gastrointestinal problems, metabolic disorders involving the liver or kidneys, and endocrine or neurovascular problems. Certain external irritants such as chemicals in skin ointments, insect bites, cold, ultra violet light, mechanical stimulation, and sweating can also be a contributing cause for urticaria. Also in some cases there is a psychosomatic component to urticaria.

Acupuncture points

Cranium—GV-20

Neck and shoulder—GV-14, GB-20, GB-21, LI-15

Back—BL-13, BL-18, BL-20, BL-23, BL-25, BL-32

Chest—LU-1

Abdomen—CV-14, CV-12, CV-4, ST-25, ST-27

Arms—LI-4, LI-10, LU-6

Legs—SP-6, SP-9, KI-3, ST-36

Treatment

Those with an allergic constitution have a predisposition toward skin conditions like eczema and urticaria. Since these problems are constitutional in nature, the whole body must be treated in acupuncture to enhance its self-regulatory function. Improving a person's constitution is something which requires much time, so it is necessary to patiently continue regular treatments over a long period.

For people with an allergic constitution, it is very common for a reaction (tenderness etc.) to appear at GV-14. Also when people have skin conditions, reactions usually appear along the lung and large intestine meridians. Therefore it is useful to needle reactive points such as LI-4, LI-15, LU-1, LU-6, and BL-13. Gentle lifting and thrusting should be applied at each point to obtain a mild sensation and then the needles can be retained for ten minutes.

Patients with eczema often complain of gastrointestinal problems such as indigestion, lack of appetite, diarrhea, or constipation. For such patients also needle points such as CV-14, CV-12, CV-4, ST-25, ST-27, ST-36, BL-20, and BL-25. In severe cases of chronic eczema, patients tend to become anxious and sensitive because of the unsightly appearance of their skin and there is loss of sleep from itching. In such cases needle GV-20, GB-20, GB-21, BL-18, BL-23, BL-32, SP-6, SP-9, and KI-3 to bring an improvement in their general condition. Care must be taken in each treatment to keep the total amount of stimulation at a moderate level. The exact amount mostly depends on the patient's sensitivity, but it should be just enough to relax the patient and make them feel better so that they sleep well that night.

Moxibustion is very effective for both acute and chronic cases of eczema and urticaria. Select several of the points listed above for treatment, also treat the local area by applying moxibustion in the center of the affected area. Moxibustion of GV-14 is particularly recommended because it is effective for patients with allergic constitutions. Three cones of moxa should be applied to each point once a day. This treatment should be applied once a day for five days in a row and then should be discontinued for two days before beginning another course.

29. Menstrual Irregularity and Dysmenorrhea

Description

Menstruation is the regular monthly bleeding caused by the shedding of the endometrium from the uterus when the egg is not fertilized after ovulation. Initially the secretion of the follicle-stimulating hormone stimulates the growth of the Graafian follicle in the ovaries and the endometrium thickens and softens (follicular phase). When the follicle matures, it expels an egg from the surface of the ovary (ovulatory phase). After this, the empty follicle in the ovary becomes a corpus luteum and secretes progesterone (secretory phase). If the egg is not fertilized, the secretion of progesterone stops in twelve to sixteen days, and the uterine epithelium breaks off and menstruation begins. This cycle of ovulation and thickening of the uterine lining is regulated by hormones secreted by the anterior lobe of the pituitary gland, the follicle-stimulating hormone, and the luteinizing hormone. The secretion of hormones from the anterior pituitary gland is in turn regulated by progesterone secreted from the corpus luteum. The mutual control of these hormones is thought to regulate ovulation and the menstrual cycle.

The period from the first day of menstruation to the day before the subsequent menstruation is known as the menstrual cycle. Generally menstruation lasts up to seven days and the normal menstrual cycle is considered to be between twenty-four and thirty-nine days. The normal amount of bleeding is hard to measure, but it should be neither too little nor excessive.

Menstrual irregularity refers to a disruption in the menstrual cycle so that the cycle either becomes too short or too long. The shortening of the menstrual cycle is often caused by inflammation of the endometrium and functional problems in the ovaries. The lengthening of the menstrual cycle occurs in cases of uterine hypoplasia and is sometimes caused by serious diseases. Most commonly the menses become late due to excessive dieting, and sometimes this can even cause amenorrhea. It is normal for a woman who is pregnant or breast-feeding to have no menses, but various psychological factors can also cause a disruption or cessation of the menstrual cycle. Also a certain amount of menstrual irregularity is normal for the young girls just beginning to have their period and for women in their late middle-ages approaching their menopause. With the exception of the above cases, menstrual irregularity can be regarded as a health problem in which there is an abnormally short or long cycle, menstrual bleeding continues over a week, or the amount of bleeding is too small or too great. The cause of menstrual irregularity must be analyzed and the root problem must be treated.

Dysmenorrhea is pain and discomfort which accompanies menstruation. It is not unusual for there to be some discomfort associated with menstruation, but dysmenorrhea refers to extreme pain and debilitating symptoms which require bed rest and cause people to miss work. Dysmenorrhea is not a disease per se, but a syndrome. Dysmenorrhea is especially common in cases of uterine hypoplasia, uterine myomas, endometriosis, pelvic inflammatory disease, and retroflexion and extreme antiflexion of the uterus, as well as for women with nervous dispositions.

The symptoms of dysmenorrhea include pain in the lower abdomen, abdominal distension, headache, low back pain, and irritability which occur shortly before and during menstruation. For those cases in which the severe symptoms appear more than a week before menstruation and disappear with the onset are known as the

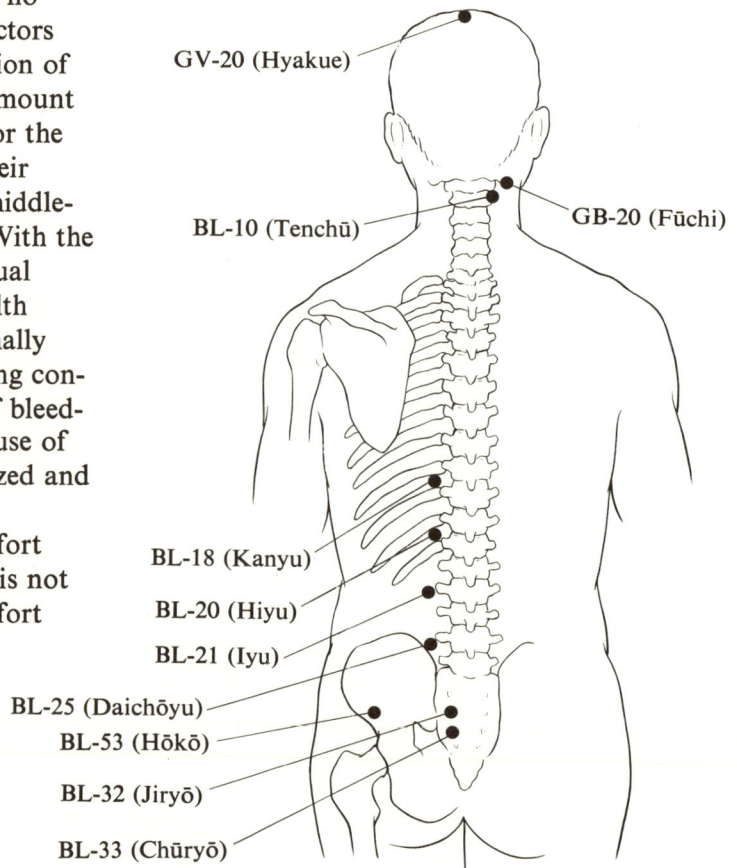

GV-20 (Hyakue)

BL-10 (Tenchū)

GB-20 (Fūchi)

BL-18 (Kanyu)

BL-20 (Hiyu)

BL-21 (Iyu)

BL-25 (Daichōyu)

BL-53 (Hōkō)

BL-32 (Jiryō)

BL-33 (Chūryō)

CV-12 (Chūkan)

CV-6 (Kikai)

SP-14 (Fukketsu)

ST-27 (Daiko)

SP-13 (Fusha)

SP-12 (Shōmon)

CV-4 (Kangen)

CV-3 (Chūkyoku)

SP-10 (Kekkai)

SP-9 (Inryōsen)

SP-6 (Saninkō)

LV-4 (Chūhō)

LV-3 (Taishō)

SP-3 (Taihaku)

ST-36 (Ashi-no-Sanri)

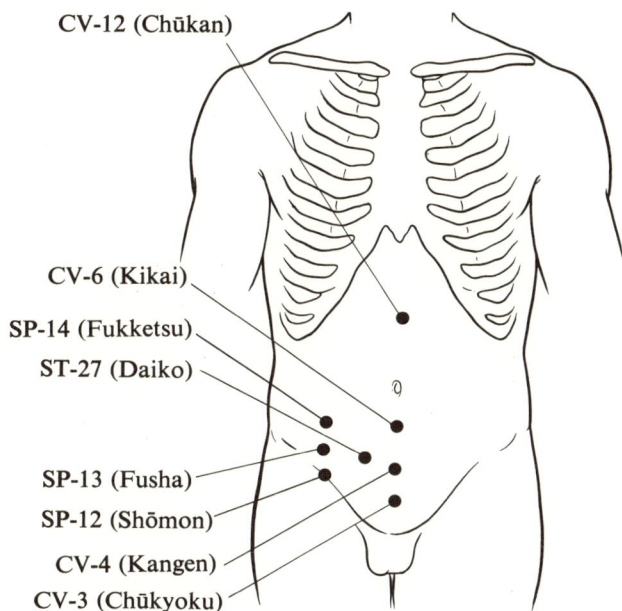

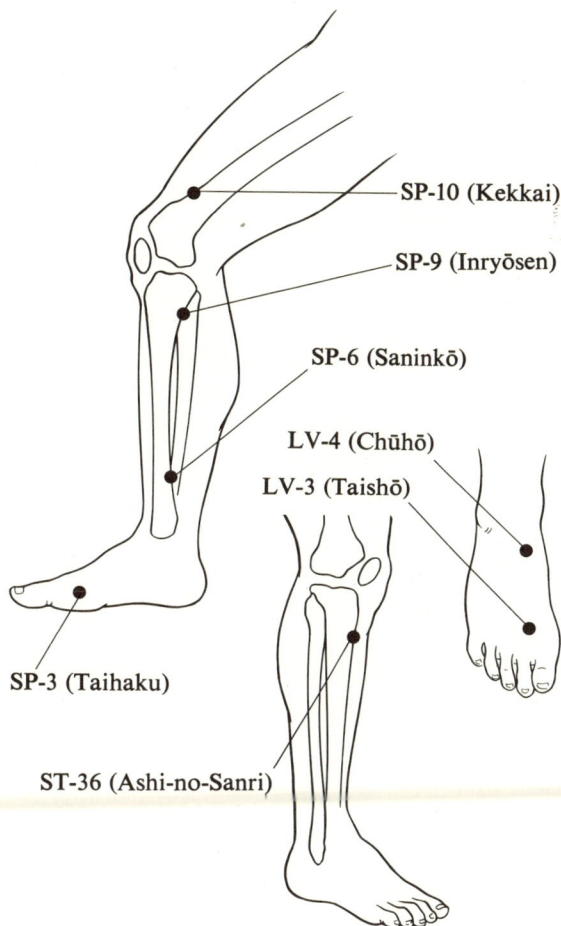

premenstrual syndrome. These symptoms are largely due to hormonal influences and all women feel them to some extent, so there is no need for concern when the symptoms are mild and transient. When there is a known cause, such as a gynecological disorders, medical treatments from a physician are necessary. In cases for which the cause of menstrual irregularity and dysmenorrhea is unclear or when these are due to functional disorders, regular acupuncture treatments over a certain period often prove effective.

Acupuncture points

Cranium and neck—GV-20, BL-10, GB-20
Back—BL-18, BL-20, BL-23, BL-25,
   BL-32, BL-33, BL-53
Abdomen—CV-3, CV-4, CV-6, CV-12,
   SP-12, SP-13, SP-14, ST-27
Legs—SP-3, SP-6, SP-9, SP-10, ST-36,
   LV-3, LV-4, GB-34

Treatment

Most gynecological disorders are related to two extra meridians: the conception vessel and the *chong* channel. For this reason the points of the conception vessel and the spleen meridian (related to the *chong* channel) are used to treat menstrual irregularity and dysmenorrhea. Needle CV-4 and CV-6 and provide mild stimulation to these points whenever there are menstrual problems. This serves to balance the energy in the conception vessel (controlling all yin meridians) and regulates blood. On the lower back, needle BL-32 and BL-53 which lie in the dermatome of the second sacral nerve. This serves to facilitate circulation in the reproductive organs and improves their function.

In cases where the menses come too early

and the flow is excessive and the blood is thick, apply comparatively strong needle stimulation to LV-3 and GB-34. These points are known to be effective in stopping bleeding. In cases where the menses tend to be late and the flow is scanty and the blood is thin, apply light stimulation to BL-20, BL-23, SP-10, and ST-36, and then retain the needles for about ten minutes.

Menstrual irregularity which manifests as a decrease in menstrual flow is considered to be a deficiency, and moxibustion is very effective for deficiencies. In this case apply three small cones of moxa consecutively on GV-20, BL-10 or GB-20, BL-18, BL-23, CV-4, SP-9, SP-6, and LV-4. Even in cases where the menses come too early and the flow is excessive, if the blood is thin in both color and consistency, it is considered to be a deficiency. Moxibustion is also effective in such cases and BL-20, BL-23, CV-12, ST-27, and LV-4 are the most useful points. Most cases of menstrual irregularity require regular treatments for about three months to show significant improvement.

For cases of dysmenorrhea needle CV-3, CV-6, SP-13, BL-25, BL-32, BL-53, and SP-6. When the pain is very strong, apply strong needle stimulation by vigorous lifting and thrusting and rotation. For those with an excessive condition also needle SP-10 and LV-3. For those with a deficient condition it is useful to needle BL-18, BL-20, and BL-23 also. Stimulation of these points serves to regulate the hormonal balance and improve the overall condition of the body.

When patients have the premenstrual syndrome, give them a treatment one week before the beginning of menstruation in the same way as explained above. At the end of the treatment imbed intradermal needles in reactive points such as SP-6, CV-3, and BL-32. Repeat this treatment over several months and once the patient becomes accustomed to acupuncture stimulation, major points such as SP-6, SP-9, and BL-32 can be stimulated electrically to yield good results.

Generally patients who complain of menstrual irregularity or dysmenorrhea have other symptoms such as headache, neck and shoulder tension, dyspepsia, and chilling in the legs. Address these symptoms in the acupuncture and moxibustion treatment and this will have a positive overall effect. In addition to mild acupuncture stimulation, it is important to provide a light massage over the whole body to relax the patient and bring deep rest and revitalization.

30. Increasing Vitality

Description
To increase vitality means to strengthen the essential drives of a human being. These are sexual desire, appetite, and the desire for physical well-being. These drives come from the most basic instincts of human beings which relate to self-preservation and preservation of the species, and these also account for the aggressive tendencies of man. These drives can be summarized as the will to live, and everyone has this most basic desire. Yet the complex and sometimes dehumanizing structure of modern society, the increase of psychological stress, the general decline in physical strength, and illnesses, not to mention the inevitable process of aging, can bring a premature decline in vitality. Since sex is an essential function, it is only natural that sexual performance is regarded as a measure of one's vitality and a major indicator of mental and physical well-being.

In Oriental medicine one's vitality is considered to be a function of the energy received at birth from one's parents (pre-natal source *ki*) and the energy taken in from one's environment after birth (post-natal source *ki*). If these two sources of energy are balanced and in abundance, a person has ample vitality, but if these are lacking in some respect, a person has low vitality which is generally associated with a kidney deficiency. If a person has ample vitality, naturally his sexual drive will be strong and he will possess the other qualities associated with vitality, such as physical energy, motivation, and ambition. Vitality is closely linked to the function of the hormonal system. A person's hormonal system normally is at its peak in the early twenties. It is known that the secretion of hormones gradually decreases with age. In the case of men, the amount of hormones declines with age as does one's physical condition. Nevertheless, the decline of hormones with age describes a sharper downward curve than the decline in physical performance.

Acupuncture points
  Back—BL-18, BL-22, BL-23, GV-4
  Chest—CV-17
  Abdomen—CV-4, CV-12, KI-16, ST-27
  Arms—TH-4
  Legs—LV-7, LV-9, LV-11, KI-1, KI-3, KI-9, KI-10

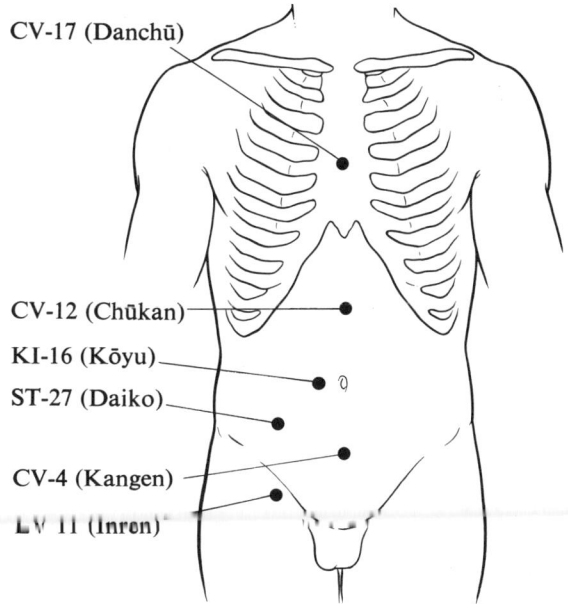

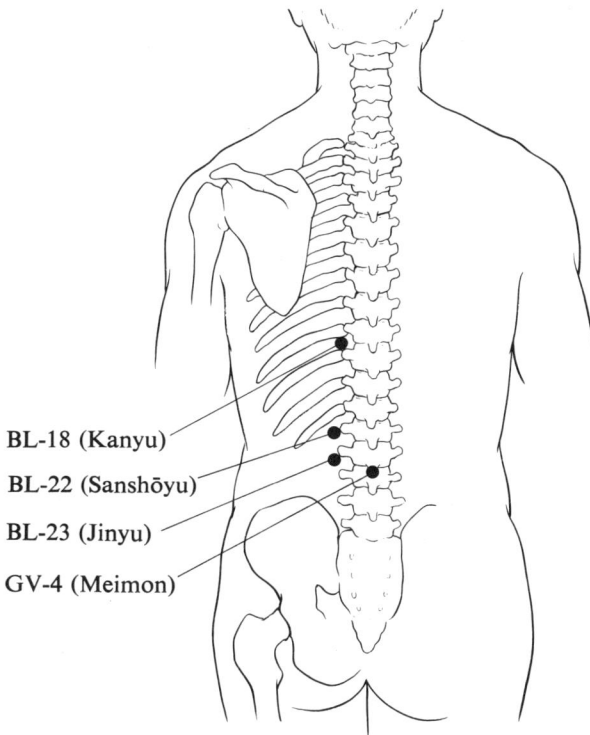

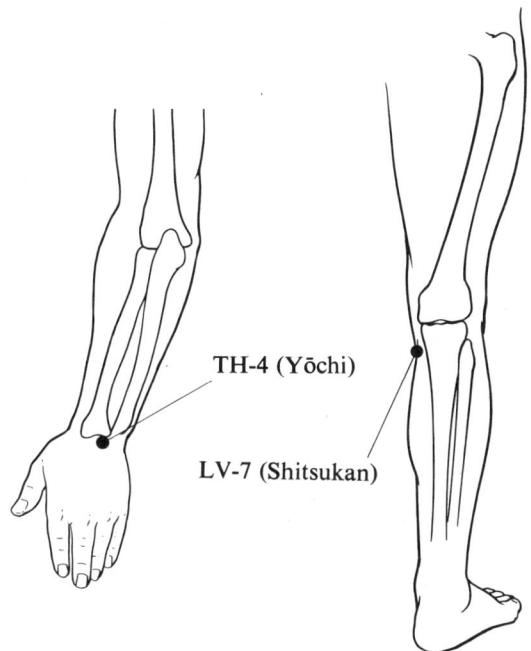

CV-17 (Danchū)

CV-12 (Chūkan)
KI-16 (Kōyu)
ST-27 (Daiko)
CV-4 (Kangen)
LV-11 (Inren)

BL-18 (Kanyu)
BL-22 (Sanshōyu)
BL-23 (Jinyu)
GV-4 (Meimon)

TH-4 (Yōchi)

LV-7 (Shitsukan)

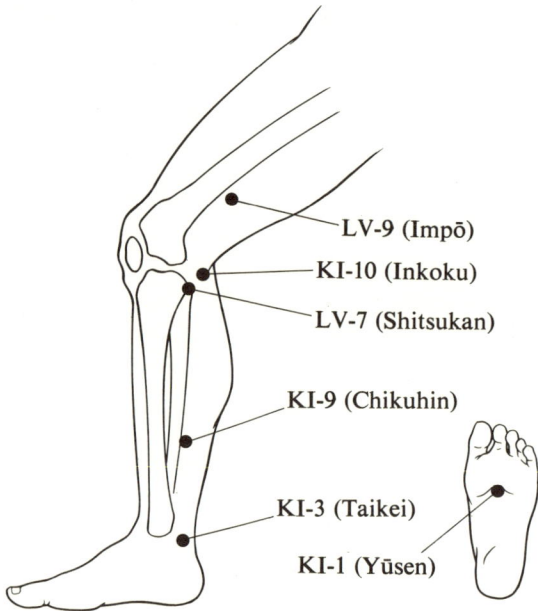

LV-9 (Impō)
KI-10 (Inkoku)
LV-7 (Shitsukan)
KI-9 (Chikuhin)
KI-3 (Taikei)
KI-1 (Yūsen)

Treatment

A general decline in vitality is usually associated with a kidney deficient condition, so the primary aim of the treatment is to tonify and raise the level of energy in the kidney meridian. One clear sign of a kidney deficiency is lack of muscle tone or a depression in the lower abdomen around CV-4. In this case, needle points related to the source *ki* and the kidney meridian such as KI-1, KI-16, GV-4, CV-4, and BL-23. Also needle some of the points listed above according to the other symptoms present. Apply needling techniques on each point to obtain a mild needle sensation and retain the needles for ten to twenty minutes. Applying an infrared lamp over the retained needles is also useful.

Those with kidney deficiency usually have tension and induration in the adductor muscles of the thigh. This area is the course of the kidney and liver meridians, so be sure to needle any reactive points and massage the area thoroughly after removing the needles.

31. Preventing the Ill Effects of Aging

Description

The phenomenon of aging is being studied extensively today. The physiological changes associated with aging are being tracked from many different angles including the increase of collagen (a fibrous protein) in cells, the calcification of bones and ligaments, atrophy of muscles, histological changes in brain cells, and the accumulation of cholesterol in the circulatory system. To live a long and healthy life has always been the wish of all people, and it is well known that a person can slow down the process of aging to some extent by leading a conscientious and active life. These days numerous diets and exercise systems are being advocated with the claim that they prevent aging. To put it simply, preventing physical problems associated with aging is primarily a matter of maintaining the vitality of the circulatory system so that an ample supply of oxygen reaches all parts of the body. This enables all organs and physical systems to operate harmoniously at an optimal level.

Acupuncture points
  Posterior neck—BL-10, GB-20, GV-14
  Shoulder—GB-21, LI-15, SI-13
  Upper back—BL-13, BL-17
  Lower back—BL-21, BL-22, BL-25
  Abdomen—CV-4, CV-12, KI-16, ST-25
  Inguinal area—GB-29
  Legs—ST-32, ST-34, ST-41, BL-36, BL-37, BL-40, BL-57, BL-60, KI-1
  Arms—LU-5, LU-9, LI-14, TH-4, TH-10, HT-7, PC-7

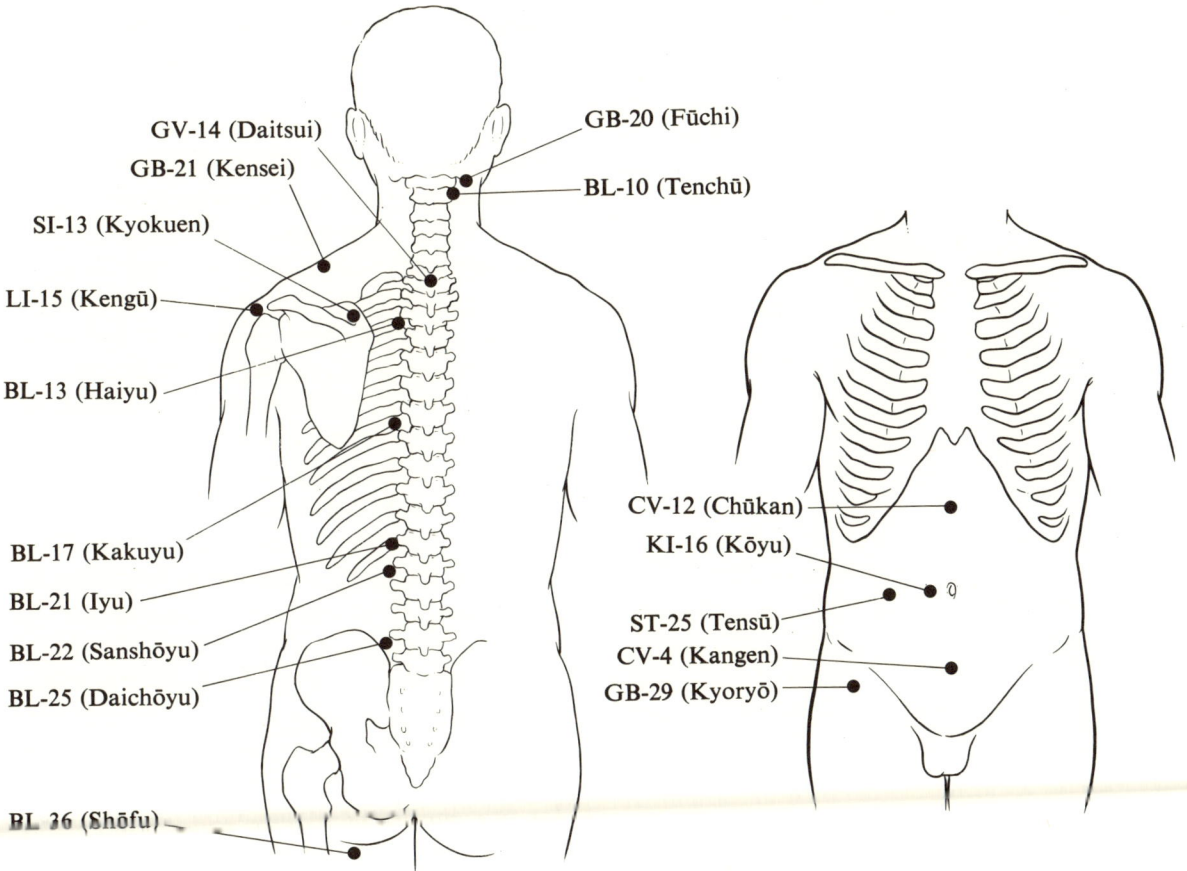

GV-14 (Daitsui)
GB-21 (Kensei)
SI-13 (Kyokuen)
LI-15 (Kengū)
BL-13 (Haiyu)

GB-20 (Fūchi)
BL-10 (Tenchū)

BL-17 (Kakuyu)
BL-21 (Iyu)
BL-22 (Sanshōyu)
BL-25 (Daichōyu)

CV-12 (Chūkan)
KI-16 (Kōyu)
ST-25 (Tensū)
CV-4 (Kangen)
GB-29 (Kyoryō)

BL 36 (Shōfu)

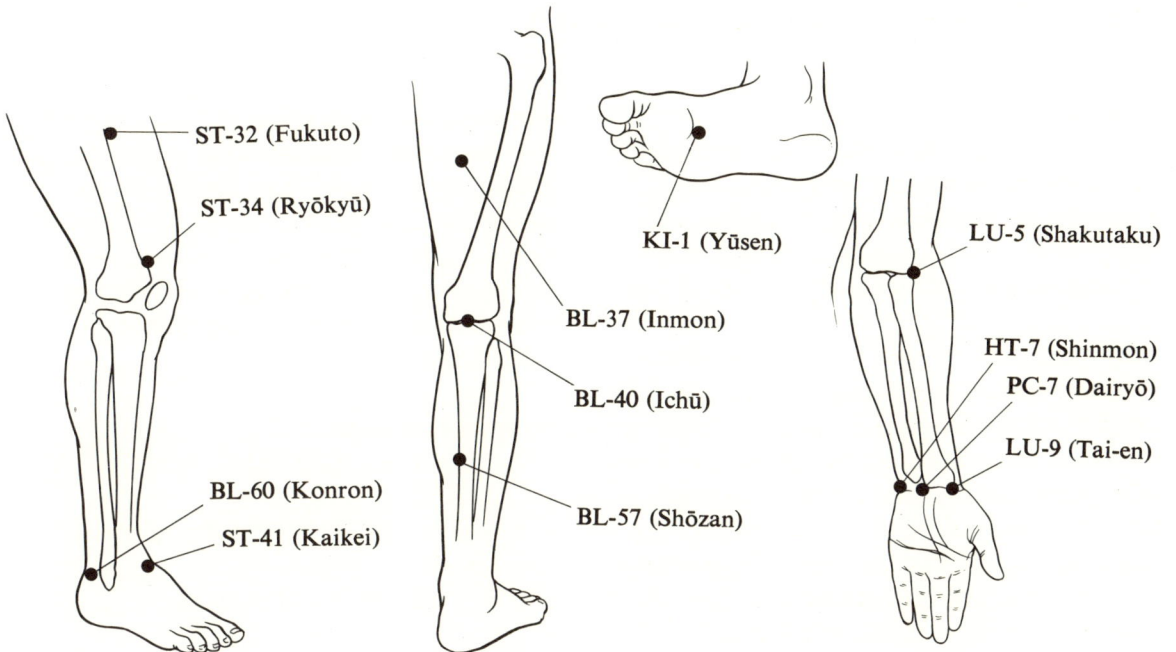

ST-32 (Fukuto)
ST-34 (Ryōkyū)

KI-1 (Yūsen)

LU-5 (Shakutaku)

BL-37 (Inmon)
BL-40 (Ichū)

HT-7 (Shinmon)
PC-7 (Dairyō)
LU-9 (Tai-en)

BL-60 (Konron)
ST-41 (Kaikei)

BL-57 (Shōzan)

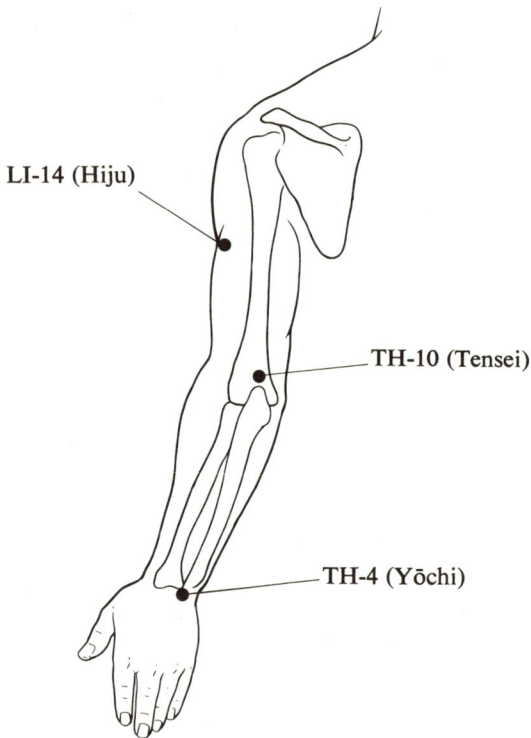

LI-14 (Hiju)

TH-10 (Tensei)

TH-4 (Yōchi)

Treatment

The first objective in giving treatments to forestall the effects of aging is to remove the tension and increase the elasticity in the paravertebral muscles in the neck and the back. The second objective is to relieve tension and improve the tone of muscles in the abdomen, pelvic area, arms and hands, hips, thighs, calves, and soles of the feet. The treatment should start with needling of points on the neck such as BL-10 and GB-20, and progress down the back to the waist and down to the feet. Needle the points listed above which show reactions and those points where the muscular tension is very strong, and apply slow lifting and thrusting and twisting on the needles to relax the muscular tension. On the abdomen needle major tonification points like CV-4, CV-12, KI-16, and ST-25 and retain the needles from ten to twenty minutes. Needling these points serves to improve the function of the digestive system and also enhances metabolic activity. Two points on the foot, ST-41, and BL-60, are known to be especially useful for preventing the ill effects of aging, so be sure to needle these points also.

32. Wrinkles in Facial Skin

Description

When reaching middle age, it is common for people to gain some weight and for excess fat to accumulate in the abdomen, upper arms, and thighs. Be that as it may, in most people not much fat appears in the facial region. Although those who are over-weight tend not to have so many wrinkles in their facial skin, gaining weight is no solution to the problem of wrinkles. The structural relationship of the muscles to skin in the facial region is very different from that in other parts of the body. In the facial region, muscles are closely intertwined with the skin, and this special structure enables us to form subtle and varied facial expressions. Those areas of facial skin which are thick and richly supplied with sebaceous glands do not wrinkle so easily. On the other hand, areas of facial skin which are thin and have fewer sebaceous glands, such as the periphery of the eyes, tend to dry out easily and are more susceptible to wrinkling.

Acupuncture points

Around eye—BL-1, BL-2, GB-1, ST-2, TH-23

Cranium—ST-4, ST-8, GB-7, GB-14, CV-24

Neck—BL-10, LI-17, CV-22

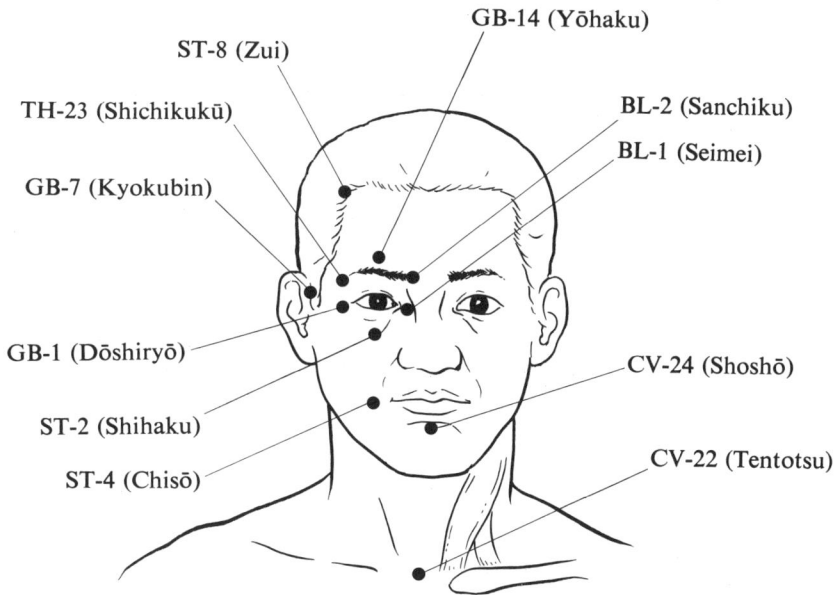

ST-8 (Zui)

GB-14 (Yōhaku)

TH-23 (Shichikukū)

BL-2 (Sanchiku)

BL-1 (Seimei)

GB-7 (Kyokubin)

GB-1 (Dōshiryō)

CV-24 (Shoshō)

ST-2 (Shihaku)

CV-22 (Tentotsu)

ST-4 (Chisō)

Treatment

The objective in treating facial wrinkles is to improve circulation in the facial muscles and skin, increase the supply of oxygen and nutrients, facilitate the removal of waste products, and raise the level of metabolic activity in the facial region. An old saying in Japan states that "the skin is the mirror (reflecting the condition) of the internal organs." Therefore, when there is an indication of problems in the visceral organs, a more holistic treatment is in order. In traditional Chinese medicine "the lungs dominate the skin," so points on the lung and large intestine meridians should be needled for the best results. Needle a number of points listed above according to the presence of cutaneous reactions, and also select the appropriate distal points to suit the patient's condition. Use very thin needles for facial points, and retain the needles for ten to fifteen minutes.

The facial region is especially sensitive to pain so take special care in the insertion and manipulation of needles. Observe the patient closely for signs of excessive pain. Also,

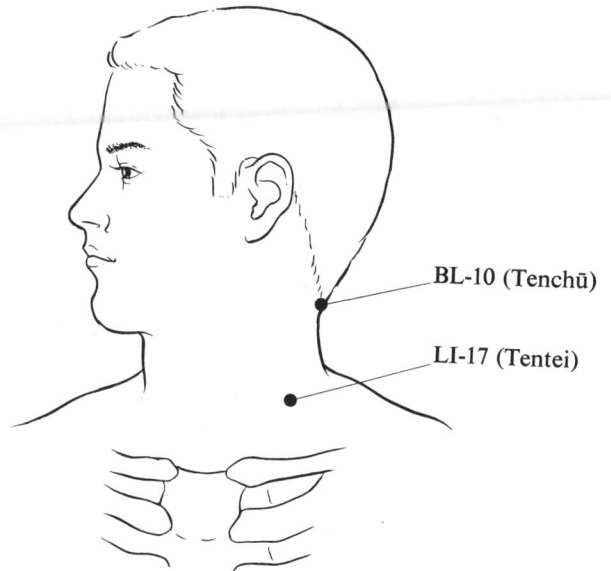

BL-10 (Tenchū)

LI-17 (Tentei)

since there is less fat in the tissues of the face and small arteries and veins lie close to the surface of the skin, there is a greater possibility of causing some bleeding or subcutaneous hemorrhage. For this reason, immediately after withdrawing the needle, press the point firmly and hold it for about half a minute. Take special care to avoid causing a subcutaneous hemorrhage which can leave an unsightly purple mark on the face.

After removing all the needles, provide a brief facial massage or acupressure treatment. A complete facial massage is the specialty of beauticians. For the conclusion to an acupuncture treatment, simply apply gentle finger pressure on the facial points shown on the figure above. Press each point for about three seconds and then slowly release the pressure, repeating about five times. Also apply kneading pressure along the hairline, scalp, and side and back of neck to thoroughly relax the muscles.

33. Blemisches and Freckles

Description

Blemishes, or darkened spots in facial skin, tend to occur just above the eyebrows, on the cheekbone, on the nose, and upper lip. These are all areas of the face which are most exposed to the sun. Blemishes sometimes appear on people in their twenties, but it most often appears in people over forty. Facial blemishes are caused by such things as pregnancy, diseases of the ovaries or uterus, dysfunctions of the adrenal cortex, liver diseases, and mental and physical stress, but in many instances a specific cause cannot be found. If blemishes are caused by an organic disease, a patient must receive appropriate medical treatment. Sometimes facial blemishes are caused by an allergic reaction to cosmetics.

Freckles are different from blemishes in that they tend to occur as numerous small spots. It is thought that in most cases freckles are caused by a congenital hypersensitive reaction to sunlight. Freckles are

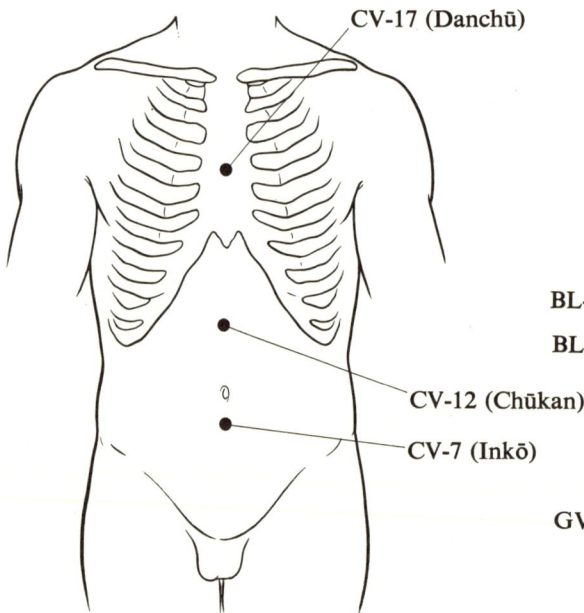

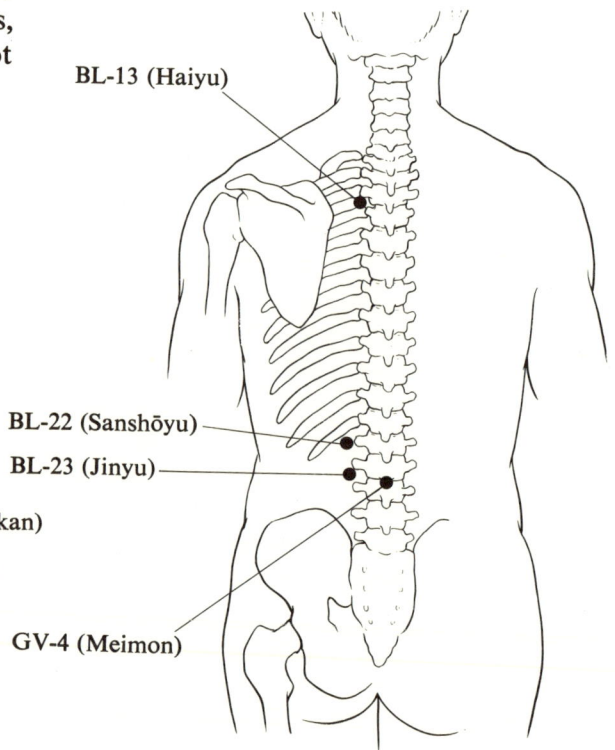

CV-17 (Danchū)

CV-12 (Chūkan)

CV-7 (Inkō)

BL-13 (Haiyu)

BL-22 (Sanshōyu)

BL-23 (Jinyu)

GV-4 (Meimon)

more common among fair skinned people and it mostly appears during adolescence. Also freckles appear most clearly during the summer. In those with extreme sensitivity to sunlight, sometimes superficial veins begin to show up on the cheeks. In this case, the skin has been severely affected by exposure to solar radiation and has become atrophied and abnormally thin. People with this condition must wear sunscreen lotions to cut down the exposure of their skin to sunlight. It is very difficult to cure a serious skin condition once it has advanced beyond a certain point. Prevention is the secret in preserving the youthful appearance of facial skin. Naturally, for this purpose, staying in the best possible physical condition is just as important as taking good care of facial skin.

Acupuncture points
  Chest—CV-17
  Back—BL-13, BL-22, BL-23, GV-4
  Abdomen—CV-7, CV-12
  Legs—KI-3
  Arms—TH-4, LI-4, PC-6, LU-9

Treatment
No acupuncture point has yet been discovered that is specifically effective in removing facial blemishes and freckles. The reason is probably because the cause of these skin conditions is due to more general imbalances in the body such as endocrine dysfunctions. Skin problems are regarded as a constitutional tendency in Oriental medicine, so performing treatments to improve a person's constitution is the best way to bring about a natural cure.

In Oriental medicine the function of the lungs is intimately related to the condition of the skin. Therefore, it is wise to first needle BL-13, the back *shu* point of the lungs. Next, for the purpose of improving the patient's physical constitution, needle BL-22, BL-23, and GV-4. Retain the needles in the back for ten to fifteen minutes. After this, to enhance the functional condition of the respiratory and circulatory systems, needle CV-17. Needle CV-12 to improve the function of the stomach, liver, and spleen. Also needle CV-7 to improve the function of the small intestine and large intestine. Insert a needle horizontally downward in

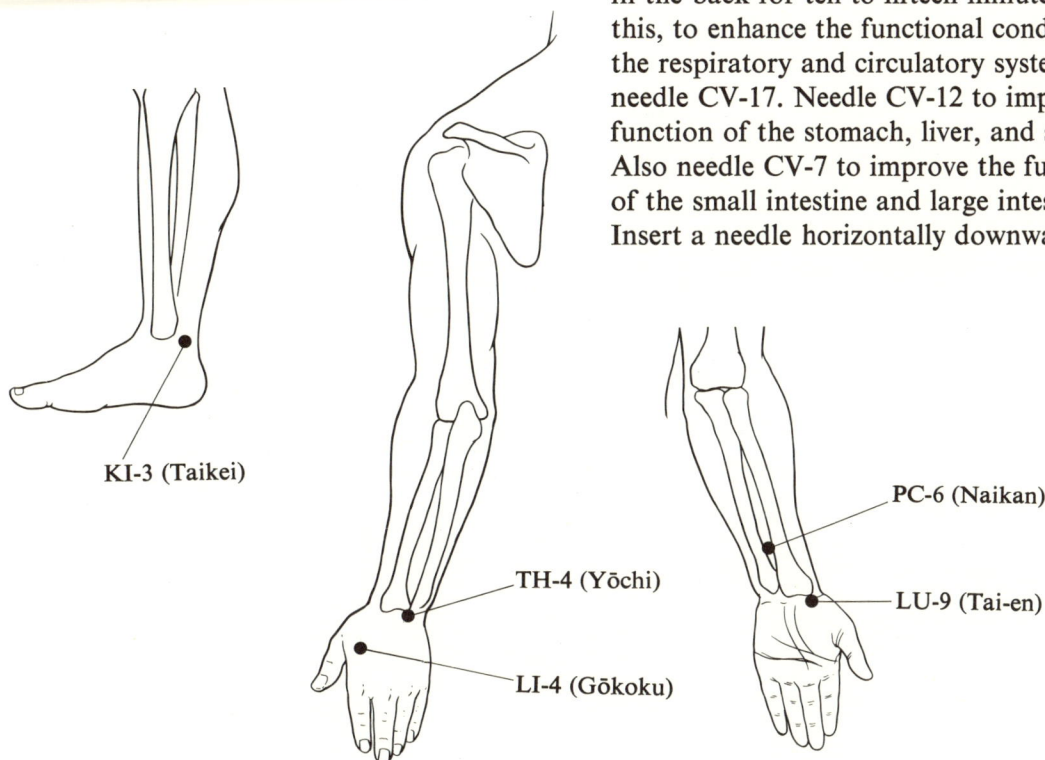

KI-3 (Taikei)

PC-6 (Naikan)

TH-4 (Yōchi)

LU-9 (Tai-en)

LI-4 (Gōkoku)

CV-17 so that the needle goes between the skin and the sternum. Insert needles vertically in CV-12 and CV-7. Retain the needles in the chest and abdomen for about ten minutes. While retaining the needles in the supine position, also needle reactive points on the arms and legs. Acupuncture points such as TH-4, LI-4, PC-6, LU-9, and KI-3 are very effective in improving the overall condition of the body.

34. Beautifying Skin

Description

Every woman wishes to stay young and beautiful as long as she can. No matter what kind of makeup, hairdos, and clothing are worn, the condition of a woman's skin gives her age away. The huge sums of money spent on basic cosmetics for keeping the skin soft and young in appearance tells us how essential the condition of the skin is in beauty.

The skin oils excreted on the epidermis by the sebaceous glands mix with dust and other impurities to form a hardened outer layer of skin with dead skin cells known as the stratum corneum. Small wrinkles can form in this surface layer when the skin is not cleansed regularly. Cleaning the skin too meticulously, however, is not good because the skin needs some oil to keep it from drying out and wrinkling. The excretion of skin oils decreases with age, so older people have to take special care to keep their skin moist. The skin glands and circulation in superficial tissues are under the control of the autonomic nervous system. Therefore, in order to keep healthy skin, a person needs to be in good condition both mentally and physically.

Acupuncture points
Neck—ST-9
Back—BL-13, BL-22, BL-23, BL-53

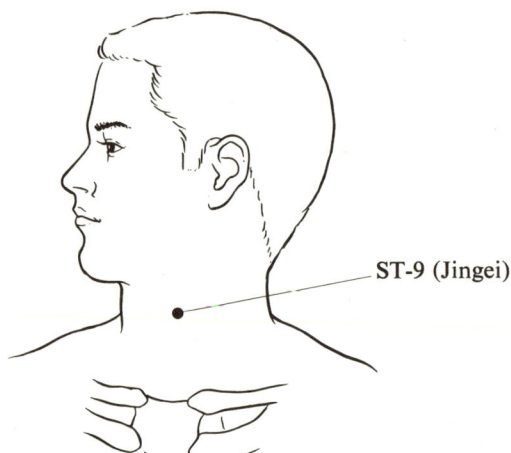

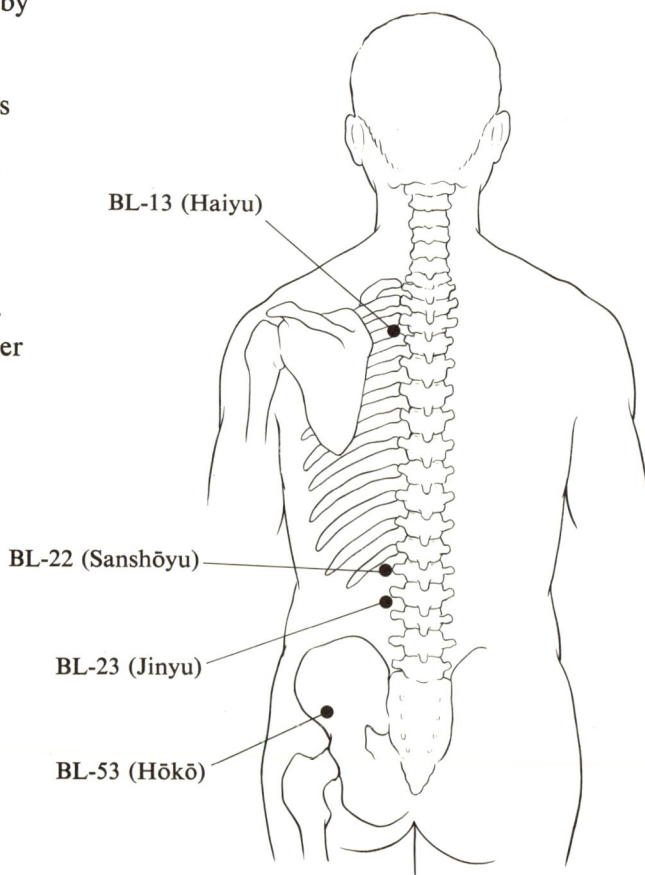

BL-13 (Haiyu)

BL-22 (Sanshōyu)

BL-23 (Jinyu)

BL-53 (Hōkō)

ST-9 (Jingei)

CV-12 (Chūkan)

CV-4 (Kangen)

LU-6 (Kōsai)

TH-4 (Yōchi)

KI-3 (Taikei)

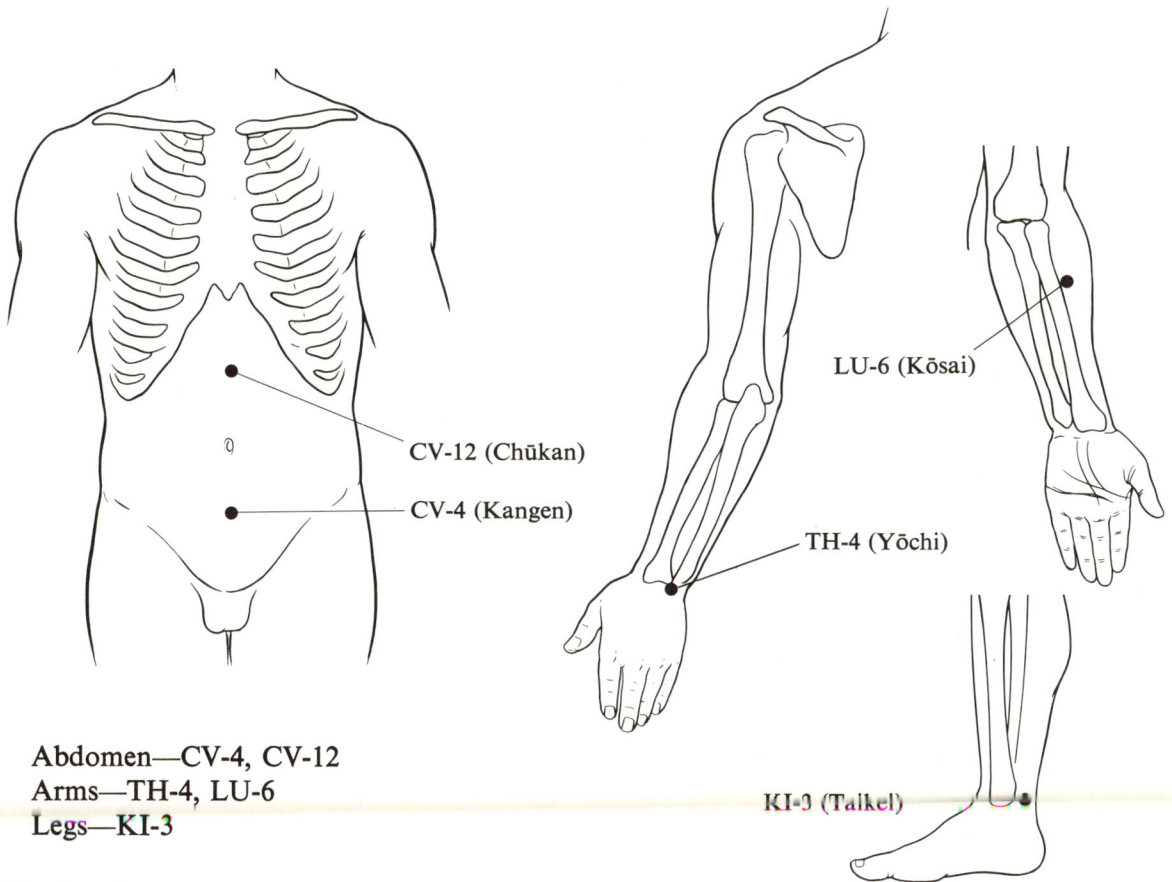

Abdomen—CV-4, CV-12
Arms—TH-4, LU-6
Legs—KI-3

Treatment

The only real way to improve the condition of the skin is to enhance the overall condition of the body. In traditional Chinese medicine the back *shu* point of the kidney meridian, BL-23, is considered to be particularly useful for improving a person's constitution. This is because the kidney is the organ where prenatal energy is stored. The postnatal energy, on the other hand, is controlled by the triple heater. Therefore BL-22 (back *shu* point of the triple heater meridian) is also very important for improving the overall condition. Also, since the lungs dominate the skin in traditional Chinese medicine, BL-13 (back *shu* point of the lung meridian) and LU-6 are important points for improving the condition of the skin. Other useful points include ST-9, CV-12, TH-4, and KI-3. Needle these points and retain the needles for up to twenty minutes. One of the biggest enemies to clear skin is constipation. For those patients who also have constipation, be sure to needle points to alleviate this problem.

Index of Tsubo

Amon, 67, 68, 149, 150
Ashi-no-Gori, 65, 66
Ashi-no-Kyō-in, 61, 64
Ashi-no-Rinkyū, 61, 64
Ashi-no-Sanri, 42, 44, 89, 134,
    163, 164, 167–70, 172, 177–79,
    182–85, 192, 194–201, 206,
    207, 209, 210
Ashi-no-Tsūkoku, 51, 54
Ashi-no-Yōkan, 61, 63
Atama-no-Kyō-in, 61, 62, 149,
    150, 178, 179
Atama-no-Rinkyū, 61, 63

Bishō, 50, 51
BL-1, 41, 50, 51, 151–53, 214,
    215
BL-2, 50, 51, 151–53, 173–75,
    214, 215
BL-3, 50, 51
BL-4, 50, 51
BL-5, 50, 51
BL-6, 50, 51
BL-7, 51, 174, 175
BL-8, 51
BL-9, 51, 149, 150
BL-10, 51, 52, 118, 149, 150,
    152–57, 159, 174, 175, 177–85,
    188–91, 208–10, 212–15
BL-11, 51, 52, 149, 150, 154,
    155, 159, 182, 183
BL-12, 51, 52, 149, 150, 154,
    159, 184, 185
BL-13, 51, 52, 161, 162, 182–87,
    205–07, 212, 213, 216–19
BL-14, 51, 52, 161, 162, 182,
    183
BL-15, 51, 52, 161, 162, 177,
    178, 184–91
BL-16, 51, 52
BL-17, 51, 52, 161, 162, 178–81,
    184, 185, 188, 189, 200, 201,
    212, 213, 220–22
BL-18, 51, 52, 161–63, 171, 172,
    177, 178, 180–83, 194–99,
    203–11
BL-19, 51, 52, 194, 195, 198–201,

203, 204
BL-20, 51, 52, 171, 172, 177,
    178, 182, 183, 194, 196, 200,
    201, 203–10
BL-21, 51, 52, 171, 172, 182, 183,
    194, 200, 201, 208, 209, 212,
    213
BL-22, 51, 52, 162, 163, 167,
    168, 171, 172, 178, 179, 196,
    198, 199, 211–13, 216–19
BL-23, 51, 52, 131, 156–58, 162,
    163, 165–68, 170–72, 177–91,
    196–207, 211, 212, 216–19
BL-24, 51, 52, 165, 166
BL-25, 51, 52, 162, 163, 165–68,
    170, 196–99, 202, 203, 205–10,
    212, 213
BL-26, 51, 52, 162, 163, 165,
    166–68
BL-27, 51, 52, 162, 163, 196–99
BL-28, 51, 52, 167, 168, 202, 203
BL-29, 51, 52
BL-30, 51, 52
BL-31, 51, 52
BL-32, 51, 52, 162, 163, 202,
    203, 205–10
BL-33, 51, 53, 208, 209
BL-34, 51, 53
BL-35, 51, 53, 202, 203
BL-36, 51, 53, 162–64, 167, 168,
    212, 213
BL-37, 51, 53, 163–68, 212, 213
BL-38, 51, 53
BL-39, 51, 53, 169, 170
BL-40, 51, 53, 167–70, 212, 213
BL-41, 51, 53
BL-42, 51, 53
BL-43, 51, 53, 182, 183
BL-44, 51, 53, 190, 191
BL-45, 51, 53
BL-46, 51, 53
BL-47, 51, 53
BL-48, 51, 53
BL-49, 51, 53
BL-50, 51, 53, 182, 183
BL-51, 51, 53
BL-52, 51, 53, 162, 163, 165–68,
    170, 184–87

BL-53, 51, 53, 162, 163, 167,
    168, 208–10, 218
BL-54, 51, 53
BL-55, 51, 53
BL-56, 51, 54, 167, 168
BL-57, 51, 54, 163–66, 202, 203,
    212, 213
BL-58, 51, 54
BL-59, 51, 54
BL-60, 51, 54, 174, 175, 212–14
BL-61, 51, 54
BL-62, 51, 54
BL-63, 51, 54
BL-64, 51, 54
BL-65, 51, 54
BL-66, 51, 54
BL-67, 51, 54
Bōkōyu, 51, 52, 167, 168, 202,
    203
Bokushin, 51, 54

Chigo-e, 61, 64
Chiki, 45, 46
Chikuhin, 55, 56, 211, 212
Chippen, 51, 53
Chizen, 186, 187
Chisō, 42, 151–53, 214, 215
Chō-e, 61, 62, 214, 215
Chōkin, 61, 63
Chōkyō, 66, 67, 202, 203
Chōkyū, 49, 151, 152, 178, 179
Chūchū, 55, 56
Chūfu, 38, 119, 156–58, 161, 162,
    184–87, 205–07
Chūhō, 65, 209, 210
Chūkan, 36, 69, 70, 162, 163,
    171, 172, 177–79, 182–85, 190–
    94, 197–201, 204–07, 209–14,
    216–19, 221, 222
Chūkyoku, 36, 69, 70, 180, 181,
    209, 210
Chūroyu, 51, 52
Chūryō, 40
Chūryō, 51, 53, 208, 209
Chūsho, 59, 178, 179
Chūshō, 57, 58
Chūsū, 67

Chūtei, 69, 70
Chūto, 65, 204
Chūtoku, 61, 63
CV-1, 69, 70
CV-2, 36, 69, 70
CV-3, 36, 69, 70, 180, 181, 209, 210
CV-4, 69, 70, 188, 189, 195–97, 205–07, 209–14
CV-5, 69, 70
CV-6, 69, 70, 209, 210
CV-7, 69, 70, 216–18
CV-8, 36, 69, 70
CV-9, 69, 70
CV-10, 69, 70
CV-11, 69, 70
CV-12, 36, 69, 70, 162, 163, 171, 172, 177–79, 182–85, 190–94, 197–201, 204–07, 209–14, 216, 219
CV-13, 69, 70
CV-14, 69, 70, 180, 181, 184, 185, 192, 200, 201, 204–07
CV-15, 69, 70, 171, 172, 177, 178, 180, 181
CV-16, 69, 70
CV-17, 59, 69, 70, 161, 162, 184, 185, 216–18
CV-18, 69, 70
CV-19, 69, 70
CV-20, 69, 70
CV-21, 69, 70
CV-22, 69, 70, 184, 185, 192, 193, 214, 215
CV-23, 69, 70
CV-24, 41, 69, 70, 214, 215

Daichōyu, 51, 52, 162, 163, 165–68, 170, 196–99, 202, 203, 205–10, 212, 213
Daigei, 41, 42, 62, 151–53
Daihō, 45, 46
Daijo, 51, 52, 149, 150, 154, 155, 159, 182, 183
Daikaku, 55, 56
Daiko, 42, 43, 177–85, 190, 191, 195–99, 202–07, 209–11
Dai-ō, 45, 46, 195–97
Dairyō, 57, 58, 154, 155, 172, 212, 213
Daishō, 55, 56
Daito, 45
Daiton, 65

Daitsui, 39, 59, 62, 66–68, 182, 183, 186, 187, 205–07, 212, 213
Danchū, 59, 69, 70, 161, 162, 184, 185, 216–18
Datan, 67, 68
Dōshiryō, 61, 62, 214, 215

Eifū, 59, 60, 133, 151–53, 177–79
E-in, 69, 70
Ekimon, 59
Eneki, 61, 63
Esō, 59, 60
Eyō, 51, 53, 202, 203

Fubun, 51, 53
Fūchi, 61, 63, 149, 150, 152–55, 159, 174, 175, 177–79, 182, 183, 205–07, 212–14
Fūfu, 66–68, 149, 150
Fugeki, 51, 53
Fuhaku, 61, 62
Fukketsu, 45, 46, 195–98
Fuku-ai, 45, 46
Fukuryū, 55, 56
Fukuto, 42, 43, 212, 213
Fūmon, 51, 52, 149, 150, 154, 159, 184, 185
Fusha, 45, 46, 209, 210
Fūshi, 61, 63, 131
Futotsu, 40, 41
Fuyō, 42, 43, 180, 181
Fuyō, 51, 54

Gaikan, 59, 60, 154, 155, 159, 160
Gaikyū, 61, 64
Gairyō, 42, 43
Ganen, 61, 62
GB-1, 61, 62, 214, 215
GB-2, 61, 62, 178, 179
GB-3, 59, 61, 62, 151–53
GB-4, 61, 62
GB-5, 61, 62, 174, 175
GB-6, 61, 62
GB-7, 61, 62, 214, 215
GB-8, 61, 62
GB-9, 61, 62
GB-10, 61, 62
GB-11, 61, 62, 149, 150, 178, 179
GB-12, 61, 62, 149, 150, 154, 155, 174, 175, 177–79

GB-13, 61, 62
GB-14, 61, 63, 214, 215
GB-15, 61, 63
GB-16, 61, 63
GB-17, 61, 63, 177, 178
GB-18, 61, 63, 177, 178
GB-19, 61, 63
GB-20, 61, 63, 149, 150, 152–55, 159, 174, 175, 177–79, 182, 183, 205–07, 212–14
GB-21, 61, 63, 118, 149, 150, 152–57, 159, 174, 175, 177–79, 182, 183, 188–91, 205–07, 212, 213
GB-22, 61, 63
GB-23, 61, 63
GB-24, 61, 63, 197–99, 204
GB-25, 61, 63
GB-26, 61, 63
GB-27, 61, 63
GB-28, 61, 63
GB-29, 61, 63, 212, 213
GB-30, 61, 63, 167, 168
GB-31, 61, 63, 131
GB-32, 61, 63
GB-33, 61, 63
GB-34, 61, 63, 149, 150, 167–70, 209, 210
GB-35, 61, 63
GB-36, 61, 64
GB-37, 61, 64
GB-38, 61, 64
GB-39, 61, 64, 167, 168
GB-40, 61, 64, 152, 154
GB-41, 61, 64
GB-42, 61, 64
GB-43, 61, 64
GB-44, 61, 64
Geikō, 40, 41
Gekan, 41–43, 133, 151–53
Gekan, 69, 70
Gekimon, 57, 58, 154, 156, 159, 160
Gekokyo, 42, 44
Geren, 40
Geryō, 51, 53
Ginkō, 67, 68
Gochō, 67, 68, 174
Gokei, 48, 49
Gōkoku, 40, 89, 134, 149, 150, 152–55, 159, 160, 172, 174, 175, 190, 191, 200, 201, 206, 207, 217, 218
Gosho, 50, 51

Gosū, 61, 63
Gōyō, 51, 53
GV-1, 66, 67, 202, 203
GV-2, 66, 67
GV-3, 67, 165, 166
GV-4, 67, 165, 166, 211, 212, 216, 217
GV-5, 67
GV-6, 67
GV-7, 67
GV-8, 67, 171, 172
GV-9, 67
GV-10, 67
GV-11, 67, 68
GV-12, 67, 68
GV-13, 67, 68
GV-14, 39, 59, 62, 66–68, 182, 183, 186, 187, 205–07, 212, 213
GV-15, 67, 68, 149, 150
GV-16, 66–68, 149, 150
GV-17, 67, 68, 149, 150
GV-18, 67, 68
GV-19, 67, 68, 174
GV-20, 67, 68, 118, 162–64, 173–75, 177, 178, 180, 181, 188–91, 202, 203, 205–10,
GV-21, 67, 68, 174, 175
GV-22, 67, 68
GV-23, 67, 68
GV-24, 67, 68, 151–53
GV-25, 67, 68
GV-26, 67, 68
GV-27, 67, 68
GV-28, 67, 68
Gyokuchin, 51, 149, 150
Gyokudō, 69, 70
Gyosai, 38, 39

Haiyu, 51, 52, 161, 162, 182–87, 205–07, 212, 213, 216–19
Hakkanyu, 51, 52
Hakko, 51, 53
Hara-no-Tsūkoku, 55, 56, 161
Heifū, 49
Henreki, 40
Hiju, 40, 41, 157–60, 212, 214
Hikan, 42, 43
Hiyō, 51, 54
Hiyu, 51, 52, 171, 172, 177, 178, 182, 183, 194, 196, 200, 201, 203–10
Hōkō, 51, 53, 162, 163, 167, 168, 208–10, 218

Honshin, 61, 62
Horō, 55, 56
Hōryū, 41, 42, 44
HT-1, 46, 47
HT-2, 47
HT-3, 47, 154, 155, 159, 160
HT-4, 47
HT-5, 47
HT-6, 47
HT-7, 47, 154, 155, 159, 160, 212, 213
HT-8, 47
HT-9, 47, 119
Hyakue, 67, 68, 118, 162–64, 173–75, 177, 178, 180, 181, 188–91, 202, 203, 205–10

Ichū, 51, 53, 118, 167–70, 212, 213
Idō, 61, 63
Iki, 51, 53
Impaku, 45
Impō, 65, 66, 211, 212
Ingeki, 47
Inkō, 69, 70, 216–18
Inkoku, 55, 56, 169, 170, 172, 211, 212
Inmon, 51, 53, 163–68, 212, 213
Inren, 65, 66, 211
Inryōsen, 45, 46, 163, 164, 169, 170, 190, 191, 206, 207, 209, 210
Inshi, 42, 43
Into, 55, 56, 161
Isha, 51, 53
Isō, 51, 53, 182, 183
Iyō, 51, 53, 169, 170
Iyu, 51, 52, 171, 172, 182, 183, 194, 200, 201, 208, 209, 212, 213

Jikan, 39, 40
Jimon, 59, 60, 178, 179
Jingei, 42, 43, 120, 121, 151–53, 177–80, 188, 189, 218, 219
Jinyu, 51, 52, 131, 156–58, 162, 163, 165–68, 170–72, 177–91, 196–207, 211, 212, 216–19
Jiryō, 51, 52, 163, 202, 203, 205–10
Jitsugetsu, 61, 63, 197–99, 204
Jōkan, 69, 70

Jōkō, 42, 44, 167, 168
Jōkokyo, 42, 44
Jōren, 40
Jōryō, 41, 52
Jōsei, 67, 68
Ju-e, 59, 60
Juyu, 48, 49

Kagai, 69, 70
Kaikei, 42, 44, 167, 168, 184, 185, 212, 213
Kakukan, 51, 53
Kakushujin, 59, 61, 62, 151–53
Kakuson, 59, 60, 178; 179
Kakuyu, 51, 52, 161, 162, 178–81, 184, 185, 188, 189, 200, 201, 212, 213
Kanchō, 61, 63, 167, 168
Kangen, 69, 70, 188, 189, 195–97, 205–07, 209–14
Kangenyu, 51, 52, 162, 163, 165, 166–68
Kankoku, 42, 44
Kankotsu, 61, 62, 149, 150, 154, 155, 174, 175, 177–79
Kanmon, 42, 43
Kanshi, 57, 58
Kanshō, 59
Kanyu, 51, 52, 161–63, 171, 172, 177, 178, 180–83, 194–99, 203–11
Karyō, 40, 41
Katsunikumon, 42, 43
Keikotsu, 51, 54
Keikyo, 38, 39
Keimon, 61, 63
Keimyaku, 59, 60
Kekkai, 45, 46, 169, 170, 209, 210
Kenchūyu, 49, 178, 179, 182, 183
Kengaiyu, 49, 182, 183
Kengū, 40, 41, 157, 159, 172, 205–07, 212, 213
Kenri, 61, 62
Kenri, 69, 70
Kenro, 61, 62, 174, 175
Kenryō, 49, 151, 152
Kenryō, 59, 60, 159
Kensei, 61, 63, 118, 149, 150, 152–57, 159, 174, 175, 177–79, 182, 188–91, 205–07, 212, 213
Kenshō, 61, 64, 167, 168
Kensū, 67

Kentei, 48, 49, 156, 157
Ketsubon, 42, 43, 161, 162
Ketsuinyu, 51, 52, 161, 162, 182, 183
KI-1, 54, 55, 163–66, 181, 188, 189, 211–13
KI-2, 55
KI-3, 55, 56, 163, 164, 172, 178, 179, 190, 191, 203, 206, 207, 211, 212, 217–19
KI-4, 55, 56
KI-5, 55, 56
KI-6, 55, 56, 172, 190, 191
KI-7, 55, 56
KI-8, 55, 56
KI-9, 55, 56, 211, 212
KI-10, 55, 56, 169, 170, 172, 211, 212
KI-11, 55, 56
KI-12, 55, 56
KI-13, 55, 56
KI-14, 55, 56
KI-15, 55, 56
KI-16, 55, 56, 161–64, 178–81, 190, 191, 197–201, 204, 211–14
KI-17, 55, 56, 161
KI-18, 55, 56
KI-19, 55, 56, 161
KI-20, 55, 56, 161
KI-21, 55, 56, 161, 162
KI-22, 55, 56
KI-23, 55, 56, 161, 162
KI-24, 55, 56, 186, 187
KI-25, 55, 56, 186, 187
KI-26, 55, 56, 186, 187
KI-27, 55, 56, 186, 187
Kikai, 69, 70, 209, 210
Kikaiyu, 51, 52, 165, 166
Kiketsu, 55, 56
Kiko, 42, 43, 149, 150
Kimon, 65, 66, 180, 181, 188, 189, 192, 193, 195, 197–99, 204
Kimon, 45, 46
Kinmon, 51, 54
Kinshuku, 67, 171, 172
Kirai, 42, 43
Kisha, 42, 43
Kishō, 42, 43
Kobō, 42, 43
Kōkan, 65
Koketsu, 69, 70, 180, 181, 184, 185, 192, 200, 201, 204–07
Kokotsu, 40, 41, 154–59, 182, 183
Kōkō, 51, 53, 182, 183

Kōmei, 61, 64
Kōmon, 51, 53
Konmon, 51, 53
Konron, 51, 54, 174, 175, 212–14
Koryō, 42, 151–53
Kōsai, 38, 39, 134, 186, 187, 202, 203, 205–07, 219
Kōshin, 55, 56
Koshi-no-Yōkan, 67, 165, 166
Kōson, 45
Kōyu, 55, 56, 161–64, 178–81, 190, 191, 197–201, 204, 211–14
Kyōhaku, 38, 156–58, 186, 187
Kyōkan, 67, 68
Kyōkei, 61, 64
Kyokkotsu, 36, 69, 70
Kyokubin, 61, 62, 214, 215
Kyokuchi, 40, 154, 155, 157–60, 172, 174, 175, 190, 191, 206
Kyokuen, 49, 152–57, 159, 174, 175, 178, 179, 182, 183, 212, 213
Kyokusa, 50, 51
Kyokusen, 65, 66, 169, 170
Kyokusen, 46, 47
Kyokutaku, 57, 58, 159, 160
Kyōkyō, 45, 46, 177, 178
Kyoryō, 61, 63, 212, 213
Kyōsha, 41–43, 62, 151, 152
Kyūbi, 69, 70, 171, 172, 177, 178, 180, 181
Kyūkyo, 61, 64, 152, 154
Kyūmyaku, 65, 66

LI-1, 39, 40
LI-2, 39, 40
LI-3, 40
LI-4, 40, 89, 134, 149, 150, 152–55, 159, 160, 172, 174, 175, 190, 191, 200, 201, 206, 207, 217, 218
LI-5, 40, 154, 155, 159, 160
LI-6, 40
LI-7, 40, 154, 155, 159, 160
LI-8, 40
LI-9, 40
LI-10, 40, 154, 155, 157–62, 177, 178, 182, 183, 196, 197, 206
LI-11, 40, 154, 155, 157–60, 172, 174, 175, 190, 191, 206
LI-12, 40
LI-13, 40
LI-14, 40, 41, 157–60, 212, 214

LI-15, 40, 41, 157, 159, 172, 205–07, 212, 213
LI-16, 40, 41, 154–59, 182, 183
LI-17, 40, 41, 151–55, 184, 185, 214, 215
LI-18, 40, 41
LI-19, 40, 41
LI-20, 40, 41
LU-I, 38, 119, 156–58, 161, 162, 184–87, 205–07
LU-2, 38, 156–58
LU-3, 38
LU-4, 38, 156–58, 186, 187
LU-5, 38, 39, 154, 155, 159, 202, 203, 212, 213
LU-6, 38, 39, 134, 186, 187, 202, 203, 205–07, 219
LU-7, 38, 39, 184, 185
LU-8, 38, 39
LU-9, 38, 39, 212, 213, 217, 218
LU-10, 38, 39
LU-11, 38, 39
LV-1, 65
LV-2, 65
LV-3, 65, 177, 178, 204, 209, 210
LV-4, 65, 209, 210
LV-5, 65
LV-6, 65, 204
LV-7, 65, 66, 169, 170, 211
LV-8, 65, 66, 169, 170
LV-9, 65, 66, 211, 212
LV-10, 65, 66
LV-11, 65, 66, 211
LV-12, 65, 66
LV-13, 64–66, 204
LV-14, 65, 66, 180, 181, 188, 189, 192, 193, 195, 197–99, 204

Meimon, 67, 165, 166, 211, 212, 216, 217
Mokusō, 61, 63

Naikan, 57, 58, 134, 154, 156, 159–62, 177, 178, 192, 194, 198, 200, 201, 217, 218
Naitei, 42, 44
Nenkoku, 55
Nōko, 67, 68, 149, 150
Nōkū, 61, 63
Nyūchū, 42, 43
Nyūkon, 42, 43, 161

Ōkotsu, 55, 56
Oku-ei, 42, 43
Onryū, 40, 154, 159, 160

PC-1, 57, 58
PC-2, 57, 58
PC-3, 57, 58, 159, 160
PC-4, 57, 58, 154, 156, 159, 160
PC-5, 57, 58
PC-6, 57, 58, 134, 154, 156, 159–62, 177, 178, 192, 194, 198, 200, 201, 217, 218
PC-7, 57, 58, 154, 155, 172, 212, 213
PC-8, 57, 58
PC-9, 57, 58

Rakkyaku, 51
Reida, 42, 44
Reidai, 67
Reidō, 47
Reikō, 65
Reikyo, 55, 56, 186, 187
Rekketsu, 38, 39, 184, 185
Rensen, 69, 70
Rōkoku, 43, 46
Rōkyū, 57, 58
Rosoku, 59, 60
Ryōkyū, 42, 43, 169, 170, 172
Ryōmon, 42, 43, 186, 187, 200, 201

Sanchiku, 50, 51, 151–53, 173–75, 214, 215
Saninkō, 45, 134, 163, 164, 167, 168, 177–79, 181, 186, 187, 190, 191, 195–203, 206, 207, 209, 210
Sankan, 40
Sanshōyu, 51, 52, 162, 163, 167, 168, 171, 172, 178, 179, 196, 198, 199, 211–13, 216–19
Sanyōraku, 59, 60
Seimei, 41, 50, 51, 151–53, 214, 215
Seirei, 47
Seirei-en, 59, 60
Sekichū, 67
Sekikan, 55, 56
Sekimon, 69, 70
Senki, 69, 70

Shakutaku, 38, 39, 154, 155, 159, 202, 203, 212, 213
Shichikukū, 59, 60, 214, 215
Shihaku, 42, 133, 151–53, 214, 215
Shi-in, 51, 54
Shikō, 59, 60
Shikyū, 69, 70
Shiman, 55, 56
Shinchū, 67, 68
Shindō, 51, 53, 190, 191
Shindō, 67, 68
Shin-e, 67, 68
Shinketsu, 36, 69, 70
Shinmon, 47, 154, 155, 159, 160, 212, 213
Shinmyaku, 51, 54
Shinpō, 55, 56, 161, 162
Shinyu, 51, 52, 161, 162, 177, 178, 184–91
Shintei, 67, 68, 151–53
Shinzō, 55, 56, 186, 187
Shisei, 48, 49
Shishitsu, 51, 53, 162, 163, 165–68, 170, 184–87
Shitoku, 59, 60
Shitsugan, 169, 170, 172
Shitsukan, 65, 66, 169, 170, 211
Shiyō, 67
Shōchōyu, 51, 52, 162, 163, 196–99
Shō-ei, 61, 63, 177, 178
Shōfu, 51, 53, 162–64, 167, 168, 212, 213
Shōfu, 47
Shōkai, 55, 56, 172, 190, 191
Shōkai, 47, 154, 155, 159, 160
Shōkai, 48, 49, 172
Shōkin, 51, 54, 167, 168
Shōkō, 50, 51
Shokutoku, 45, 46
Shōkyoku, 55, 56, 161
Shōkyū, 45
Shōkyū, 42
Shōman, 42, 43
Shōmon, 45, 46, 209
Shōmon, 64–66, 204
Shōrei, 61, 63, 177, 178
Shōreki, 59, 60, 157
Shōshō, 41, 69, 70, 214, 215
Shōshō, 47, 119
Shōshō, 38, 39
Shōtaku, 48, 49, 119
Shōyō, 41, 42, 44

Shōyō, 39, 40
Shōzan, 51, 54, 163–66, 202, 203, 212, 213
Shū-ei, 45, 46
SI-1, 48, 49, 119
SI-2, 48, 49
SI-3, 48, 49
SI-4, 48, 49
SI-5, 48, 49, 154, 155
SI-6, 48, 49, 154, 155
SI-7, 48, 49
SI-8, 48, 49, 172
SI-9, 48, 49, 156, 157
SI-10, 48, 49
SI-11, 49, 154–57, 159
SI-12, 49
SI-13, 49, 152–57, 159, 174, 175, 178, 179, 182, 183, 212, 213
SI-14, 49, 182, 183
SI-15, 49, 178, 179, 182, 183
SI-16, 49
SI-17, 49, 149, 154, 155
SI-18, 49, 151, 152
SI-19, 49, 151, 152, 178, 179
Sokkoku, 61, 62
Sokkotsu, 51, 54
Soryō, 67, 68
SP-1, 45
SP-2, 45
SP-3, 45, 209
SP-4, 45
SP-5, 45
SP-6, 45, 134, 163, 164, 167, 168, 177–79, 181, 186, 187, 190, 191, 198–203, 206, 207, 209, 210
SP-7, 45, 46
SP-8, 45, 46
SP-9, 45, 46, 163, 164, 169, 170, 190, 191, 206, 207, 208, 210
SP-10, 45, 46, 169, 170, 209, 210
SP-11, 45, 46
SP-12, 45, 46, 209
SP-13, 45, 46, 209, 210
SP-14, 45, 46, 195–98
SP-15, 45, 46, 195–97
SP-16, 45, 46
SP-17, 45, 46
SP-18, 45, 46
SP-19, 45, 46, 177, 178
SP-20, 45, 46
SP-21, 45, 46
ST-1, 42
ST-2, 42, 133, 151–53, 214, 215

ST-3, 42, 151–53
ST-4, 42, 151–53, 214, 215
ST-5, 41, 42, 62, 151–53
ST-6, 41–43, 62, 151, 152
ST-7, 41–43, 133, 151–53
ST-8, 36, 41–43, 151–53
ST-9, 42, 43, 120, 121, 151–53,
    177–80, 188, 189, 218, 219
ST-10, 42, 43
ST-11, 42, 43
ST-12, 42, 43, 161, 162
ST-13, 42, 43, 149, 150
ST-14, 42, 43
ST-15, 42, 43
ST-16, 42, 43
ST-17, 42, 43
ST-18, 42, 43, 161
ST-19, 42, 43, 180, 181
ST-20, 42, 43
ST-21, 42, 43, 186, 187, 200, 201
ST-22, 42, 43
ST-23, 42, 43
ST-24, 42, 43
ST-25, 42, 43, 171, 172, 180–87,
    192–203, 205–07, 212–14
ST-26, 42, 43
ST-27, 42, 43, 177–85, 190, 191,
    195–99, 202–07, 209–11
ST-28, 42, 43
ST-29, 42, 43
ST-30, 42, 43
ST-31, 42, 43
ST-32, 42, 43, 212, 213
ST-33, 42, 43
ST-34, 42, 43, 169, 170, 172
ST-35, 42, 44
ST-36, 42, 44, 89, 134, 163, 164,
    167–70, 172, 177–79, 182–85,
    192, 194–201, 206, 207, 209,
    210
ST-37, 42, 44
ST-38, 42, 44, 167, 168
ST-39, 42, 44
ST-40, 41, 42, 44
ST-41, 42, 44, 167, 168, 184,
    185, 212, 213
ST-42, 41, 42, 44
ST-43, 42, 44
ST-44, 42, 44
ST-45, 42, 44
Suibun, 69, 70
Suidō, 42, 43

Suikō, 67, 68
Suisen, 55, 56
Suitotsu, 42, 43

Tai-en, 38, 39, 212, 213, 217, 218
Taihaku, 45, 209
Tai-itsu, 42, 43
Taikei, 55, 56, 163, 164, 172,
    178, 179, 190, 191, 202, 203,
    206, 207, 211, 212, 217–19
Taimyaku, 61, 63
Taishō, 65, 177, 178, 204, 209,
    210
Taiyō, 172–75
Tanyu, 51, 52, 194, 195, 198–201,
    203, 204
Tenchi, 57, 58
Tenchū, 51, 52, 118, 149, 150,
    152–57, 159, 174, 175, 177–85,
    188–91, 208–10, 212–15
Tenkei, 45, 46
Te-no-Gori, 40
Te-no-Sanri, 40, 154, 155, 157–
    62, 177, 178, 182, 183, 196,
    197, 206
Tenpu, 38
Tenryō, 59, 60, 154, 182, 183
Tensei, 59, 60, 212, 214
Tensen, 57, 58
Tenshō, 61, 62
Tensō, 49, 154–57, 159
Tensō, 49
Tensū, 42, 43, 171, 172, 180–87,
    192–203, 205–07, 212–14
Tentei, 40, 41, 151–55, 184, 185,
    214, 215
Tentotsu, 69, 70, 184, 185, 192,
    193, 214, 215
Tenyō, 49, 149, 154, 155
Tenyō, 59, 60, 177–79
TH-1, 59
TH-2, 59
TH-3, 59, 178, 179
TH-4, 59, 60, 154, 155, 159, 172,
    211, 212, 214, 217–19
TH-5, 59, 60, 154, 155, 159, 160
TH-6, 59, 60
TH-7, 59, 60
TH-8, 59, 60
TH-9, 59, 60
TH-10, 59, 60, 212, 214

TH-11, 59, 60
TH-12, 59, 60, 157
TH-13, 59, 60
TH-14, 59, 60, 159
TH-15, 59, 60, 154, 182, 183
TH-16, 59, 60, 177–79
TH-17, 59, 60, 133, 151–53,
    177–79
TH-18, 59, 60
TH-19, 59, 60
TH-20, 59, 60, 178, 179
TH-21, 59, 60, 178, 179
TH-22, 59, 60
TH-23, 59, 60, 214, 215
Tōdō, 67, 68
Tokubi, 42, 44
Tokuyu, 51, 52
Tsūri, 47
Tsūten, 51, 174, 175

Unmon, 38, 156–58

Wakuchū, 55, 56, 186, 187
Wankotsu, 48, 49
Waryō, 59, 60

Yintang, 173–75
Yōchi, 59, 60, 154, 155, 159,
    172, 211, 212, 214, 217–19
Yōhaku, 61, 63, 214, 215
Yōho, 61, 64
Yōkei, 40, 154, 155, 159, 160
Yōkō, 61, 63
Yōkō, 51, 53
Yōkoku, 48, 49, 154, 155
Yōrō, 48, 49, 154, 155
Yōryōsen, 61, 63, 149, 150,
    167–70, 209, 210
Yōsō, 42, 43
Yōyu, 66, 67
Yufu, 55, 56, 186, 187
Yūmon, 55, 56, 161, 162
Yūsen, 54, 55, 163–66, 181, 188,
    189, 211–13

Zenchō, 67, 68, 174, 175
Zenkoku, 48, 49
Zui, 36, 41–43, 151–53

General Index

abdominal distension, 200, 208
abdominal pain, 117, 198
abnormal moisture level, 107
abnormal temperature, 107
abscesses, 91
acetycholine, 89
acupuncture analgesia, 89, 90
acute arthritis, 139
acute diarrhea, 197
acute eczema, 205
acute enterocolitis, 139
acute gastritis, 139
acute muscular rheumatism, 139
acute tonsillitis, 121
AIDS, 119, 141
alcoholism, 173
allergies, 185, 206, 207, 216
amenorrhea, 208
analgesic effect, 85, 89, 139
Anatomical Locations of Carotid
　Sinus, 120
Anatomical Location of the
　Stellate Ganglion, 121
anemia, 119, 177, 189, 201
anesthesia, 89
aneurysms, 151
angina pectoris, 119, 188
Ankyō, 18
anorectal fistulas, 201, 202
anorexia, 171, 172, 185, 196,
　198, 200
anxiety attacks, 196
aortic aneurysm, 160
apoplexy, 188
appendicitis, 193, 195
analgesic effect, 139
anemia, 177, 189, 201
angina pectoris, 188
anorexia, 185, 196, 198, 200
Areas of Stimulation in Pediatric
　Acupuncture, 117
arrhythmia, 126
Artemesia vulgaris, 94
arteriosclerosis, 139, 166, 177,
　180, 188
arthritis, 81, 121
　of the knee, 115
asthenic constitutions, 117, 179,

190
asthma, 121, 187
atherosclerosis, 120, 121
atonic constipation, 195
atopic dermatitis, 205
atrophic gastritis, 199
atrophy of the thymus gland, 81
auditory nerve tumor, 178
auricular acupuncture, 122
Auricular Acupuncture Points,
　124
Autonomic Dermatomes, 77, 78
autonomic dysfunction, 134, 154
autonomic dystonia, 177
autosensitive dermatitis, 205
Average Depth of Insertion, 102

Back *Shu* Point, 32, 33, 78, 108,
　110
Bainbridge reflex, 80
Beautifying Skin, 218, 219
Bei Ji Qian Jin Fang, 20
Bei Jin Qian Jin Yao Fang, 20
belching, 191
Bianque, 19
bianshi, 91
Bladder Meridian, 51
bleeding hemorrhoids, 201, 202
Blemishes, 216–18
blemishes, 107
Boesher, D., 88
bone cancer, 160
Brachialgia, 158–60
Brachial Neuralgia, 158–60
bradycardia, 190
brain tumors, 151, 193
Bronchial Asthma, 185–87
bronchial asthma, 117, 139, 190
bronchiectasis, 185
bronchitis, 186
bronze figure, 20

cancer, 87
Cannon, Walter, 80
Cao Yuanfung, 20
cardiac asthma, 186

cardiac neurasthenia, 139
caries, 149
carotid sinus stimulation, 120
catarrheal inflammation of the
　digestive organs, 138
cautery moxibution, 102
cerebral anemia, 177
cerebral arteriosclerosis, 173
cerebral hemorrhage, 145, 193
cerebral hyperemia, 119, 138,
　174, 175
cerebral hypoxia, 193
cervicobrachial syndrome, 160
cervicobrachialgia, 121, 127, 181
cervicothoracic ganglion, 121
chilling, 64
　　in the extremities, 114, 191,
　　　122
　　in the feet, 153, 179, 189
　　in the legs, 44, 164, 187, 201,
　　　210
　　in the lower extremities, 118
chinetsu-kyū, 103
choleithiasis, 173
chronic arthritis, 139
Chronic Bronchitis, 183–85
chronic bronchitis, 139, 185
chronic diarrhea, 197
chronic eczema, 205
chronic enteritis, 195
Chronic Gastritis, 199–201
chronic gastritis, 139, 191
chronic headaches, 118
Chronic Hepatitis, 203, 204
chronic muscular rheumatism,
　139
chronic nephritis, 139
Chronic Rheumatoid Arthritis,
　171–73
chronic rhinitis, 134
chronic urticaria, 206
cicatrical stenosis of the rectum,
　195
circulatory diseases, 177
cirrhosis, 203
climacteric disorders, 134, 177,
　181
cluster needle, 116

colds, 149, 171, 201
collagenosis, 171
command points, 32
compatibility relationship, 28
Conception Vessel, 69
conductive tinnitus, 178
Confucius, 23
congestive headaches, 144
Constipation, 195–97
constipation, 44, 139, 173, 175, 179, 181, 200, 203, 204, 207, 219
contact dermatitis, 205
Contact Needling, 100, 101
Contrast of Tendencies in Western Medicine and Oriental Medicine, 16
Controlling Cycle, 28
controlling relationship, 28
contusions, 139
convulsions, 137
convulsive fits, 140
coolness and hotness, 107
Correlation of Fetus to Auricular Points, 121
coughing, 37, 180
cramping of calf muscle, 50
cun, 36
cupping, 119
Cupping by Use of Manual Pump, 119
cutaneovisceral reflex, 72, 76, 78
cybernetics, 82, 83
cystitis, 139
cystospasm, 139

dai vessel, 110
danō-kyū, 102
dashin technique, 22
deafness, 179
denaturation, 140
Depression, 106,
dermatomes, 78, 89
diabetes, 166, 173, 177
diabetes millitus, 166
diagnosis, 105
Diarrhea, 197–99
diarrhea, 44, 54, 64, 114, 139, 180, 207
Direct Insertion Technique, 95
direct moxibustion, 105
distension in the abdomen, 203
dizziness, 139, 140, 154, 155,

175, 181, 188, 189, 196
on standing, 54
Dō-In, 18
dorsal raphe nuclei, 87–89
dryness and dampness, 107
duodenal ulcer, 191
Dysmenorrhea, 207–10
dyspepsia, 210

Eczema, 205–07
eczema, 115, 187
edema, 82, 139, 203
Electroacupuncture, 126
electroacupuncture, 125–27
emaciation, 140
emphysema, 185
encephalitis, 173
encephaloma, 173
endocrine disorders, 179
endometriosis, 208
endorphin, 86
enkephalin, 86, 88
enterocolitis, 198
epidemic meningitis, 173
epilepsy, 175
epistaxis, 39, 41, 50
Erector Spinae Muscles in the Lumbar Region, 128
Eructation, 191, 192
erysipelas, 140
erythema, 123
esophageal paralysis, 139
esophageal spasm, 139
essential hypertension, 121, 139, 187
essential hypotension, 189, 190
extra meridian, 30, 110
extreme antiflexion of the uterus, 208
eyestrain, 127, 177

Facial Nerve, 133, 134
facial paralysis, 129
Features of High Quality Moxa and Low Quality Moxa, 94
febrile diseases, 140
feedback systems, 82, 83
fever, 81, 119, 198, 203
feverishness, 61, 64
filiform needle, 92, 93
Five Element Correlations, 27
five element theory, 23, 25, 28

Freckles, 216–18
freckles, 107, 123
Front Mu and Back Shu Points and Sensory Dermatomes, 78
Front Mu Point, 32, 33, 78, 110
Frozen Shoulders, 156–58
frozen shoulders, 114
fu, 25
Full-moon Hold, 98
Fuxi, 18

Gallbladder Meridian, 61
gallstone, 193
gastric neurosis, 139, 191
gastritis, 193, 201
gastroasthenia, 191
gastroatony, 139
gastrointestinal disorders, 114, 120, 175
gastrospasms, 121, 139
gate control theory, 85, 89
general fatigue, 81
general malaise, 134, 173, 191
giddiness, 175
Governor Vessel, 67

habitual constipation, 195
Half-moon Hold, 98
haozhen, 92
Headache, 173–75
headaches, 60, 81, 121, 139, 149, 154, 177, 181, 185, 188, 189, 193, 196, 203, 209, 210
heartburn, 191
heart disease, 68, 191
Heart Meridian, 47
heaviness of the head, 48, 175, 185, 188, 196
hemophilia, 140
hemoptysis, 54
Hemorrhoids, 201–03
hemorrhoids, 50, 139
hepatic constipation, 139
hepatitis, 173
Hepatitis B, 141
Herniated Disk in Lumbar Vertebrae, 165, 166
herniated disks, 162, 166
herniation of intervertebral disks, 154
high blood pressure, 140, 173, 177, 183, 187

high fever, 140
hives, 187, 206
homeostasis, 80, 81, 83
Horizontal Insertion, 101
hotness of the head, 119, 196
Huangdi Nei Jing, 18–20, 23, 91
Huangfu, Mi, 19
Hua Shou, 20
hyperemia, 118, 120, 138, 145
Hypertension, 187–89
hypertension, 118, 119
hypertrophic gastritis, 199
hypertrophy, 140
    of the adrenal glands, 81
hypesthesia, 107, 137, 144, 165, 167
hypoglycemia, 175
Hypotension, 189–91
hypotension, 119, 177
hysteria, 139

I-Ching, 18, 23
idiopathic gynecological symptoms, 134
idiopathic trigeminal neuralgia, 151–53
Imbedded Intradermal Needles, 115
Increasing Vitality, 210–12
indigestion, 207
Indirect Moxibustion, 103
Induration, 106
infectious diseases, 149, 151, 166, 199
influenza, 166
insertion tubes, 93, 94
insertion tube technique, 96
Insomnia, 180, 181
insomnia, 44, 139, 172, 179, 196, 203
Intercostal Neuralgia, 160–62
intermittent insertion, 100
interscapular pain, 139
inter-transforming relationship of yin and yang, 24
intestinal atony, 139
intestinal disorders, 120
intestinal obstruction, 193
intradermal needling, 115
irritability, 117, 179, 209
ischemia, 162
Ishimpō, 21
Ishizaka, Sōtetsu, 22

itching, 203, 205, 207

Japanese Filiform Needle, 92
jaundice, 44, 203
Jianzhen, 21
Jin Kui Yao Lue Fang Lun, 19
Jivaka, 18
Ju Fang Xue, 20

Keeping Hair Healthy, 220–22
ketsu, 29
ki, 25
Kidney Meridian, 55

lack of appetite, 54, 204, 207
lacrimation, 154
Large Intestine Meridian, 40
laryngitis, 134
Lasègue's test, 164, 167, 169
lassitude, 139
lateral humeral epicondylitis, 158
legally designed communicable diseases, 140
Lei Jing, 20
leprosy, 140
levator scapulae muscle, 127
Liebeskind, J.C., 87
lifting and thrusting, 100
Ling Shu, 19, 32, 35, 91, 98
Liver Meridian, 65
localized anemia, 138
loss of appetite, 81, 203
loss of hearing, 48, 177
low back pain, 64, 114, 118, 127, 170, 203, 209
low blood pressure, 173, 175, 177
lower lumbar plexus, 131
low vitality, 211
lumbago, 139, 162, 164, 168
lwmbago-sciatica syndrome, 166
Lumbar Plexus and Femoral Nerves, 131
Lumbar Plexus and Sciatic Nerve, 132
lung cancer, 185
Lung Meridian, 38
Luo Connecting Point, 32

Mai Jing, 19
mandibular neuralgia, 151, 153

maxillary neuralgia, 151, 153
Mechanism of Analgestic Effect Caused by Stimulation of the Periaqueductal Gray Matter, 88
mechanism of pain, 84
Median Nerve, 130
Melzack, Ronald, 85
Ménière's disease, 177, 178
Menstrual Irregularity, 207–10
menstrual irregularity, 114, 118, 140
metal needle, 18
microacupuncture, 111, 118
migraine headaches, 60, 139, 175
Minor and Major Rhomboideus Muscles, 128
Misono, Isai, 22
morphine, 85–87
moxa
    production of, 94
    quality of, 94
mu points, 33
muscle atrophy, 138
muscular tension in the neck and shoulders, 115
Myotomes, 75
myotomes, 76, 78

naloxine, 87
Nan Jing, 19
Nan Jing Ben Yi, 20
nasal congestion, 50, 134
nasal discharge, 39
Nausea, 193–95
nausea, 44, 64, 154, 155, 176, 181, 192, 196, 200, 203
neck and shoulder stiffness, 127, 182
Neck and Shoulder Tension, 181–83
neck and shoulder tension, 139, 210
necrosis, 140
neoplasms, 140
nervous cardialgia, 139
nervous indigestion, 139
nervous palpitation, 139
nettle rash, 206
neuralgia, 114, 126, 129, 137, 139, 154, 162, 168
    of the median nerve, 160
    of the radial nerve, 160

of the ulnar nerve, 160
neurasthesia, 134, 139
neurogenic cervicobrachialgia, 129
neuromuscular scoliosis, 167
neuropathy, 160
night terror, 140
Nine Traditional Needles, 91
nocturnal enuresis, 117, 140, 188
Nogier, Paul, 122
non-scarring moxibution, 102, 103
noradrenalin, 88
numbness in the extremities, 129

Oblique Insertion, 101
occipital headaches, 118
Occipital Neuralgia, 149, 150
occlusion of arteries, 162
ocular pain, 154
on-kyū, 103
Onodera Point, 166
opthalmic trigemeinal neuralgia, 151
orthopathic hypotensive asthenia, 175
orthostatic hypotension, 189, 190
Osteoarthritis of the Knee Joint, 169, 170
Osteorarhritis of the Lumbar Vertebrae, 162–64
otitis interna, 178
otitis media, 177
overweight, 214

pain and stiffness in the intra-scapular region, 128
pain and tension in the lumbar and sacral region, 129
pain and tension in the lumbar area, 129
Pain and Tension in Occipital Region, 149
pain in the occipital region, 127
pain in the shoulders, 154
palpatory examination, 107
palpitations, 37, 57, 140, 155, 188, 189
paraditis, 139
paralysis, 129, 137–39, 153
parasites, 140

paresthesia, 107, 144, 154, 164
partial paralysis, 137
Path of the Old and New Spinothalamic Tracts, 88
patterning theory, 84
pediatric acupuncture, 116
pediatric dyspepsia, 140
pelvic inflammatory disease, 208
penetrating moxibution, 102
peptic ulcers, 81, 190, 191, 193, 199, 201
periaqueductal gray matter, 87, 89
Pericardium Meridian, 57
peritonitis, 193, 195
pharyngitis, 134
pigmentation, 107
piles, 201
plum blossom needle, 116
pneumothorax, 128
poisoning, 178
polio, 144
polyuria, 181
poor hearing, 58
presbycusis, 178
pressure points, 106
Preventing the Ill Effects of Aging, 212–14
Productive Cycle, 28
productive relationship, 28
psychological strain, 180
psychological stress, 177
pulmonary tuberculosis, 184, 186
purpura, 140
Pyrosis, 191, 192

Quadratus Lumborum Muscle, 129

Radial Nerve, 130
Raynaud's disease, 121
rectal caner, 195
regular meridian, 30
Reilly, J., 83
Reilly phenomenon, 83, 84
Reinold, D.V., 87
renal hypertension, 121
retaining the needle, 100
retroflexion of the uterus, 208
rheumatoid arthritis, 166, 169
rheumatoid fever, 171
rhomboideus muscles, 128

ringing in the ears, 177, 179
roller needle, 116
Ryōdo-Raku acupuncture, 125

sanitation, 141
Scapulohumeral Periarthritis, 156–58
scarring moxibution, 102
Sciatica, 166–69
sciatica, 50, 118, 129, 165, 167
Sciatic Nerve, 132
scrofula, 60
scurvy, 140
seasickness, 193
secondary hypertension, 187
secondary hypotension, 189, 191
Selye, Hans, 81
Sensory Dermatomes, 74, 78
sensory tinnitus, 178
serotonin, 88
Shang Han Lun, 19
Shangshu, 23
Shen Nong, 18
Shen Nong Ben Cao Jing, 18
Shirota, Bunshi, 120
Shi si Jing Fa Hui, 20
shō, 15
shock, 119
shortness of breath, 37, 54, 188
shōshaku-kyū, 102
shoulder stiffness, 183
shoulder tension, 114, 118
shu points, 33, 120
Siebold, Phillip, 22
Simple Insertion and Withdrawal, 99, 100
sinusitis, 134, 151
skin diseases, 140
skin rashes, 173, 206
Slipped Disk, 165, 166
Small Intestine Meridian, 49
sore throat, 48, 54, 66, 119, 185
Source points, 125
sparrow pecking, 100
spasms, 139
spastic constipation, 195
specilization theory, 84
Spinal Cord, 73
Spinal Dermatomes, 73
spinal dermatomes, 76, 78, 108–10
Spleen Meridian, 45
sprains, 139

stellate ganglion stimulation, 121
sterilization, 141
stiffness in the neck and
    shoulders, 127, 154, 179
stimulation produced analgesia
    (SPA), 87 89
stomachaches, 200
stomach cancer, 191, 199
Stomach Meridian, 42
stone needle, 18
stressors, 81, 82
stress theory, 81
subjugation relationship, 28
subluxations in the cervical
    vertebrae, 158
Sugiyama, Waichi, 22
superficial gastritis, 199
Superficial Tension, 106
supprative moxibustion, 102
Surface Anatomy of the Auricle,
    124
Su Weng, 19
sympathetic dermatome, 76,
    109, 110
symptomatic constipation, 195
symptomatic trigeminal
    neuralgia, 151, 152
synergistic action, 79
syphilis, 140, 160, 166

tachycardia, 121
Tai Ji, 23
Tamba, Yasunari, 21
tapping in, 97
telansiectasis, 118
Tender Point, 106
Tennis Elbow, 158–60
tenosynovitis, 158
TENS (Transcutaneous Electrical
    Nerve Stimulation), 125
tension headaches, 121
tension in the neck and
    shoulders, 127
tension in the occipital region,
    127
testitis, 139
tetanus, 140
tetany, 139
Three Edged Needle, 118
Tinnitus, 177–79
tinnitus, 121, 139, 154, 155

tōnetsu-kyū 102, 144
*Tong Ren Shu Xue Zhen Jiu Tu
    Jing*, 20
tonification and dispersion
    techniques, 111, 112
tonsillitis, 117, 134
toothache, 39
Trauma to Vervical Vertebrae,
    154, 155
Trigeminal Nerve, 133
Trigeminal Neuralgia, 151–53
trigeminal neuralgia, 129
Triple Heater Meridian, 59
tuberculosis, 160
tumors, 120, 149
Twelve Meridians and Their
    Relationships, 34
Twisting and Rotating, 99, 100

Ulnar Nerve, 130, 131
upper lumbar plexus, 131
Upper Portion of Levator
    Scapulae, 128
Upper Portion of Trapezius, 127
uremia, 173, 188
uremic asthma, 186
urethral inflammation, 139
Urticaria, 205–07
uterine hypoplasia, 208
uterine myomas, 208
uterospasms, 140

varicose veins, 118
varicosities, 201
Varieties of Intradermal Needles,
    115
Varieties of Pediatric
    Needles, 117
Various Insertion Tubes, 94
vascular headaches, 121
vascular reflex, 109
venesection, 118
vertex headaches, 118
Vertical Insertion, 101
Vertigo, 175–77
vertigo, 121
Vibration, 100, 101
Visceroautonomic Reflex, 77
visceroautonomic reflex, 72, 76,
    79, 109

viscerocutaneous reflex, 72, 79,
    110
Visceromotor Reflex, 75
visceromotor reflex, 72, 76, 78,
    109, 110
Viscerosensory Reflex, 74
viscerosensory reflex, 72, 76, 78,
    110
viral hepatitis, 119
Vomiting, 193–95
vomiting 174, 176, 198, 200, 203

Wai Tai Mi Yao, 20
Wall, Patrick, 85
Wang Shuhe, 19
Wang Tao, 20
Wang Weiyi, 20
warming moxibustion, 103, 111
weight loss, 54, 171, 203
"well" points, 119
Whiplash Injury, 154, 155
Wiener, Nobert, 82
Winkles in Facial Skin, 214–16
wormwood plant, 94
writer's cramp, 139

Xi Cleft Point, 32
Xingli, 20

*Yellow Emperor's Classic of
    Internal Medicine, The*, 18–20,
    23, 91
Yin-Yang Relationship of the
    Zang-Fu, 29
yin-yang theory, 23–25
Yuan Source Point, 32

zang, 25
Zen Jin Jia Yi Jing, 19
Zhang Jiebin, 20
Zhang Zhong Jing, 19
Zhen Jia Shu Yao, 20
Zhen Jiu Ju Ying, 20
Zhicong, 21
Zhu Bing Yuan Hou Zong Lun,
    20